The Politics of Chinese Medicine under Mongol Rule

Under the rule of the descendants of Chinggis Khan (1167–1227), China saw the development of a new culture in which medical practice came to be considered a highly respected occupation for elite men. During this period, further major steps were also taken towards the codification of medical knowledge and promotion of physicians' social status.

This book traces the history of the politics, institutions, and culture of medicine of China under Mongol rule, through the eyes of a successful South Chinese official Yuan Jue (1266–1327). As the first comprehensive monograph on history of medicine in China under the Mongols, it argues that this period was a separate moment in Chinese history, when a configuration of power different from that of previous and succeeding periods created its own medical culture. *The Politics of Chinese Medicine under Mongol Rule* emphasizes the impact of the political and institutional changes caused by the Mongols and their collaborators on the social and cultural history of medicine, which culminated in the medical theory of Zhu Zhenheng (1282–1358), still influential in East Asian medicine. Using a variety of Chinese-language sources including gazetteers, legal texts, biographies, poems, and medical texts, it analyses the roles of the Mongols and West and Central Asians as cultural brokers and also as unifiers of China. Further, it views North and South Chinese elites as agents of historical change rather than as victims of Mongol oppression.

Underlining the complexity of the history of China under the Mongols and the significance of time and geography for the study of this history, this book will be of great interest to students and scholars of Chinese medical history, Chinese social and cultural history, and medieval global history.

Reiko Shinno is Professor at the Department of History, the University of Wisconsin-Eau Claire, USA.

Needham Research Institute Series
Series Editor: Christopher Cullen

Joseph Needham's "Science and Civilisation" series began publication in the 1950s. At first it was seen as a piece of brilliant but isolated pioneering. However, at the beginning of the twenty-first century, it became clear that Needham's work had succeeded in creating a vibrant new intellectual field in the West. The books in this series cover topics that broadly relate to the practice of science, technology and medicine in East Asia, including China, Japan, Korea and Vietnam. The emphasis is on traditional forms of knowledge and practice, but without excluding modern studies that connect their topics with their historical and cultural context.

Celestial Lancets
A history and rationale of acupuncture and moxa
Lu Gwei-Djen and Joseph Needham
With a new introduction by Vivienne Lo

A Chinese Physician
Wang Ji and the Stone Mountain medical case histories
Joanna Grant

Chinese Mathematical Astrology
Reaching out to the stars
Ho Peng Yoke

Medieval Chinese Medicine
The Dunhuang medical manuscripts
Edited by Vivienne Lo and Christopher Cullen

Chinese Medicine in Early Communist China, 1945–1963
Medicine of revolution
Kim Taylor

Explorations in Daoism
Medicine and alchemy in literature
Ho Peng Yoke

Tibetan Medicine in the Contemporary World
Global politics of medical knowledge and practice
Laurent Pordié

The Evolution of Chinese Medicine
Northern Song dynasty, 960–1127
Asaf Goldschmidt

Speaking of Epidemics in Chinese Medicine
Disease and the geographic imagination in Late Imperial China
Marta E. Hanson

Reviving Ancient Chinese Mathematics
Mathematics, history and politics in the work of Wu Wen-Tsun
Jiri Hudecek

Agriculture and the Food Supply in Premodern Japan
The place of rice
Charlotte von Verschuer with Wendy Cobcroft

The Politics of Chinese Medicine under Mongol Rule
Reiko Shinno 秦 玲子

The Politics of Chinese Medicine under Mongol Rule

Reiko Shinno 秦 玲子

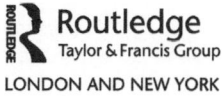
Routledge
Taylor & Francis Group

LONDON AND NEW YORK

First published 2016
by Routledge
2 Park Square, Milton Park, Abingdon, Oxon OX14 4RN

and by Routledge
711 Third Avenue, New York, NY 10017

First issued in paperback 2017

Routledge is an imprint of the Taylor & Francis Group, an informa business

British Library Cataloguing in Publication Data
A catalogue record for this book is available from the British Library

Library of Congress Cataloging-in-Publication Data
Shinno, Reiko.
The politics of Chinese medicine under Mongol rule / Reiko Shinno.
pages cm. — (Needham Research Institute series)
Includes bibliographical references and index.
1. Medicine, Chinese—Political aspects—Mongolia. 2. Medicine—Political
aspects. I. Title.
R628.N37 2016
610.9517—dc23
2015022608

ISBN 13: 978-1-138-09932-6 (pbk)
ISBN 13: 978-1-138-78119-1 (hbk)

Typeset in Times New Roman
by Swales & Willis Ltd, Exeter, Devon

To Kazuko, Tsutomu, and Masako Shinno

Contents

Illustrations

Acknowledgments

This book is an extensive revision of my doctoral dissertation submitted to the History Department of Stanford University in 2002. Without my mentor Harold Kahn's superb guidance, I simply could not have completed the dissertation. Through my advisor Ellen Neskar's excellent graduate research seminar, I found Yuan Jue's gazetteer and the topic for this project. Another dissertation reader of mine, Timothy Brook, listened to me patiently as I tried to make sense of the sources that I had gathered and encouraged me throughout the project. Charlotte Furth kindly agreed to be the external reader of the dissertation, read the draft chapters carefully, and advised me how I ought to wrap up my dissertation as well as how I should revise it as a book. I also benefitted greatly from the courses and workshops offered at Stanford University and in Palo Alto by Clifford Barnett, Albert Dien, Peter Duus, Gordon Chang, Estelle Freedman, Jeffrey Mass, Morris Rossabi, Laura Smoller, Lyman Van Slyke, and Roger Thompson. I am so grateful to Dorothy Ko and Susan Mann for recommending me to study at the university.

Friends who studied Chinese history and culture in the Bay Area at the same time as I did—Lisa Claypool, Hilde De Weerdt, Shari Epstein, Siyen Fei, Max Ko-wu Huang, Jin Jiang, Pauline Lee, Sonya Lee, Zwia Lipkin, Yongling Lu, Ya-zhen (Maya) Ma, Yun-chiu Mei, Tobie Meyer-Fong, Ruth Mostern, M. Colette Plum, Shannon Sweeney, Mark Swislocki, Zhaohua Yang, Juan Wang, and Erica Yao—have offered me tremendous intellectual and moral support. So did Andrew Jenks, Michael Kahan, Benjamin Lawrence, Christopher Lee, Caitlin Murdock, Nancy Stalker, and Sarah Sussman, as members of the History Department dissertation reading group. A great role model and mentor, Emiko Mashiko Moffitt, took me to wonderful concerts and told me stories of her fascinating life. One of the very few Japanese faculty members at Stanford University at the time, Takeshi Amemiya, sometimes took me out for lunch and quietly made sure that I survived the doctoral program all right. Other friends of mine, including Catherine Bae, Miki and Alex Bay, Thomas Conlan, Robert Eskildsen, Kara Gardner, Rajat Garg, Brian Goldsmith, Kenji Hasegawa, Robert Hellyer, Angus Lockyer, Daniel Mah, Ming-Yuen Meyer-Fong, Miho Nagasawa, Yoshimi Ohshima, Christine Pajak, Ethan Segal, Vickie Sherman, Michiko Suzuki, Roderick Wilson, Judy Tzu-Chun Wu, helped me make Palo Alto my home.

While I focused on political, institutional, and social history of medicine in my dissertation, I have added a chapter on the history of medical books and theories in this book. I was able to do so thanks to Kosoto Hiroshi's and Mayanagi Makoto's guidance. Also, Hasebe Eiichi, my former classmate at the University of Tokyo, helped me learn to read medical texts by organizing a group to translate and annotate Zhu Zhenheng's *Further Views on Extended Knowledge* (Gezhi Yulun). A couple of years ago we were finally able to publish the annotated translation as Kakuchi yoron *chūshaku* (Tokyo: Iseisha, 2014). I am grateful to him, Onda Hiromasa, Matsushita Michinobu, Uemura Asami, and other past participants of the reading group.

I am also indebted to many other scholars and friends in Japan. In particular, Ōshima Ritsuko has inspired me through her pioneering articles on the Yuan policies and through face-to-face conversations. I thank the members of *Yuan dianzhang* reading group at Waseda University, especially the organizer Funada Yoshiyuki. I am grateful to the faculty and staff members at the University of Tokyo, where I completed my master's degree in Chinese philosophy in 1990. Mizoguchi Yūzō and Togawa Yoshio taught me the rigor required when reading premodern Chinese texts. Shiba Yoshinobu and Satō Shin'ichi opened my eyes to English-language scholarship on Chinese history. Ikeda Tomohisa, Ishikawa Hiroshi, Kawahara Hideki, and Kojima Tsuyoshi have always welcomed me back whenever I needed to look at the books in the *Kanseki konā*. Yokote Yutaka and my *sempai* Mabuchi Masaya have given me precious advice on intellectual history and history of religions of the Yuan period. Suzuki Kōichirō also assisted me when I was back in Japan for dissertation research. Yanagida Setsuko, the first Japanese female historian studying Song-Jin-Yuan China, was a conscientious scholar and caring mentor for me. I am also grateful to Fujiwara Yoshiko, Kasagi Yasufumi, Kawashima Yasushi, Kohama Masako, Ohmura Yoshiaki, Sakamoto Hiroko, Suetsugu Reiko, and Yamaoka Seiichirō for their friendship and support.

I first became interested in Chinese medical history while I was studying Chinese language and history in Taiwan from 1991 to 1993. I am grateful to all my Chinese-language teachers at the Inter-University Program in Taipei and the professors whose courses I took as a special student (*xuandu sheng*) at the National Taiwan University: Lin Wei-hong, Liu Ts'ui-jung, Wang De-yi, and Wu Mi-cha. Lin's course on Chinese women's history and the conversations with my classmate Chen Yuan-Peng opened my eyes to medical history as a way to explore Chinese history. Liu Ching-cheng, Wu Jen-shu, and Neil Katkov helped me connect to Taiwanese academia. It was also a great privilege to become friends with Kim Taik-kyun, Catherine Stuart, and Jeff Wong there. When I returned to Taiwan in 2007, Li Jianmin kindly hosted my stay at Academia Sinica.

During my fieldwork in mainland China in the late 1990s, Zheng Jinsheng and Zhu Jianping of the China Academy of Traditional Chinese Medicine, Chen Gaohua and Yu Heping of the Chinese Academy of Social Sciences, Yang Shengmin of Minzu University of China, Chen Dezhi and Hua Tao of Nanjing University, and Zhang Jishun and Yao Dali of Fudan University all kindly shared with me their insights and knowledge on my topic. Wu Yiye spent a whole afternoon showing me around Nanjing and introducing me to Chinese scholarship on *Hui* history. Xian Yuechong and Gong Lijun working for the city government as well as Xu Liangxiong and Xu Jiongming of Tianyige Library took me around

Ningbo, the home city of my protagonist Yuan Jue seven centuries earlier. I also appreciated Chang Minyi, a doctor and medical historian of Ningbo, for discussing with me the medical history of the city.

I have been fortunate to be allowed to present parts of this study in the following venues: the University of Southern California, the University of Tokyo, Center for Chinese Studies in Taibei, the University of Oxford, the University of Cambridge, the Kluge Center, the Association for Asian Studies, the Japanese Society for the History of Medicine, and the International Conference on History of Science in East Asia. I greatly appreciated the questions and comments from the organizers, participants, and audiences of all the events. Part of the dissertation has been published as "Medical Schools and the Temples for the Three Progenitors in Yuan China: A Case of Cross-Cultural Interactions," in *Harvard Journal of Asiatic Studies* 67.1 (2007): 89–133. Johanna Handlin Smith's and Shigehisa Kuriyama's comments have been incorporated into the article and this book. I thank Michael Brose, the Needham series editor Christopher Cullen, Sarah Schneewind, Yi-Li Wu, and the two anonymous reviewers of this book for their thorough comments on the manuscript. Christopher Atwood, Patricia Ebrey, and John Moffitt helped me with maps, and Ming Poon with an illustration. Michael and Christopher Atwood also assisted me with transliteration of Central and West Asian names. Peter Bol and Angela Leung have also offered me great support. I am also grateful to Joe McDermott and Susan Bennett for their advice while I was at the Needham Institute. Bruce Tindall and Rachel Schneewind painstakingly proofread the manuscript. I thank Hannah Mack, Rebecca Lawrence and Thomas Newman for their excellent editorial support.

At the University of Wisconsin-Eau Claire (UW-EC), Thomas Miller made sure that I went back to scholarly activities when I was pulled in multiple directions as a new assistant professor, and Jane Pederson has long urged me to complete the book as soon as possible. Janice Bogstad, Maria DaCosta, Selika Ducksworth-Lawton, Steve Gosh, Bob Gough, Karen Havholm, Donna Kuklinski, Paulis Lazda, Manuel Lopez-Zafra, Scott Lowe, John McCrackin, Ron Mickel, Helaine Minkus, Eugenio Pinero, Teresa Sanislo, Rick St. Germaine, Judy Stitt, Matt Waters, Kim Wellnitz, and many other colleagues supported my scholarly and other professional activities. My graduate student Xuyuan Sui checked the transliteration of Chinese and Japanese words. Friends in Eau Claire—Eberth Alarcon, Saori Braun, Janet Carson, Charlotte Hubert, Chiayu Hsu, Sooyun Im, David Jones, Eunsook Jung, Tomomi Kakegawa, Paul Kaldjian, Esther and Antonio Lazcano, Roberta Lewis, Gerardo Licon, Mikako Matsunaga, Mary Mickel, Tarique Niazi, Meg Nord, Mafumi Ohmura, Joe Orser, Hiroko Saigo, Asha Sen, Simei Tong, Ka Vang, Charles Vue, Nobuyoshi Yasuda, and many others—have kindly helped and enlightened me in different ways.

Various grants generously funded the different stages of this book: the Kluge Fellowship, Andrew W. Mellon Foundation Research Fellowships for US-based Scholars at the Needham Research Institute, Research Grant to Assist Foreign Scholars in Chinese Studies, UW-EC Sabbatical Grant, UW-EC University Research and Creative Activity Grants, "Maritime Cross-Cultural Exchange in East Asia and the Formation of Japanese Traditional Culture" Project Team,

James Birdsall Weter Fellowship, Grants-in-Aid for Scientific Research from the Japan Society of the Promotion of Science, and a Stanford University Ph.D. Fellowship. I appreciate the great assistance that staff members and librarians offered to me while I was a visiting scholar at the Kluge Center (the Library of Congress), the Needham Research Institute, the Center for Chinese Studies in Taiwan, and Academia Sinica.

Finally, my deepest gratitude goes to my family in Japan. A determined feminist, former scientist at a national lab, and professional translator, my mother Kazuko has always encouraged my sister and me to pursue our own careers since our childhood. My father Tsutomu was a gentle and reliable breadwinner, who trusted his wife's judgments about everything, especially their daughters' education. My sister Masako is the best sister one could ever hope for. I also thank her partner Suetsugu Akira and their two children Yō and Shun for lighting up our lives.

Despite the support that I have received from numerous people mentioned here and from those I failed to mention, I am solely responsible for all the errors that remain in this book.

Chinese dynasties referenced in this book

Shang 商: 16th–11th century BCE
Zhou 周: 11th century–256 BCE
Qin 秦: 221–207 BCE
Han 漢: 202 BCE–220 CE
    Former Han 前漢: 202 BCE–9 CE
    Later Han 後漢: 25–220
Wei 魏: 220–265
Western Jin 西晉: 265–316
Nan-Bei chao 南北朝: 420–589
    Liu-Song 劉宋: 420–479
    Northern Wei 北魏: 386–534
    Northern Zhou 北周: 557–581
Sui 隋: 581–618
Tang 唐: 608–907
Liao 遼: 916–1125
Song 宋: 960–1276
    Northern Song 北宋: 960–1127
    Southern Song 南宋: 1127–1276
Jin 金: 1115–1234
Yuan 元: 1260–1368 (Mongol Empire: 1206–1368)
Ming 明: 1368–1644
Qing 清: 1644–1912

Abbreviations

Beitu	Beijing tushuguan guji zhenben congkan 北京圖書館古籍珍本叢刊.
CSJC	Congshu jicheng 叢書集成.
Huikan	Yuanren wenji zhenben huikan 元人文集珍本彙刊. Taibei: Guoli Zhongyang tushuguan.
Qingrong	Yuan Jue 袁桷. *Qingrong jushi ji* 清容居士集. SKQS.
Sanshiqi	Song-Yuan difangzhi sanshiqi zhong 宋元地方志三十七種. Taibei: Guotai wenhua shiye youxian gongsi.
SBCK	Sibu congkan 四部叢刊.
SKQS	Wenyuange siku quanshu 文淵閣四庫全書.
SKQSZB	Siku quanshu zhenben 四庫全書珍本.
SYD Xubian	Song-Yuan difangzhi congshu xubian 宋元地方志叢書續編. Taibei: Dahua shuju.
Tsūsei (1)	Kobayashi Kōshirō 小林高四郎 and Okamoto Keiji 岡本敬二, eds. *Tsūsei jōkaku no kenkyū yakuchū* 通制條格の研究譯注, vol. 1.
Tsūsei (2)	Okamoto Keiji 岡本敬二, ed. *Tsūsei jōkaku no kenkyū yakuchū* 通制條格の研究譯注, vol. 2.
Tsūsei (3)	Okamoto Keiji 岡本敬二, ed. *Tsūsei jōkaku no kenkyū yakuchū* 通制條格の研究譯注, vol. 3.
TYG Xubian	Tianyige cang Mingdai fangzhi xuankan xubian 天一閣藏明代方志選刊續編. Shanghai: Shanghai shudian.
TZTG	*Tongzhi tiaoge* 通制條格. Reprint, Nanjing: Zhejiang guji chubanshe, 1986.
WKIS	*Wakoku kanseki isho shūsei* 和刻漢籍医書集成. Tokyo: Entapraizu Shuppanbu, 1992.
YDZ	*Da Yuan shengzheng guochao dianzhang* 大元聖政國朝典章. Taibei: Guoli Gugong bowu yuan, 1976.
YRCK	Yuanren wenji zhenben congkan 元人文集珍本叢刊. Taibei: Xinwenfeng gongsi.
ZGFZCS	Zhongguo fangzhi congshu 中國方志叢書. Taibei: Chengwen chubanshe.

Note on transcription and translation

This book in principle adopts the *Hanyu pinyin* system and the Hepburn romanization system to transcribe Chinese and Japanese terms respectively into the Latin alphabet. In cases of modern scholars' names, however, I have tried to preserve the spellings of their own choosing. I have referred to Christopher Atwood's *Encyclopedia of Mongolia and the Mongolian Empire* (New York: Facts on File, 2004) to transcribe Mongolian as well as other Central and West Asian names and words. When translating the names of governmental offices, I have consulted David M. Farquhar's *Government of China Under Mongolian Rule: A Reference Guide* (Stuttgart: Steiner, 1990) and Charles O. Hucker, *A Dictionary of Official Titles in Imperial China* (Taibei: Nantian shuju, 1988).

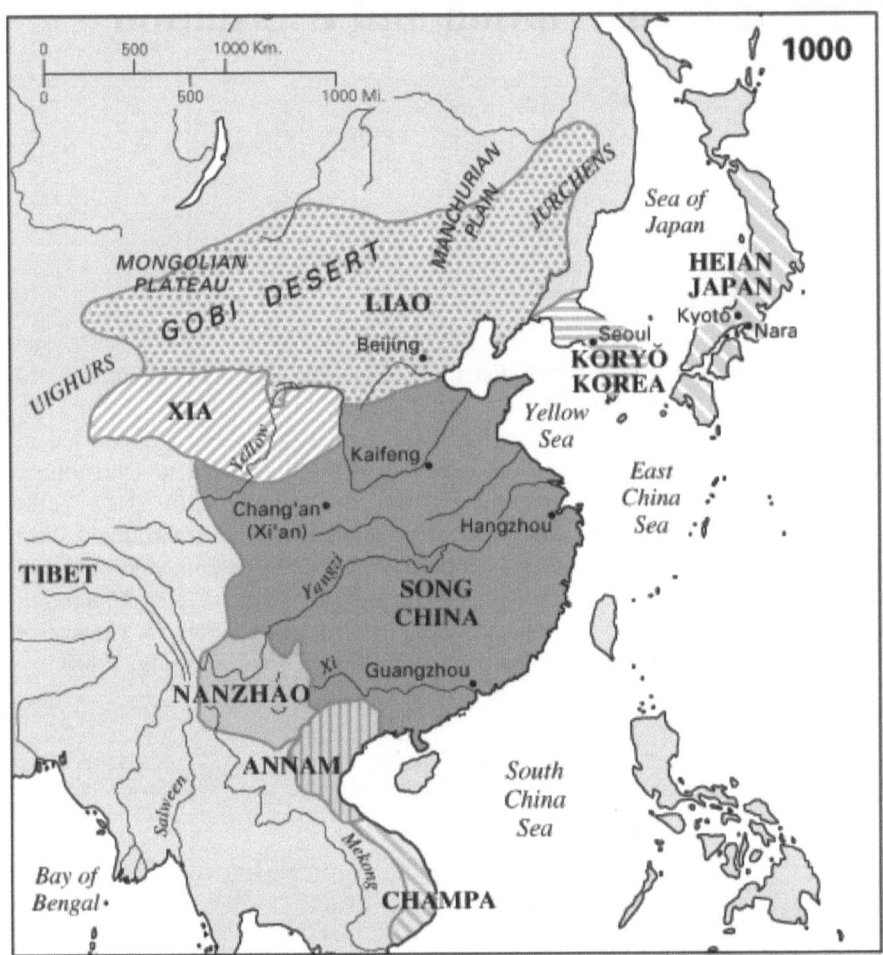

Map 0.1 China under Northern Song

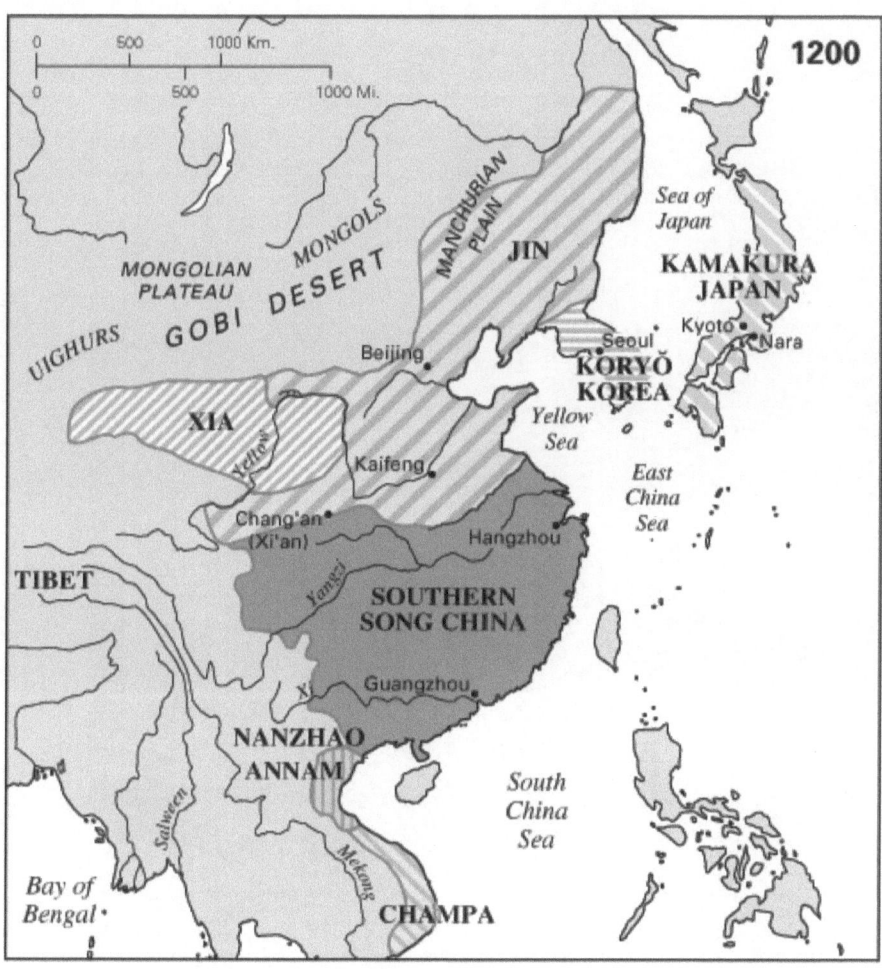

Map 0.2 China under Jin and Southern Song

From Patricia B. Ebrey, *China: A Cultural, Social, and Political History.* 1E. © 2006 Wadsworth, a part of Cengage Learning, Inc. Reproduced by permission. www.cengage.com/permissions.

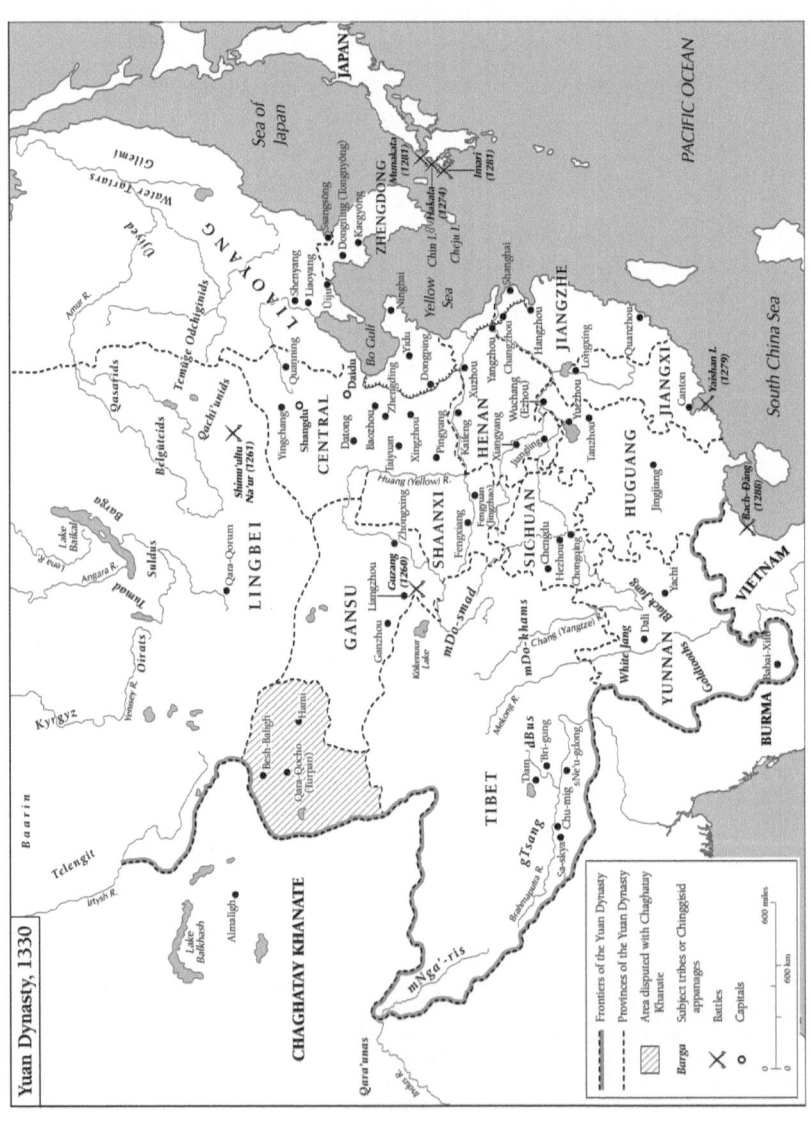

Map 0.3 Yuan dynasty, 1330

From Christopher Atwood, *Encylopedia of Mongolia and the Mongol Empire.* Copyright © 2004 by Infobase Learning. Reprinted with permission of the publisher.

Prologue

This book relates the history of the politics, institutions, and culture of medicine in China under Mongol rule through the eyes of Yuan Jue 袁桷 (1266–1327, *zi* Bochang 伯長, and *hao* Qingrong jushi 清容居士), a scholar-official from a prominent family in Yin county 鄞縣 of Qingyuan circuit 慶元路 (present Ningbo 寧波). I "met" him when I was a graduate student. At the time, I was going through local gazetteers (*difangzhi* 地方志) of the circuit, trying to learn how I might be able to use this genre for my research on medical history. Historians consider local gazetteers excellent primary sources because they give local and central administrators' overviews of the areas under their supervision. They were also vehicles for local elites to express pride.[1] I chose Ningbo as a focus of my preliminary study because prior to the twentieth century it was one of the most important commercial and cultural centers of China, and as such it produced some of the earliest extant gazetteers.[2] This region compiled three gazetteers in the Song period and two in the Yuan period.

Yuan Jue attracted my attention because of an editorial decision that he made for the gazetteer that he compiled, *Records of Siming in the Yanyou Era* (*Yanyou Siming zhi* 延祐四明志, preface in 1320). Unlike the three preceding gazetteers from the same region, the literary name of which is Siming, Yuan's provided a nineteen-page description of local medical schools (*yixue*) and the halls in those schools dedicated to the Three Progenitors (*Sanhuang* 三皇, i.e., Fuxi 伏羲, Shennong 神農, and Huangdi 黃帝).[3] In the introductory paragraph of the "Medical School in This Circuit" section, he wrote:

> Medical school. In the third year of the Zhongtong 中統 era [1262], [we] received an edict ordering [us] to establish the schools and build the Halls of the Three Progenitors. [The edict ordered that we should] annually practice rituals on the third day of the third month and the ninth day of the ninth month. Goumang 勾芒, Zhurong 祝融, Fenghou 風后, and Limu 力牧 should also be worshiped [along with the Three Progenitors].[4]

Yuan Jue then discussed changes in the location of the circuit medical school and cited commemorative writings inscribed on the walls of the building. He also recorded the dimensions of the paddy field to support the school, the sizes of the rooms in the building, the ritual tools and the books that the school owned, and the titles of the instructors affiliated with the institution.[5] This entry on the circuit medical school was followed by descriptions of prefectural medical schools and temples.

Yuan Jue's editorial decision was later followed by Wang Housun 王厚孫 (1300–76), the author of the second gazetteer, the *Continued Records of Siming in the Zhizheng Era* (*Zhizheng Siming xuzhi* 至正四明續志), compiled in 1342. Wang Housun was the grandson of Yuan Jue's teacher Wang Yinglin 王應麟 (1223–96), and he shared the same mentors as Yuan Jue. Wang Housun maintained Yuan Jue's structure for the gazetteer and provided information on what happened in Qingyuan circuit after Yuan's gazetteer was completed.[6] According to Wang's gazetteer, the circuit medical school was renovated twice, in 1333 and 1342, after the completion of Yuan Jue's gazetteer. The renovations resulted in several additional rooms and a gate named "Stone Gate for the Elite Star" (*shi lingxingmen* 石櫺星門).[7] The circuit Confucian school had built a "Gate for the Elite Star" in 1238 and reconstructed it in 1320.[8] In other words, by 1342 both the circuit Confucian school and the circuit medical school had gates that symbolized the elite status of the students and the instructors.

These discoveries made me curious about Yuan Jue and the ways medical history intersected with his life. Why did he write so much about medical schools? What were the Halls or the Temples of the Three Progenitors? Did he have any personal reasons for caring about medicine? Did his editorial decision have anything to do with the Mongol rule of the time? How about the Learning of the Way (*Daoxue* 道學), which was becoming the dominant philosophical trend in China? What impact did it have on the medical innovations that had been going on since the Northern Song period (960–1127)? The following pages will show that Yuan had personal and social reasons to include medical schools in his gazetteer.

By the time Yuan Jue was born in 1266, Mongols had been engaged in attempts at world conquest for sixty years. Chinggis Khan (Temujin, Taizu 太祖, 1167–1227, r. 1206–27) unified the tribes of the Mongol Plain in 1206, and his descendants reached as far as the Adriatic Sea by 1241. The Mongol empire gradually expanded into China as well, completing in 1234 the conquest of North China (an area north of the Huai River 淮河 and the Qinling Mountains 秦嶺山脈), which had been ruled by the Jin dynasty since 1127. Mongols brought in Central and West Asians (*Semu* 色目) and North Chinese (*hanren* 漢人, or *beiren* 北人) elites, who helped them govern the former Jin territory. The Southern Song dynasty, which had occupied South China since 1127, officially surrendered to the Mongols in 1276.[9] This was when Yuan Jue was ten years old, or in Chinese counting, about eleven *sui* 歲. He and his family witnessed and took part in the great transition that South China went through as the South Chinese (*nanren* 南人) explored how they could survive and thrive as newcomers to the empire led by Mongol rulers and their advisers from Central and West Asia and North China.

As the first comprehensive monograph on medicine in China under the Mongols, this book argues that this period was a separate moment in Chinese history, when a configuration of power different from the Song, Jin, or Ming periods created its own medical culture. In other words, I emphasize the impact of the political and institutional changes caused by the Mongols and their collaborators on the social and cultural history of medicine. This book also points to the complexity of the history of China under Mongol rule and to the significance of time and geography for the study of this complex history. I use a variety of Chinese-language sources—gazetteers, legal texts, biographies, poems, and medical texts—to analyze the roles of the Mongols and Central and West Asians as cultural brokers and also as unifiers of China. I see North and South Chinese elites as agents of historical change rather than as victims of Mongol oppression. Physicians and their clients in China had certainly experienced major changes in the previous dynasties, and they went through substantial changes under the Mongols as well.

This book is comprised of six chapters. The first chapter looks at Yuan Jue's personal life. It shows that family tragedies partially explained why he believed that medicine was an important field of study, in addition to political, institutional, and cultural reasons explained in the chapters to follow. Chapters 2 to 4 use legal texts such as *Institutions in the Sagely Administration of the Great Yuan* (*Da Yuan shengzheng guochao dianzhang* 大元國朝聖政典章, also called *Yuan dianzhang* 元典章) to explore the political processes that shaped the medical institutions of the Yuan period.[10] These three chapters are in chronological order: 1206 to 1276 ("The Mongol conquest and the new configuration of power"); 1276–1300 ("The reunification of China"); and 1300–1368 ("The South Chinese participation in imperial politics"). The fifth chapter focuses on prose and poetry that five literati patients wrote about medicine and doctors. Chapter 6 looks at the history of medical books and theories from the Northern Song until the end of Mongol China.

This book is in line with recent studies on the history of science, technology, and medicine in China and Eurasia under Mongol rule. Thomas T. Allsen's *Culture and Conquest in Mongol Eurasia* has used primary and secondary sources in multiple languages to show the significance of the Mongols as cultural brokers, who had the power to decide which elements of Islamic civilization should be brought to China and vice versa.[11] Translating two important books from fourteenth-century China—*Correct Summary of Drinking and Eating* (*Yinshan zhenyao* 飲膳正要) and *Islamic Pharmacology* (*Huihui yaofang* 回回藥方)—Paul Buell and Eugene Anderson uncovered West Asia's strong influence on the palace culinary culture and medical prescriptions used at the Office of Broad Grace (*Guanghui si* 廣惠司), institutions in the Yuan capitals that provided West Asian medical services. This was an important discovery because the fourteenth-century books, on the surface, explained the values of the culinary and medical recipes using Chinese medical terms.[12]

While Allsen, Buell, and Anderson have made important contributions using multilingual sources, a growing number of scholars have employed Chinese-language sources to explore the history of medicine in China from the tenth to the fourteenth century. In the 1960s, Miyashita Saburō wrote a pioneering work dedicated to the Song-Yuan institutional history of medicine.[13] Okanishi Tameto showed the significance of the so-called "Four Great Masters of Medicine of the

Jin-Yuan Period" (*Jin-Yuan dasijia* 金元大四家) in the history of pharmacology.[14] Wai-kam Ho was the first historian to point to "the rise of medical and fortune-telling professions" in the Yuan dynasty and argue that "the fourteenth century is probably the only period in Chinese literature in which mention of Confucian turned physician is commonplace."[15]

The number of scholars interested in this topic increased dramatically after Robert Hymes' 1988 article reinforced Ho's point by introducing primary sources that were new to medical historians at the time, collections of literati writing (*wenji* 文集).[16] Despite the changes in the number of physicians with elite backgrounds in the Yuan, Hymes argued that physicians were seen as "not quite gentlemen," and that their social status was not considered as high as elite men in other occupations, such as government officials or tutors. Using more *wenji* materials than Hymes did, however, Chen Yuan-Peng disagreed with him. Chen argued that the major changes in medical culture occurred from the Tang to the Northern Song and that what we see in the Yuan medical culture simply "reinforced" what had happened earlier. In particular, he paid attention to the emergence of elite medical amateurs (*shangyi shiren* 尚醫士人) and coinage of the term "Confucian physicians" (*ruyi* 儒醫) in the Northern Song.[17] Angela Leung accepted Chen Yuan-Peng's notion that the Northern Song was the beginning of the new medical culture and pointed to the three factors that influenced the transmission of medical knowledge from the Song to the Ming: popularization of printing, civil service examinations as the primary methods of governmental recruitment, and the rise of Neo-Confucianism.[18] Catherine Despeux reinforced the point of view that the Song was the starting point for the new medical culture by analyzing medical innovations that occurred in the Northern Song period and by showing that Northern Song doctors had made important contributions before the Four Great Masters of Medicine came up with their medical theories, which physicians of later periods valued greatly.[19] Asaf Goldschmidt expanded on this point in his first English-language monograph devoted to Song medical history, paying close attention to the history of medical institutions, illnesses, and medical theories.[20] Charlotte Furth substantiated what Angela Leung called the "bifurcation" of medical practitioners, by focusing on the development of medicine for women (*fuke* 婦科). She also discussed the complex ways in which Yuan medical and intellectual histories intersected with each other in her analysis of Zhu Zhenheng 朱震亨 (1282–1358), the last of the Four Great Masters of Jin-Yuan medicine.[21]

Independently from the above-mentioned works conducted by Taiwanese and English-language scholars, Kosoto Hiroshi, Mayanagi Makoto, and Urayama Kika in Japan have researched histories of a large number of medical books from this period, some of which were extant only in libraries outside of China.[22] Ding Guangdi and Liu Shijue in mainland China wrote books dedicated to the Jin-Yuan Masters and Southern Song physicians, respectively.[23] More historians have recently written dissertations and articles on Chinese medical history from the tenth to the fourteenth century.[24]

To understand the political, institutional, and social context of the history of medicine, my study relies heavily on numerous recent studies on politics, society, and culture under the Mongols. To name a few, Elizabeth Endicott-West, Ōshima Ritsuko, Sugiyama Masaaki, Uematsu Tadashi, Funada Yoshiyuki, and Miya Noriko have explored the dynamism and complexities of the Mongol empire.[25] Whether adopting multilingual sources or focusing on Chinese-language sources, they have shown Mongols as significant contributors of cultural legacies in Yuan China, even though some Chinese people later might have discredited their contributions. While using excellent previous studies on Yuan society and culture to contextualize my discoveries, I will show that medicine was an integral component of Mongol China and that we cannot study this period without paying attention to what happened to doctors and medical institutions.

The present study will also speak to the growing number of works on the history of the Learning of the Way. Although scholars in the field still debate issues such as the proper terms for this intellectual trend and its definitions, they agree that historians should look beyond philosophical theses and annotations to Confucian classics to understand the development of this intellectual trend. Following Hilde de Weerdt, I define the Learning of the Way as a version of Confucian learning as organized by Zhu Xi 朱熹 (1130–1200), which became socially influential in South China by the time of his passing. Zhu's annotations to the Four Books (*Sishu* 四書, i.e., the *Great Learning*, *Analects*, *Mencius*, and *Doctrine of the Mean*) were adopted as the primary texts for the civil service examination when it was revived by the Yuan government 100 years later.[26] Peter Bol's groundbreaking work clarified the process through which literati from the Tang to the Northern Song periods came to value the Way (*Dao* 道), as opposed to their literary tradition (*wen* 文). To explore the activities of *Daoxue* members in the thirteenth century, Hoyt Tillman, for example, analyzed Zhu Xi's and his contemporary philosophers' letters, Ellen Neskar temple inscriptions, and Hilde de Weerdt the civil service examination questions and answers.[27] I will suggest that in order to understand the history of the Learning of the Way in the Yuan period, scholars should also analyze the inscriptions dedicated to medical institutions, biographies of doctors, and medical texts.

Following conventions in present-day English-language studies, I use the terms "China under the Mongols," "Mongol China," or the "Mongol Period" for the period between 1206 (unification of tribes in the Mongol plain) and 1368 (the Mongols' surrender to the Ming dynasty) and "the Yuan dynasty" for the period between 1260 (Qubilai Khan's ascendance to the throne) and 1368. Qubilai's ascendance to the throne, in Christopher Atwood's words, "created a power center in North China that differed significantly from the earlier reigns of the Mongol khans."[28] Note, however, that there are some disagreements about these terms in the field. Elizabeth Endicott-West, for example, defines the Yuan period broadly from 1206 to 1368.[29] Sugiyama, Miya, and Funada suggest that historians should use "The Great Yuan" (*Dayuan* 大元), not the "Yuan," because Mongols declared the former as their country's name (*guohao* 國號) in 1271, because it came from a phrase in the *Book of Changes*, and because it was probably associated with the Mongol concept of *tenggeri* (heaven).[30] English-language authors might follow Sugiyama, Miya, and

Funada in the future, just as some Japanese authors have, but this book will follow current English-language conventions.

I will also follow current conventions regarding the terms that refer to Chinese philosophical and religious traditions. I use specific words such as the Learning of the Way or the Complete Reality Sect (*Quanzhen zong* 全眞宗) whenever my primary sources allow me, but I sometimes cannot avoid using broader terms, such as Confucianism and Daoism. I am certainly aware that some recent scholars of Chinese religions and philosophies have expressed concerns about the English word Confucianism as the translation of the Chinese words *rujia* 儒家 and *rujiao* 儒教. Mark Czikszentmihalyi, for example, says that the English term "mistakenly suggests a tradition that grew out of the foundational teachings of one person." To decentralize Confucius from this tradition, he uses the term "the Ru tradition," instead of Confucianism, in his analysis of excavated materials from early China.[31] He also uses Kongzi 孔子 ("Master Kong"), a commonly used Chinese appellation for Kong Qiu 孔丘, instead of "Confucius," the sixteenth-century Jesuits' rendering of another Chinese appellation, Kong fuzi 孔夫子.[32] Czikszentmihalyi is certainly making an important point, but by the Yuan period, the centrality of Confucius in the *Ru* tradition had long been established.[33] Nathan Sivin's 1978 article did not problematize Daoism as a translation of the Chinese words *Daojia* 道家 or *Daojiao* 道教 but cautioned against the tendency in the field that, in his view, had tried to see Daoism as one entity and establish links between history of the religion and history of science and medicine in East Asia without much research or thought.[34]

While using the conventional translations for the names of East Asian philosophical and religious traditions, I remind the readers that they were highly inclusive and that they often coexisted in the society and in one person's life. Although Chinese words like *rujiao* 儒教 (Confucianism) and *daojiao* 道教 (Daoism) existed at the latest by the late Six Dynasties period to be juxtaposed to *fojiao* 佛教 (Buddhism), the Chinese language did not have words equivalent to the English words "religion" and "philosophy" until the 1870s, when the Japanese began using words such as *shūkyō* 宗教 (Chinese *zongjiao*) and *tetsugaku* 哲學 (*zhexue*) as translations of the Western concepts and the Chinese adopted them.[35] In the minds of middle-period Chinese people, Confucianism and Daoism were "teachings" (*jiao* 教), and it was normally acceptable for a literatus to learn from multiple teachings.[36]

I have made a difficult decision to adopt "Confucian physician" as my translation of the term *ruyi* 儒醫, even though I see the merits of other translations such as "literati physicians" and "scholar-physicians."[37] Adopting the last translation, Yi-Li Wu explains the meaning of *ru* 儒 as follows:

> At the most basic level, the scholar (*ru*) was a man who had mastered a canon of books comprising the teachings of Confucius, the major commentaries on the same, and books that the Sage had deemed essential for the proper nurturing of worthy men: odes and poetry, histories, rituals and government regulations from model states, and yin-yang cosmology.[38]

As Peter Bol and Benjamin Elman have shown, participation, not necessarily success, in the civil service examinations defined who belonged to the elite stratum of the society in the Song as well as in the Ming-Qing period, and the examinations primarily tested the candidates' knowledge of Confucian texts.[39] Thus elite men, by definition, were all familiar with Confucian texts. The translations "literati physicians" and "scholar-physicians" highlight the facts that *ruyi* came from the elite families and that they were highly educated, but do not show the contents of the education that they received from childhood on.

This book adopts "Confucian physician," or "Confucian doctor," as the translation of *ruyi* because I think "literati physician" and "scholar-physician" are too broad to convey the nuances of the word in the Jin and Yuan periods. Due to the political and institutional developments described in Chapters 2 through 4, *yi* alone was a respectful term, juxtaposed vis-à-vis *ru* in the Yuan household and school systems. China under Mongols was different from Song or Ming-Qing China when the civil service examinations were *the* "ladder of success," to use an expression that Ping-ti Ho used in his classic study of the examinations during this period.[40] Under Mongols, the civil service examinations were held only sporadically, and elites had other ladders of success into the government, such as medicine. Moreover, the Learning of the Way was still a relatively new intellectual movement attracting passionate followers, and it was not a stale orthodoxy, so to say, like the one Wang Shouren 王守仁 (1472–1529, *hao* Yangming 陽明) and other Ming philosophers tried to overcome.[41] As Bol says, Neo-Confucians, "people who identified themselves as participants in the intellectual streams that emerged from the philosophical teachings of the eleventh-century brothers Cheng Yi and Cheng Hao," "associated being a Ru with a commitment to ideology."[42] As I will show in Chapter 5, it was the members of this intellectual stream who called a learned physician *ru* or *ruyi* in the Jin and Yuan periods. I thus believe that we would best be able to look at the complex interactions between Chinese political, intellectual, and medical history by retaining the word "Confucian" in our translation of *ruyi*.

Notes

1 See Joseph Dennis, "Early Printing in China Viewed from the Perspectives of Local Gazetteer," in *Knowledge and Text Production in an Age of Print: China, 900–1400*, ed. Lucia Chia and Hilde de Weerdt (Leiden: Brill, 2011), in particular 107–11.
2 For the economic development of this area, see, for example, Shiba Yoshinobu, *Sōdai Kōnan keizaishi no kenkyū* (Tokyo: Kyūko shoin, 1988), in particular "Kōhen: Nei-Sho achiiki no keizai keikyō 後編: 寧紹亜地域の経済景況."
3 Yuan Jue, *Yanyou Siming zhi*, ZGFZCS (vol. 578), 14.12b–21b.
4 Yuan Jue, *Yanyou Siming zhi*, 14.12b.
5 Yuan Jue, *Yanyou Siming zhi*, 14.12b–17a.
6 For Wang Housun's biography, see Bei Qiong, *Qingjiang Bei xiansheng ji*, SBCK chubian, 30.4b–7b. He wrote the *Continued Records* and let the official author be Wang Yuangong 王元恭, the director-general of the Qingyuan circuit at the time.
7 Wang Yuangong, *Zhizheng Siming xuzhi* (Beijing: Zhonghua shuju, Song-Yuan fangzhi congkan, 1990), 8.2a.

8   Yuan Jue, *Yanyou Siming zhi*, 13.23b.
9   For an overview of the Mongol expansion, see Herbert Franke and Denis Twitchett, *The Cambridge History of China, vol. 6: Alien Regimes and Border States, 907–1368* (Cambridge: Cambridge University Press, 1994), in particular chapter 4; and Christopher Atwood, *Encyclopedia of Mongolia and the Mongol Empire* (New York: Facts on File, 2004), in particular 365–69 and 601–12.
10 As Yuan specialists readily acknowledge, the language used in *Sagely Administration* is challenging. There are two reasons for this difficulty. First, each entry is a mixture of two different kinds of information—information about the content of edicts or regulations and information about the legislative processes through which they were proposed, debated, and approved. (Tanaka Kenji, "*Gen tenshō* bunshō no kōsei," *Tōyōshi kenkyū*, 23.4 [March, 1965]: 452–77).

   Second, *Sagely Administration* is difficult because it was written in three different styles. The first style is so-called *guwen* (old style). The second style is named "Chinese clerical style (*Kanbun ritokutai*)" by some Japanese historians. Yoshikawa Kōjirō pointed out that in this style, the writers tenaciously stick to phrases composed of four or six Chinese characters and use rather colloquial words to maintain the rhythm ("*Gen Tenshō* ni mieta Kanbun ritoku no buntai," in Yoshikawa Kōjirō and Tanaka Kenji, *Gen Tenshō no buntai*, a supplement [*furoku*] to Iwamura Shinobu and Tanaka Kenji, *Kōteibon Gen Tenshō keibu dai 1 satsu*, 1964). The third style is named the "style of direct translation from Mongolian (*Mōbun chokuyaku tai*)" by Japanese historians and "a sort of translationese Chinese in Mongolian word-order" by Herbert Franke (cited in Elizabeth Endicott-West, *Mongolian Rule in China: Local Administration in the Yuan Dynasty* [Cambridge, MA: Harvard Council on East Asian Studies, 1989], 22). Tanaka showed the richness of the information contained in the documents written in this style and deciphered the unique linguistic structure and vocabulary ("*Gen tenshō* ni okeru Mōbun chokuyakutai no bunshō," in *Gen Tenshō no buntai*; and "Mōbun chokuyakutai ni okeru hakuwa ni tsuite: *Gen tenshō* oboegaki," *Tōyōshi kenkyū*, 19.4 [1961]: 483–501).
11 Thomas T. Allsen, *Culture and Conquest in Mongol Eurasia* (Cambridge: Cambridge University Press, 2001).
12 See, for example, Paul D. Buell and Eugene N. Anderson, *A Soup for the Qan: Second Revised and Expanded Edition* (Leiden: Brill, 2010), part A, chap. 1; and Paul D. Buell, "How Did Persian and Other Western Medical Knowledge Move East, and Chinese West? A Look at the Role of Rashīd al-Dīn and Others," *Asian Medicine: Tradition and Modernity* 3.2 (2007): 279–95. For other areas of the history of science in China under the Mongols, see, for example, Nathan Sivin, *Granting the Seasons: the Chinese Astronomical Reform of 1280, With a Study of Its Many Dimensions and an Annotated Translation of Its Records* (New York: Springer, 2010).
13 Miyashita Saburō, "Sō-Gen no iryō," in *Sō-Gen jidai no kagaku gijutsu shi*, ed. Yabuuchi Kiyoshi (Kyoto: Kyoto daigaku jinbun kagaku kenkyūjo, 1967), 123–70.
14 Okanishi Tameto, "Chūgoku honzō no dentō to Kin-Gen no honzō," in *Sō-Gen jidai no kagaku gijutsu shi*, ed. Yabuuchi Kiyoshi (Kyoto: Kyoto daigaku jinbun kagaku kenkyūjo, 1967): 171–210.
15 Sherman E. Lee and Wai-kam Ho. *Chinese Art Under the Mongols: The Yüan Dynasty (1279–1368)* (Cleveland, OH: Cleveland Museum of Art, 1968), 83.
16 Robert Hymes, "Not Quite Gentlemen? Doctors in Sung and Yuan," *Chinese Science* 8 (1988): 9–76.
17 Chen Yuan-Peng, *Liang-Song de "shangyi shiren" yu "ruyi": jianlun qizai Jin-Yuan de liubian* (Taibei: Guoli Taiwan daxue wenshi congkan, 1997).
18 Angela Ki Che Leung, "Medical Learning from the Song to the Ming," in *The Song-Yuan-Ming Transition in Chinese History*, ed. Paul Smith and Richard von Glahn (Cambridge, MA: Harvard University Asia Center, 2003), 374–98.

19 Catherine Despeux, "The System of the Five Circulatory Phases and the Six Seasonal Influences (*wuyun liuqi*), a Source of Innovation in Medicine Under the Song (960–1279)," in *Innovation in Chinese Medicine*, ed. Elizabeth Hsu (Cambridge: Cambridge University Press, 2002), 121–65.

20 Asaf Goldschmidt, *The Evolution of Chinese Medicine: Song Dynasty, 960–1200* (London: Routledge, 2009).

21 Charlotte Furth, "The Physician as Philosopher of the Way: Zhu Zhenheng (1282–1358)," *Harvard Journal of Asiatic Studies*, 66.2 (2006): 423–59. Also see her *Flourishing Yin: Gender in China's Medical History, 960–1665* (Berkeley: University of California Press, 1999).

22 See the bibliography for the list of their works.

23 Ding Guangdi, *Jin-Yuan yixue pingxi* (Beijing: Renmin weisheng chubanshe, 1999); and Liu Shijue, *Yongjia yipai yanjiu* (Beijing: Zhongguo guji chubanshe, 2000).

24 For example, relatively recent dissertations on the Song medical history include Chen Junkai, "Songdai yizheng zhi yanjiu" (Ph.D. diss., Guoli Taiwan Shifan Daxue, 1996); T.J. Hinrichs, "The Medical Transforming of Governance and Southern Customs in Song Dynasty China (960–1279 C.E.)" (Ph.D. diss., Harvard University, 2003); and Hsiao-wen Cheng, "Traveling Stories and Untold Desires: Female Sexuality in Song China, 10th–13th Centuries" (Ph.D. diss., University of Washington, 2012). Dissertations that discuss medical history under Mongols include Reiko Shinno, "Promoting Medicine in the Yuan Dynasty (1206–1368): An Aspect of Mongol Rule in China" (Ph.D. diss., Stanford University, 2002); Wu Xianglan, "Yuandai yizheng yanjiu" (Ph.D. diss., Jinan Daxue, 2008); Fabien Simonis, "Mad Acts, Mad Speech, and Mad People in Late Imperial Chinese Law and Medicine" (Ph.D. diss., Princeton University, 2010); Huang Junda, "Yuandai yishi zhidu yanjiu" (MA thesis, Guoli Qinghua Daxue, 2011); and Zhang Xueqian, "Yuan-Ming ruyi sixiang yu shijian de shehuishi: yi Zhu Zhenheng ji 'Danxi xuepai' wei zhongxin" (Ph.D. diss., Xianggang Zhongwen Daxue, 2012). Recent articles on medicine under Mongol rule include, Miya Noriko, "Mongoru ōzoku to kitai no gijutsu shugi shūdan," in *Gakumon no katachi: mōhitotsu no Chūgoku shisōshi*, ed. Kominami Ichirō (Tokyo: Kyūko shoin, 2014), 177–222.

25 Endicott-West, *Mongolian Rule in China: Local Administration in the Yuan Dynasty*; Ōshima Ritsuko, *Mongoru no seifuku ōchō* (Tokyo: Daitō shuppansha, 1992); Uematsu Tadashi, *Gendai Kōnan seiji shakaishi kenkyū* (Tokyo: Kyūko shoin, 1997); Sugiyama Masaaki, *Mongoru teikoku to Daigen urusu* (Kyoto: Kyoto daigaku gakujutsu shuppannkai, 2004); and Miya Noriko, *Mongoru jidai no shuppan bunka* (Nagoya: Nagoya daigaku shuppankai, 2006).

26 Hilde de Weerdt, *Competition over Content: Negotiating Standards for the Civil Service Examinations in Imperial China (1127–1276)* (Cambridge, MA: Harvard University Asia Center, 2007), 25–42.

27 Peter Bol, *"This Culture of Ours": Intellectual Transitions in T'ang and Sung China* (Stanford, CA: Stanford University Press, 1992); Hilde de Weerdt, *Competition over Content*; Hoyt Tillman, *Confucian Discourse and Chu Hsi's Ascendancy* (Honolulu: University of Hawai'i Press, 1992); and Ellen Neskar, "The Cult of Worthies: A Study of Shrines Honoring Local Confucian Worthies in the Sung Dynasty (960–1279)" (Ph.D. diss., Columbia University, 1993). Also see Bol's *Neo-Confucianism in History* (Cambridge, MA: Harvard University Asia Center, 2008).

28 Atwood, *Encyclopedia of Mongolia and Mongol Empire*, 601.

29 Elizabeth Endicott-West, *Mongolian Rule in China*, 1.

30 Song Lian et al., *Yuanshi* (Beijing: Zhonghua shuju, 1976), 7.138. Sugiyama, *Mongoru teikoku to Daigen urusu*, 14. Miya Noriko, *Mongoru jidai no shuppan bunka*, 15–16, note 1. Funada Yoshiyuki, review of Sugiyama Masaaki's *Mongoru teikoku to Daigen urusu*, *Shigaku zasshi* 113.11 (2004): 100–10.

31 Mark Czikszentmihalyi, *Material Virtue: Ethics and the Body in Early China* (Leiden: Brill, 2004). His quote comes from p. 15.

32 Lionel M. Jensen, *Manufacturing Confucianism: Chinese Traditions and Universal Civilization* (Durham, NC: Duke University Press, 1998), is a highly controversial analysis of the Jesuits' writings on Confucianism. See Czikszentmihalyi's, Kai-wing Chow's, and R. Po-chia Hsia's reviews of the book (*Journal of the American Academy of Religion*, 67.3 (1999): 678–81; *American Historical Review*, 104.5 (1999): 1645–46; and *History of Religions*, 41.1 (2001): 71–73).

33 For example, during the Yuan period, localities built *Ruxue* 儒學 (the Ru schools, or Confucian schools) accompanied by Xuansheng Temples (*xuansheng miao* 宣聖廟). Xuansheng was an honorary name given to Confucius. An imperial edict ordered the members of *ruhu* 儒戶 (Ru, or Confucian, households) to go there every fifteen days to pray to Confucius. See "*Miaoxue*" section of Chapter 3.

34 Nathan Sivin, "On the Word 'Taoist' as a Source of Perplexity, with Special Reference to the Relations of Science and Religion in Traditional China," *History of Religions*, 17.3/4 (1978): 303–30. The quote is on p. 319.

35 Kobayashi Masayoshi, *Rikuchō dōkyō shi kenkyū* (Tokyo: Sōbunsha, 1990), 511–21 discusses the history of the terms *rujiao*, *daojiao*, and *fojiao*. For history of the words *shūkyō* and *zongjiao*, see Isomae Jun'ichi, *Kindai Nihon no shūkyō gensetsu to sono keifu* (Tokyo: Iwanami shoten, 2003), 29–38; Viren Murthy, "On the Emergence of New Concepts in Late Qing China and Meiji Japan: the Case of Religion," *Sino-Japanese Transculturation: From the Late Nineteenth Century to the End of the Pacific War*, ed. Richard King, et al. (Lanham, MD: Lexington Books, 2012), 71–97; and Sun Jiang, "Fangyi zongjiao," in *Yazhou gai'nian shi yanjiu, di 1 ji*, ed. Sun Jiang and Liu Jianhui (Beijing: Shenghuo, Dushu, Xinzhi Sanliang shudian, 2013), 84–108. For history of *tetsugaku* and *zhexue*, see Takano Shigeo, "*Meiroku zasshi* no goi kōzō: niji kango o chūshin ni (sono 1)," *Jinbungaku kenkyūjo hō* (Kanagawa Daigaku), 34 (2001), in particular p. 43; his "*Meiroku zasshi* no wasei kango: gendaigo ni natta go to shōmetsu shita go," in Meiroku zasshi *to sono shūhen* (Tokyo: Ochanomizu shobō, 2004), ed. Kanagawa Daigaku Jinbungaku Kenkyūjo, in particular 200–01; Sang Bing, "Kindai 'Chūgoku tetsugaku' no kigen," trans. Murata Ei, in *Kindai Higashi Ajia niokeru honyaku gainen no tenkai*, ed. Ishikawa Yoshihiro and Hazama Naoki (Kyoto: Kyoto daigaku jinbun kangaku kenkyūjo fuzoku Chūgoku kenkyū sentā, 2013), 143–66; and Kawajiri Fumihiko, "'Zhexue' zai jindai Zhonguo: yi Cai Yuanpei de 'zhexue' wei zhongxin," in *Yazhou gai'nian shi yanjiu, di 1 ji*, 66–83.

36 For example, as shown in Chapter 5, Wu Cheng (1249–1333), a leading Neo-Confucian philosopher in the Yuan period, stayed in a Daoist temple during the time of transition from the Southern Song to the Yuan and later wrote an annotation to *Laozi*. Chapter 6 will show that a prominent physician and medical theorist, Liu Wansu (b. 1126–32), said, "In the Zhou dynasty, Mr. Lao elaborated on the Great Way to specifically create *daojiao*; Confucius elaborated on the Normal Way to specifically create *rujiao*" 老氏以精大道，專爲道教; 孔子以精常道，專爲儒教.

37 Yüan-ling Chao (*Medicine and Society in Late Imperial China: A Study of Physicians in Suzhou, 1600–1850*, New York: Peter Lang International Academic Publishers, 2009) and Angela Leung ("Medical Learning from the Song to the Ming") translate the term "Confucian physicians"; Furth (*Flourishing Yin*) and Goldschmidt (*The Evolution of Chinese Medicine*) "literati physicians"; Volker Scheid (*Currents of Tradition in Chinese Medicine 1626–2006*, Seattle, WA: Eastland Press, 2007) and Yi-Li Wu (*Reproducing Women: Medicine, Metaphor, and Childbirth in Late Imperial China*, Berkeley: University of California Press, 2010) "scholar-physicians."

38 Yi-Li Wu, *Reproducing Women*, 39.

39 Peter Bol, "The Sung Examination System and the *Shih*," *Asia Major*, third series, 3.2 (1990): 149–71. Benjamin Elman, "Political, Social, and Cultural Reproduction via

Civil Service Examinations in Late Imperial China," *Journal of Asian Studies*, 50.1 (1991): 7–28.
40 Ping-ti Ho, *The Ladder of Success in Imperial China: Aspects of Social Mobility, 1368–1911* (New York: Columbia University, 1962).
41 Mabuchi Masaya, "Gen-Minsho seirigaku no ichi sokumenn: Shushigaku no biman to Son Saku no shisō," *Chūgoku tetsugaku* 4 (1992): 60–131.
42 Bol, *Neo-Confucianism in History*, 78 and 80.

1   Yuan Jue and his family

Yuan Jue's story gives us an excellent example of some of the ways in which South Chinese elites accommodated themselves to Mongol rule. His story is of course only one of many stories surrounding the medical culture of the Yuan period, but thanks to the relatively extensive available sources on him, his family, and his home county, it reveals reasons why some felt compelled to participate in an empire-wide movement to promote medicine. His life reminds us that although historians tend to focus on a male actor's experiences in his public sphere when they try to understand the reasons for his social decisions, his experiences in the private sphere were equally important.

Family status

Yuan Jue was born in 1266, ten years prior to the fall of the Song dynasty, from an alliance between two nationally eminent descent groups from Qingyuan.[1] At that time, three families were considered most eminent: the Shi 史, the Lou 樓, and the Yuan 袁.[2] The first family, the Shi, the most prominent descent group throughout the Southern Song realm, produced Yuan Jue's mother, Shi Diqing 史棣卿 (1246–66), while the third one, the Yuan, produced his father, Yuan Hong 袁洪 (1245–98).

The prominence of the Shi descent group was unquestionable. A Qingyuan gazetteer dating from the Southern Song praises the Shi for having produced four generations of men who became grand councilors and vice-grand councilors (*sishi zaizhi* 四世宰執), a pair of brothers who both became imperial attendants (*xiongdi shicong* 兄弟侍從, rank 4b or above), and four brothers who simultaneously won *jinshi* 進士 degrees (*xiongdi tongbang* 兄弟同榜).[3] Shi Diqing was a daughter of one of the imperial attendants, Shi Binzhi 史賓之 (1190–1251), as well as a great-granddaughter and grandniece of the grand councilors, Shi Hao 史浩 (1106–94) and Shi Miyuan 史彌遠 (1164–1233) (See Figure 1.1). The latter was particularly influential in Southern Song politics because he served as grand councilor for twenty-two years, longer than any other grand councilor during this period. Diqing's sister married into the Xie 謝 family, whose members included an empress.[4]

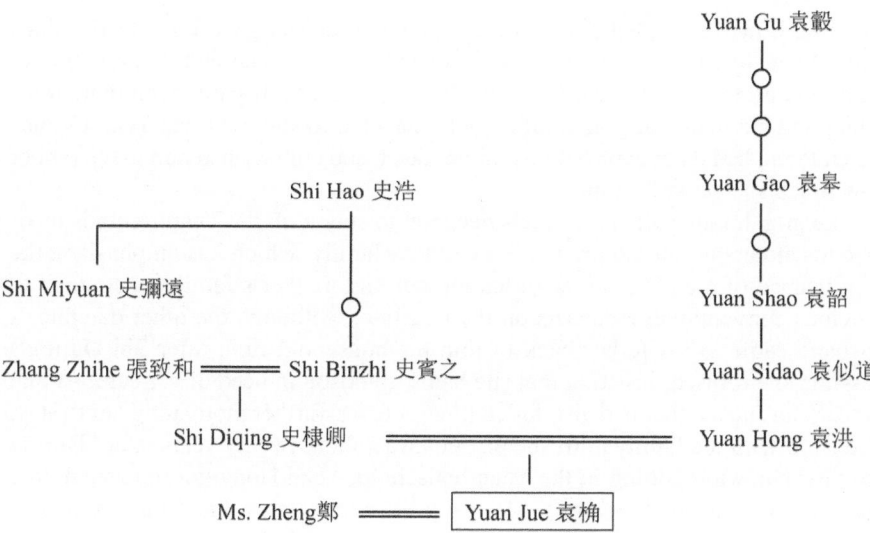

Figure 1.1 Yuan Jue's maternal and paternal families

The Yuan descent group had been prominent in Qingyuan by 1061, when they produced their first *jinshi*, Yuan Gu 袁轂.[5] He and his descendants lived in Kaifeng 開封, the capital of the Northern Song, or in its vicinity, until the Jin army invaded North China and Yuan Gu's great-grandson Yuan Gao 袁皋 returned to Qingyuan in the first half of the twelfth century. Yuan Gao's grandson, Yuan Shao 袁韶, passed the civil service examination in 1187, became a Participant in Determining Governmental Affairs (*canzhi zhengshi* 參知政事, rank 2a) in 1228, and was posthumously given the title of Grand Preceptor (*taishi* 太師, rank 1a). Both his son, Yuan Sidao, and grandson, Yuan Hong, benefited from Shao's political success and entered officialdom through his *yin* 蔭 privilege.[6]

In 1251, when both Shi Diqing's father Binzhi and Yuan Hong's father Yuan Sidao 袁似道 were back in Qingyuan from the capital, Binzhi fell ill. After sharing with Sidao, who was paying a visit, his concern that none of his two sons and two daughters were married, Binzhi proposed the match between six-*sui* Shi Diqing, a daughter of his concubine Zhang Zhihe 張致和 (1213–87), and seven-*sui* Yuan Hong. Sidao gladly accepted the proposal, saying that "the son [to be born out of this marriage] would carry [the honors of] the two families!" and arranged the children's engagement. The couple got married in 1261 and Diqing moved in with her husband, who was serving in the central government at that time. Diqing's mother sometimes lived with her, and at other times with her elder sister's marital household.[7] Diqing appeared to have found the happiness that her father had hoped to pass down to her, as she was the wife of an elite man, enjoyed her mother's frequent company, and gave birth to two daughters and a son in the four years following her wedding.

Mother's death

Her life, however, ended abruptly seven days after she gave birth to her third child, Yuan Jue, in 1266. She was only twenty-one *sui*. The fact that his mother died right after his own birth left Yuan Jue with a sense of guilt, even though his father and his maternal grandmother, who decided to stay with the Yuan to raise the children, had other explanations for her death and only wished him to remember how much she cared for him.

The grandmother Zhang Zhihe's decision to stay with the Yuan reminds us of recent scholarship on the premodern Chinese family, which has emphasized the significance of a child's ties with his mother and mother's family in contrast to previous conventional emphasis on the patriline.[8] Although the other daughter's husband came to invite her back to join his household right after Shi Diqing's passing, she refused, insisting that she had a grandson in need of her care. At that time, Yuan Jue's father had also fallen ill with fever, further motivating her to stay. She lived with the family until she passed away about twenty years later.[9] During the time she was residing in the Yuan household, Yuan Hong got remarried, to a woman from a local elite family, Ms. Yang 楊. Interestingly, the daughter she had with Yuan Hong eventually married a member of the Shi family.[10] Also, Yuan Jue wrote a funerary inscription for Diqing's second cousin as late as in 1323.[11] In other words, the relationship between the Shi and Yuan families was not affected by Diqing's passing.

Yuan Jue seems to have thought that he was responsible for the death of his mother. Several decades later, he wrote her biographical account (*xingshu* 行述) to request his friend Yuan Mingshan 元明善 (1269–1322) to draft the text to be inscribed onto his birth mother's new gravestone.[12] It was common practice at this time for a family member to write a several-page biography of the deceased to be used as source material for a respected individual to compose a funerary inscription. The biography of Shi Diqing started with a confession: "Oh! Merely seven days after I was born, I already caused an unfilial disaster. My mother's voice and appearance were gone forever, and my guilt may never be forgiven."[13]

He expressed a similar sense of guilt in his prayer essay (*jiwen* 祭文) for his maternal grandfather, Shi Binzhi. After explaining how his grandfathers arranged his parents' marriage, he said, "[Binzhi's daughter] gave a birth to an unfilial son called Jue and passed away seven days later."[14]

Certainly, neither Yuan Jue's father nor maternal grandmother thought the mother's death was his fault. Yuan Jue's biography of Shi Diqing says:

> Whenever I served my father, he told me, "The year you were born was extremely hot. It was a year of *bingyin* 丙寅, the year of Fire, so the celestial stem and terrestrial branch contributed [to the weather and your mother's illness]. People living in the capital suffered greatly, gasping for breath without stopping. Seats and tables were hot as if burning. Your mother had generally been weak. One evening, she suddenly suffered severe diarrhea and we could not give her any medicine. The light was fading from her eyes, but she still

looked at you in infant clothes and sadly said, 'Jue, come here.' Her feelings for you reached this level. How could [we] forget?" I record this [episode] with tears in my eyes.[15]

The year of Shi Diqing's death, the second year of the Xianchun 咸淳 era (1266–67), was a year of *bingyin*. The summer might have been hot as the official history of the Song dynasty records that the government held a ceremony to pray for rain in the seventh month.[16] *Bing* in the calendrical system was one of the ten celestial stems (*tiangan* 天干) and represented Fire in the Five Phases Theory (*wuxing* 五行). *Yin*, one of the twelve terrestrial branches (*dizhi* 地支), represented summer heat (*shu* 暑).[17] Yuan Hong was not of course making an academic argument based on the complex theory of calendrical influences on human beings, but was trying to convey that his wife's death was beyond anyone's control.

Those of us living in the West in the twenty-first century might suspect that at least by the time he was an adult, Yuan Jue must have known that he was not responsible for an event that had happened when he was only seven days old. We might even be tempted to argue that he intentionally feigned a sense of guilt. He was, however, a Neo-Confucian scholar whose most important moral duty was to take good care of his parents until they had enjoyed long and healthy lives. His sense of guilt might have been more real than we like to think. We can at least say that, because his maternal grandmother continued living with the family, he did not have the option of forgetting his mother's passing and the reasons for it.

Primary education

Glancing at a large number of the biographical essays and poems written for Yuan Jue,[18] one quickly notices that he was praised as a well-rounded literatus, strongly trained in Confucian classics and talented in various arts. In 1295, when he was thirty *sui*, Dai Biaoyuan 戴表元 (1244–1310), his teacher and his father's friend, said, "[Yuan Jue] deeply understands the principles of various arts (*zhuyi* 諸藝) such as zither (*qin* 琴), calligraphy, medicine, and pharmacology."[19] Yuan Jue was also famous for his poems, and was later named one of the five most important Chinese poets at court.[20] His family members (maternal grandmother and father) took care of his primary education and later hired three teachers outside of his family.

His grandmother, Zhang Zhihe, was born into a musician's family, employed by the Zhao 趙 family in the Song imperial clan. According to Yuan Jue's funerary inscription for her, she was already well trained in music by the time she was seven. Her future mother-in-law met her at the Zhaos' and liked Zhihe so much that she returned home with the girl, asking her to take care of her young son, Shi Binzhi. When both of them grew up, she became his concubine. Having been raised in an elite musical household, Zhang also had a distinguished taste for music. Yuan Jue's funerary inscription for her mentions how she looked down on music "nowadays" for being less sophisticated than in the past. Furthermore, the inscription goes into detail about the singing methods that she thought were proper.[21]

In addition to having talent in music, Zhang Zhihe was a strict person well versed in books. Yuan Jue's biographical account said that even after she became Shi Binzhi's concubine, she lectured him when he lost his temper. Yuan Jue also referred to her moral character by mentioning that she did not enjoy the extravagant lifestyle of the Xie family, into which her first daughter married.[22] Given that it was a common practice for parents and sometimes grandparents to collaborate to educate their children, particularly when they were small, we can safely assume that she participated in Yuan Jue's moral and music education, as well as his literary education.[23]

His father, Yuan Hong, was also a talented man. He excelled in various kinds of arts and was particularly good at writing letters, playing chess, and playing a zither.[24] He studied with Wang Xu 王鎔 (*jinshi* 1202), who was known for his deep understanding of Neo-Confucian ideas.[25] Qingyuan in the Song and Yuan dynasties had been a center of the Neo-Confucian movement and produced the "Four Masters of Siming 四明 in the Chunxi 淳熙 Period [1174–89]," namely, Yang Jian 楊簡 (1141–1226), Yuan Xie 袁燮 (1144–1224), Shen Huan 沈煥 (1139–91), and Shu Lin 舒璘 (1136–99). Their philosophies and the overall intellectual tradition of Qingyuan that they fostered were "influenced by a variety of philosophical schools of the time, including not only the ideas of Zhu Xi (1130–1200) and Lu Jiuyuan 陸九淵 (1139–92), but also those of Lü Zuqian 呂祖謙 (1137–81) from neighboring Jinhua."[26] One of the Four Masters, Yuan Xie, was a distant relative and the teacher of Yuan Jue's great-grandfather, Yuan Shao. He left the bureaucracy at the same time as his teacher Yuan Xie was purged in the Jiatai 嘉泰 era (1201–04) with other followers of Zhu Xi, and stayed in Qingyuan until the purge was cancelled in the Jiading 嘉定 era (1208–24).[27]

Yuan Hong provided an environment that exposed Yuan Jue to the literary heritage from an early stage and aided him in cultivating his own versatility and facility in letters. While denying his excellence in any single specific field, Yuan Jue modestly acknowledged that he had read widely from the family's collection of books.[28] References to the family's library are found in several sources. In the preface to the catalog of the Yuans' old library, Jue mentions that when his great-grandfather studied for the civil service examination, the family was too poor to own many books so he had to memorize them; but once he became an official, he bought books in the capital.[29] When this old library was destroyed by fire in 1289,[30] Yuan Hong and Jue quickly built a new library.[31] When, later, he was assigned to write the official histories of the Song, Liao, and Jin dynasties as a member of Hanlin and National Academy during the reign of Ayurbawada (Renzong 仁宗, 1285–1320, r. 1311–20), he made great use of the books in the family library. Unfortunately this project was interrupted, but when the government finally managed to restart it twenty years after the death of Yuan Jue, his descendants donated a large number of books.[32]

Post-primary education

According to Yuan Jue's biographical account of his father, the latter liked entertaining guests, and rarely spent a day without them.[33] Many of them were prominent scholar-officials who had seen service in the capital during the Southern Song but who had returned to Qingyuan around the time of the Mongol conquest in the mid-1270s.[34] Their and his father's daily conversations must have been stimulating for young Yuan Jue. Moreover, the father asked three of his guests—Dai Biaoyuan, Shu Yuexiang 舒嶽祥 (1217–1301), and Wang Yinglin—to teach his son.

A year younger than Yuan Jue's father, Dai Biaoyuan entered the National University (*taixue* 太學) in 1269 and was granted the *jinshi* degree in 1271. He worked as the instructor (*jiaoshou* 教授) of the governmental school in Jiankang super prefecture 建康府 (present-day Nanjing) when Yuan Jue's father was the controller-general of the locality. They paid visits to each other's house almost every day. Upon their return to Qingyuan, Yuan Hong asked Dai Biaoyuan to teach Yuan Jue who was about ten *sui* at that time. While teaching Yuan Jue, Dai himself became a disciple of Shu Yuexiang and Wang Yinglin, who were also in Yuan Hong's circle. Dai's main academic concern was that "the vital energy (*qi* 氣) of the literary compositions (*wenzhang* 文章) and the rhetoric (*ci* 辭) was bent as the Song period withered." He made it his responsibility to promote "This Culture of Ours" (*siwen* 斯文), in which writing was the primary marker of the civilization.[35]

Shu Yuexiang and Wang Yinglin, the two teachers of Dai Biaoyuan and Yuan Jue, were, respectively, in their late fifties and early sixties when they began teaching Yuan Jue. Most likely, they did not interact with Yuan Jue as often as Dai, who was in his thirties, but gave guidance to the young instructor and his pupil. It was common for an elite family to have a junior tutor for the daily instruction of their sons while requesting a senior scholar to set the framework and goals for the education.[36]

Shu Yuexiang was from Ninghai county 寧海縣, Taizhou 台州 prefecture, and had attained the *jinshi* degree at age twenty in the 1230s. His talent had attracted attention since he was young, particularly from Wu Ziliang 吳子良 (b. 1197), a Song literatus, who compared him to Jia Yi 賈誼, a prodigy in the Han dynasty. After the surrender of the Song dynasty, he lived in Fenghua 奉化, a prefecture of Qingyuan.[37] Yuan Jue's talent in poetry was attributed to Shu's teaching.[38]

Born in Qingyuan in 1223, Wang Yinglin passed the civil service examination in 1241, and became well known to his contemporaries by passing a special exam entitled "Extensive Learning and Resonant Prose" (*boxue hongci* 博學宏詞) in 1256. It was a particularly difficult examination, taken both by *jinshi* degree-holders and by non-degree-holders seeking promotion to offices that required an especially high level of literary competence and knowledge of history and letters for the drafting of imperial documents. This examination "required the memorization of all classics, histories, works of science, and literature, which had ever been compiled, and of course, the commentaries to these works as well."[39] The renowned *Yuhai* 玉海 encyclopedia was in fact Wang's "study book" that he had compiled as part of his preparation for this examination. No one had passed the examination for forty-eight years before him; he and his brother were the last ones to pass it in the Southern Song.[40] After serving several offices and having been twice purged from the government because of political conflicts, Wang was appointed director of the Board of Rites in 1264, and played a significant role in the drafting of imperial edicts concerning the imperial funeral. He also lectured to Emperor Duzong 度宗 (1240–74, r. 1264–74) as a Hanlin Academy Reader. In 1275, he was what Langley calls a "heroic document officer," writing numerous documents to praise military and civil officials in the war against the Mongols and proclamations addressing the desperate military situation.[41]

Wang traced his intellectual lineage back to Lü Zuqian, a leader of the Neo-Confucian movement, through his father's mentor, Lou Fang 樓昉 (1170–1227),[42] and to Zhen Dexiu 眞德秀 (1178–1235), another Neo-Confucian leader, through his own mentor, Wang Ye 王埜 (c. 1194–1260).[43] In his preface to the *Yuhai*, Wang says, "Lü Zuqian and Zhen Dexiu bequeathed that which I emulate."[44] The biographers of his descendants have also noted that Neo-Confucianism was an integral part of the Wang family's education.[45] However, in her study of Southern Song encyclopedias, Hilde de Weerdt points out that Wang mentions Zhu Xi in his *Yuhai* only to comment on philological and bibliographic matters and not on philosophy.[46] Wang did not share the new exclusivist trend among *Daoxue* scholars, nor did he focus solely on moral cultivation as the goal of his study.[47] Characteristics of his scholarship lay in its breadth, and the practicality which a scholar-official needed to serve in the government.[48]

Yuan Jue did not have a teacher who specialized in medicine, but Wang's teaching included knowledge of medical concepts and books. Wang's elementary primer, *Purple Pearls of Primary Education* (*Xiaoxue ganzhu* 小學紺珠) had a section, "On Human Matters" (*Renshi lei* 人事類), in which he listed names of parts of the human body and methods of maintaining health for his pupils to memorize.[49] His study book for the *boxue hongci* examination, the *Yuhai*, included a section called "Arts" (*yishu* 藝術), and there he gave detailed information on fifteen medical books.[50]

Other friends of Yuan Hong's also had good knowledge of medicine. In Yuan Jue's letter to a young doctor, he said, "Elite families in Yin [county] flourish most [in the empire]. In their hometown, their houses are next to one another and [the elites] often discuss medicine."[51] A modern historian, Chen Yuan-Peng, has argued that medical knowledge was a part of elite culture in the Northern and Southern Song dynasties.[52] Yuan Jue was certainly a beneficiary of this culture.

Marriage and family deaths in adulthood

Yuan Jue was married only once, to a woman surnamed Zheng 鄭 (1270–98), whose first name we do not know, and lost her in his early thirties. They appeared to have had a loving relationship, and her early death, followed by his father's death just eight days later, was a great shock to him. He later cited the two family deaths as a reason why he thought medicine was important as a specialized study.

Ms. Zheng was born into and raised by another elite family in Qingyuan. An elder brother of her great-grandfather, Zheng Qingzhi 鄭清之 (1176–1251, *jinshi* 1217) was a grand councilor during the reign of Lizong 理宗 (1205–64, r. 1224–64) of the Southern Song. Her great-grandfather, grandfather, and father all served in the Southern Song government. Her father resigned from the central government when Jia Sidao 賈似道 (1213–75) came into power because, for some reason, they did not get along well. Her father became good friends with Yuan Hong, who was also purged from the central government by Jia, and who had returned to Qingyuan. Visiting her family, Yuan Hong had seen and liked her as a small child, joking that she might make a good daughter-in-law for him someday. In 1273, right before Yuan Hong left for Jiankang, her father formally proposed an engagement between his daughter and Yuan Jue. Soon afterwards, both of her parents passed away. When Hong came back to Qingyuan in 1275, he talked to the relative who had been taking care of her, and married his ten-*sui* son and the six-*sui* girl. The education she needed to be a proper wife in an elite household was given by Yuan Jue's grandmother. No record, of course, mentions when the couple consummated their marriage, but they eventually had three sons and four daughters.[53]

A year after Yuan Jue took up his first official position, Ms. Zheng passed away. She gave birth to their fourth daughter in late 1297, fell ill, and then died at age twenty-nine *sui* a month after the delivery. In the biography that Yuan Jue wrote for her seventeen years after her death, he says, "[When I heard the news that she was gravely ill,] I was in Hangzhou administering my maternal nephew's marriage. I came back quickly, but when I saw her, it was too late." Furthermore, adding to his grief, his father passed away eight days later.[54]

There is a good chance that he had a close bond with his wife. They were together from childhood, married for twenty-three years, so she was like a younger sister to him. In her biography of his writing, he repeatedly mentioned that his father loved her as if she had been his own daughter, and described how lovely she was as a child.[55] Yuan Jue might have been projecting his own feelings onto his father. Moreover, although Yuan Jue became a widower at thirty-four, still in his prime, and lived until he was sixty-two *sui*, he never remarried. Seventeen years later when his colleagues asked him the reasons for this decision, he replied, "The manners in which my deceased wife supported me and served my father never violated the family rites. She died eight days before my father passed away. So I cannot tolerate the thought of it."[56]

His decision not to get remarried might partly have been a result of his desire to strictly follow the Neo-Confucian morality, whose adherents considered celibacy after the death of their first spouse praiseworthy. They advocated the idea that in a family shrine a man should be worshipped with only one wife; if he had married twice, confusion would result: which of the two wives should be treated as his wife in the shrine?[57] So when a Northern Song Neo-Confucian proponent, Cheng Yi 程頤 (1033–1107), said "It is better that a woman starve than remarry," he did not pronounce against only female remarriages, as modern critics believed, but also against male remarriages, for the sake of order and propriety in ancestral worship.[58]

However, the reality was that many Song men and women practiced remarriage, so Zhu Xi was flexible on this matter.[59] In fact, Yuan Jue did not express any sense of shame or reservation about his father's remarriage. That was why his colleagues were curious about Yuan Jue's decision not to get married despite the fact that "[Even] a sage would find it hard."[60] Thus, morality alone cannot explain Yuan's decision not to remarry. Could it have been that he avoided going through another round of marriage and childbirth because he lost both his mother and wife due to postpartum exhaustion?

Whatever the true reason for his decision not to remarry might have been, Yuan Jue later claimed that the shock of losing his wife and father at once made him realize the significance of practical learning like medicine. When he wrote a preface to the book called *Ten Points on Medical Matters* (*Yishu shishi* 醫書十事) by Gao Yiqing 高一清, a doctor from a prominent Qingyuan family, he said:

> I once said that if we order all the intentions under heaven, all the affairs under heaven will be ordered. [The affairs under the Heaven means] Hard labor that cracks one's hand, the famine that Confucius went through in the state of Chen, hunger, coldness, difficulties, and pains. Even if one dies nine times, one does not regret [if one does the right things].[61] Just when I had risen to official position, I went through mourning after mourning. Talking about the emptiness of human nature and fate, while neglecting the reality of principles of things, I lacked something important![62]

The only goal he was expected to achieve in this preface was to praise Gao and his medical text. As long as he fulfilled this goal, Yuan Jue did not need to refer to his family's deaths. In other words, it was Yuan Jue's choice to connect the deaths of his family members and his support for medicine. Clearly he regretted not fulfilling his duty as a good son and husband to prevent his father's and wife's deaths.

Conclusion

As this chapter has shown, Yuan Jue was from an elite family in South China and received top-level education, despite the political turmoils of the Song–Yuan transition. His teachers were talented in various kinds of art and boasted broad knowledge, including medicine. At the same time he was distressed as a result of feeling at least partially responsible for his parents' and wife's deaths. He also lost two of his three sons in his lifetime.[63] These family members' deaths were obviously a force behind his support for medicine.

However, Yuan Jue was certainly not the first man to experience the unexpected losses of his family members. A lot of elite men in the Song, for example, were interested in medicine not just for the sake of their own lives but also their families', even though their interest did not materialize in the forms of local medical schools or the accompanying Temples of the Three Progenitors. We should now leave Yuan Jue's private sphere and explore the political, institutional, and intellectual context that shaped his specific actions.

Notes

1 This area was named Mingzhou in the Northern Song period, Qingyuan fu (Superior prefecture) in Southern Song, Qingyuan circuit in Yuan, Ningbo fu in Ming and Qing. Siming is the name of a mountain in Qingyuan and the literary name for the area.

2 Sutō Yoshiyuki, *Sōdai kanryōsei to daitochishoyū* (Tokyo: Nihon Hyōronsha, 1950), 67–68. Ihara Hiroshi, "Sōdai Meishū ni okeru kanko no kon'in kankei," *Chūō daigaku daigakuin kenkyū nenpō*, 1 (March 1972): 157–68. Linda Ann Walton-Vargö, "Education, Social Change, and Neo-Confucianism in Sung-Yuan China: Academies and the Local Elite in Ming Prefecture (Ningpo)" (Ph.D. diss., University of Pennsylvania, 1978) and Huang Kuanzhong, "Songdai Siming Yuanshi jiazu yanjiu," in *Zhongguo jinshi shehui wenhuashi lunwenji*, ed. Zhongyang yanjiuyuan lishi yuyan yanjiusuo chubanpin bianji weiyuanhui (Taibei: Zhongyang yanjiuyuan lish yanjiusuo, 1992), 105–31.

3 Luo Jun et al., *Baoqing Siming zhi*, cited in Sutō, *Sōdai Kanryōsei*, 68. See also Richard L. Davis, "Political Success and the Growth of Descent Groups: The Shih of Ming-chou during the Sung," in *Kinship Organization in Late Imperial China 1000–1940*, ed. Patricia B. Ebrey and James L. Watson (Berkeley: University of California Press, 1986), 62–94; and Davis, *Court and Family in Sung China, 960–1279: Bureaucratic Success and Kinship Fortunes for the Shih of Ming-chou* (Durham, NC: Duke University Press, 1986).

4 *Qingrong*, 33.20a–23b.

5 *Qingrong*, 33.5a. For the year that Yuan Gu passed the civil service examination, see Chang Bide et al., *Songren zhuanji ziliao suoyin* (Taibei: Dingwen shuju, 1974–84), 3.1858.

6 *Qingrong*, 33.5a–6b.

7 *Qingrong*, 33.1b–2a and 20a–b.

8 See, for example, Beverly Bossler, "A Daughter is a Daughter All Her Life: Affinal Relations and Women's Networks in Song and Late Imperial China," *Late Imperial China* 21.1 (2000): 77–106, and Patricia Ebrey, *Inner Quarters: Marriage and the Lives of Chinese Women in the Sung Period* (Berkeley: University of California, 1992), 103 and 244–45. Benjamin Elman, *Classicism, Politics, and Kinship: The Ch'ang-chou School of New Text Confucianism in Late Imperial China* (Berkeley: University of California Press, 1990), 59–73, discusses the relation between literati education and affinal ties.

9 *Qingrong*, 33.21a–b and 27a–b.

10 *Qingrong*, 33.13a.

11 *Qingrong*, 30.8b–10a.

12 See, for example, Bettine Birge, "Chu Hsi and Women's Education," in *Neo-Confucian Education: the Formative Stage*, ed. Wm. Theodore de Bary and John W. Chaffee (Berkeley: University of California Press, 1989), 328–29, on the relation between a biographical account and a funerary inscription (*muzhiming*).

13 *Qingrong*, 33.20a.

14 *Qingrong*, 43.15a.

15 *Qingrong*, 33.20a.

16 Tuotuo et al., *Songshi* (Beijing: Zhonghua shuju, 1977), 46.896.

17 Catherine Despeux, "The System of the Five Circulatory Phases and the Six Seasonal Influences (*wuyun liuqi*), a Source of Innovation in Medicine Under the Song (960–1279)." *Innovation in Chinese Medicine*, ed. Elizabeth Hsu (Cambridge: Cambridge University Press, 2001), 123 and 126.

18 The biographical materials about Yuan Jue are indexed in Wang Deyi et al., *Yuanren zhuanji ziliao suoyin* (Taibei: Xinwenfeng chuban gongsi, 1979–82), 2: 950–52.

19 Dai Biaoyuan, *Shanyuan wenji*, SKQS, 12.19b.

20 Yoshikawa Kōjirō, *Sō-Min shi gaisetsu* (Tokyo: Iwanami shoten, 1963), 112–14, and Maeno Naoaki, ed., *Chūgoku bungakushi* (Tokyo: Tokyo daigaku shuppankai, 1975), 174–76.

21 *Qingrong*, 33.27b–28a.

22 *Qingrong*, 33.27b–28a.

23 Birge, "Chu Hsi and Women's Education," 348–52. Ebrey, *Inner Quarters*, 185–86.

24 *Qingrong*, 33.12b.

25 *Qingrong*, 33.13b–14a.

26 Linda Walton, "The Institutional Context of Neo-Confucianism: Scholars, Schools, and *Shu-yüan* in Sung-Yüan China" (1989), in *Neo-Confucian Education*, ed. de Bary and Chaffee, 468, and Ichiki Tsuyuhiki, *Shu Ki monjin shūdan keisei no kenkyū* (Tokyo: Sōbunsha, 2002), 326–53.

27 *Qingrong*, 33.5b. Neo-Confucianism was banned in the years between 1195 and 1202, and its honor was gradually recovered afterwards. James T.C. Liu, *China Turning Inward: Intellectual-Political Changes in the Early Twelfth Century* (Cambridge, MA: Council on East Asian Studies, Harvard University, 1988), 143–47.

28 *Qingrong*, 22.11b–12b.

29 *Qingrong*, 22.11a.

30 Dai, *Shanyuan wenji*, CSJC, 30.467.

31 *Qingrong*, 22.13a.

32 Su Tianjue, *Zixi wengao* (Beijing: Zhonghua shuju, 1997), 9.136.

33 *Qingrong*, 33.12a.

34 See *Qingrong*, 33.13b–23a for the list of Yuan Hong's teachers and friends.

35 *Qingrong*, 18.12a–14a; Song Lian et al., *Yuanshi* (Beijing: Zhonghua shuju, 1976), 190.4336.

36 C. Bradford Langley, "Wang Ying-lin (1223–1296): A Study in the Political and Intellectual History of the Demise of the Sung," (Ph.D. diss., Indiana University, 1980), 464–68 and 518–19 (note 64).

37 Chang et al., *Songren zhuanji*, 4.3062; *Qingrong*, 33.18b.

38 Su, *Zixi wengao* (Zhonghua shuju), 9.134.

39 Langley, "Wang Ying-lin," xxiv–xxv.

40 On the *boxue hongci* examination, see Langley, "Wang Ying-lin," chap. 2.

41 Langley, "Wang Ying-lin," 383–85.

42 Langley, "Wang Ying-lin," 35–40.

43 Langley, "Wang Ying-lin," 171–75.

44 Langley, "Wang Ying-lin," 176.

45 Langley, "Wang Ying-lin," 473–76.

46 Hilde de Weerdt, "Aspects of Song Intellectual Life: A Preliminary Inquiry into Some Southern Song Encyclopedias," *Papers on Chinese History* 3 (1994): 16.

47 De Weerdt, "Aspects," 23.

48 On Wang's scholarship, also see Lin Sufen, "Boshi yi zhiyong: Wang Yinglin xueshu de zai pingjia" (Master's thesis, Guoli Taiwan Daxue, 1994).

49 Wang Yinglin, *Xiaoxue ganzhu*, CSJC, 3.107–13.

50 Wang Yinglin, *Yuhai* (Taibei: Hualian Chubanshe), 63.14b–25b.

51 *Qingrong*, 44.18b.

52 Chen Yuan-Peng, *Liang-Song de "shangyi shiren" yu "ruyi": jianlun qizai Jin-Yuan de liubian* (Taibei: Guoli Taiwan daxue wenshi congkan, 1997).

53 *Qingrong*, 33.23b–26b; Yu Ji, *Daoyuan xuegulu*, SKQS, 19.26a–28a. The former only mentions two sons and four daughters, but the latter says she had three sons. One of the sons probably died so young that Yuan Jue did not feel the need to mention him in his biography of his wife.

54 *Qingrong*, 33.25b; Yu, *Daoyuan xuegulu*, 19.26a–28a.

55 *Qingrong*, 33.24b.

56 Yu, *Daoyuan xuegulu*, 19.26a.

57 Reiko Shinno, "Sōdai kōgōsei kara mita Chūgoku kafuchōsei," in *Ajia joseishi: hikakushi no kokoromi*, ed. Ajia joseishi kokusai shimpojūmu jikkō iinkai (Tokyo: Akashi shoten, 1997), 297–311. Also female remarriages in premodern China have been studied thoroughly. See, for example, Ebrey, *Inner Quarters*, 204–12; Lau Nap-yin,"Qiantan Songdai funü de shoujie yu zaijia," *Xin shixue* 2.4 (1991): 37–76; Bettine Birge, *Women, Property, and Confucian Reaction in Sung and Yuan China, 960–1368* (Cambridge: Cambridge University Press, 2002); and Fei Si-yen, *You dianfan dao guifan: cong Mingdai zhenjielienü de bianshi yu liuzhuan kan zhenjie guannian de yangehua* (Taibei: Guoli Taiwan daxue wenshi congkan, 1996).

58 Cheng Hao and Cheng Yi, *Henan Er-Cheng quanji*, Sibu beiyao, 22 *xia*. 4a and 6b.

59 Shu Jingde comp., *Zhuzi Yulei*, Yingyuan shuyuan collection (1872), 83.23b and 128.3a–3b.

60 Yu, *Daoyuan xuegulu*, 19.26a.

61 "The famine that Confucius went through in the state Chen" refers to an incident mentioned in *The Analects*, chap. 15. See D. C. Lau's translation (Harmondsworth: Penguin Books, 1979), 132. "Even if one dies nine times, one does not regret" comes from Qu Yuan 屈原, "Li Sao" 離騷 in *Chu Ci* 楚辞, SBCK chubian, 1.15a.

62 *Qingrong*, 21.22a–22b.

63 In addition to the son who died in his childhood (see note 53), Yuan Jue lost another son who reached maturity (*Qingrong*, 43.28a–b).

2 The Mongol conquest and the new configuration of power, 1206–76

By 1276, when Yuan Jue was eleven *sui* and the Mongols captured the capital city of the Southern Song dynasty, roughly seventy years had passed since Chinggis Khan unified the Mongol tribes and embarked on world conquest. Also, it had been forty years since they conquered Kaifeng 開封, the Jin dynasty capital. South Chinese people like Yuan Jue were newcomers in the empire, which had already been shaped by Mongols, West and Central Asians, and North Chinese. His father's contemporary, a *nanren* Zheng Sixiao 鄭思肖 (1241–1318), wrote in 1282:

> According to the Tartars' laws (*dafa* 韃法), the first [rank goes to] officials, the second clerks, the third Buddhist monks, the fourth Daoist monks, the fifth physicians, the sixth craftsmen, the seventh hunters, the eighth ordinary people, the ninth Confucians, and the tenth beggars.[1]

Although it was an emotional statement by an angry Southern Song loyalist, Zheng was right to point out that the status order in the new empire was different from that in earlier dynasties. Mongols gave physicians privileges in return for their service. They created a taxation category called, "medical household" (*yihu* 醫戶), to assign special privileges and duties. To continue Zheng's observation: "Each [occupational group] has an office to supervise them. Buddhist monks become Buddhist officials and supervise Buddhist monks. Daoist monks become Daoist officials and supervise Daoist monks."[2]

By the same token, some doctors became government officials and supervised doctors. This chapter will look at the new configuration of power that the Mongols created, from the medical point of view.

The *jasaq* and recruitment of doctors

It is not exactly clear which laws Zheng was referring to when he said the "Tartars' laws," but we can find abundant evidence that the laws and policies of the Mongol empire privileged physicians. Mongols first articulated such privileges as part of the *jasaq*. They later sent down edicts repeating their interest in physicians as they conquered different parts of China.

In 1206, after the Mongol diet (*quriltai*) had elected Temujin as their leader and he had assumed the title Chinggis Khan, "Ocean Leader," he began sending out ordinances (*jasaq*).³ One of them said:

> He (Jenghis Khan [Chinggis Khan]) decided that no taxes or duties should be imposed upon the descendants of Ali [ʿAlī]-Bek and Abu-Ta-leb [Abū Ṭālib], without exception, as well as upon fakirs, readers of the Al-Koran [Qurʾān], lawyers, *physicians*, scholars, people who devote themselves to prayer and asceticism, muezzins and those who wash the bodies of the dead [brackets and italics mine].⁴

This ordinance gave tax exemptions based on occupations, and physicians were among those given privileges. In return, they were expected to provide the Khan with medical services.

As the Mongol army penetrated China, they sought out and supported religious practitioners and physicians as they had in central and western Eurasia. In 1234, Chinggis's son, Ögedei (Taizong 太宗, 1186–1241, r. 1229–41), selected craftsmen, Confucians, Buddhist monks, Daoist monks, physicians, and diviners, sent them to live all over Hebei, and required officials to give them stipends.⁵ In 1235, when the emperor attempted his first attack on the Southern Song, he ordered an official, Yao Shu 姚樞 (1203–80), "to seek Confucians, Daoist monks, Buddhist monks, physicians, and fortune-tellers for [his] armies."⁶ In 1261, after capturing Xichuan 西川, part of the Sichuan basin, Qubilai Khan (Shizu 世祖, 1214–94, r. 1260–94) sent Wang You 王祐 to "examine physicians, Confucians, Buddhist monks, and Daoist monks."⁷ In 1262, he also commanded the Vietnamese king to send "three Confucians, physicians, fortune-tellers, and craftsmen,"⁸ along with various special products of the region, to join his triennial official embassies. During the conquest of Jiangnan 江南 in 1275, Qubilai additionally sent envoys to look for "Confucians, physicians, Buddhist monks, Daoist monks, and fortune-tellers, et cetera."⁹ As a result, many of the doctors from various ethnic backgrounds followed the rulers and princes on military campaigns and administrative tours.¹⁰ Others were expected to serve the medical needs of their locality.

The Mongols recruited specialists, including physicians, for two reasons. The Mongols, just like other nomads, were thinly dispersed over a large territory, which dictated that individuals should be capable of carrying out many different tasks without necessarily being skilled in one specific art. Having thus become generalists themselves for ecological reasons, the Mongols needed specialists to help them conquer and manage developed agrarian societies. So they recruited specialists when they advanced beyond the Mongol Plains and confronted sedentary societies such as China and Iran. Second, by gathering talented individuals in their courts and armies, the Mongols tried to create an "aura of majesty" and to "mobilize and monopolize the spiritual forces of the realm." The Mongols like other Central Asians considered that talented individuals commanded not just technical skills, but also magical power. If these specialists came from afar they appeared even more mysterious, and thus more spiritually powerful, to the Mongols and their subjects.[11]

In this context, talents in specialized arts became important ways for men from the conquered areas to convince Mongols that they would make good imperial subjects. A good example is Yelü Chucai 耶律楚材 (1190–1244), the ninth descendant of the first emperor of the Liao dynasty, Yelü Abaoji 耶律阿保機 (872–926, r. 907–26). Upon the fall of the Liao dynasty to the Jin, Chucai's grandfather, Deyuan 德元, began serving the Jin government, and Chucai's father, Lü 履 (1130–90), was the Assistant Director of the Right in the Department of State Affairs (*shangshu youcheng* 尚書右丞) at the end of his career.[12] Chucai was granted an audience with Chinggis Khan in 1214, right after the latter had pushed the emperor of the Jin dynasty away to Kaifeng. Yelü's handsome appearance, mentioned by all of his biographers, might have played a part in attracting Chinggis Khan's attention, but Yelü was, at the same time, no intellectual lightweight: he had read widely. Particularly in the early stage of his career, he built his reputation with a thorough and precise knowledge of astronomy. Furthermore, he was versed in medicine. His medical knowledge was demonstrated and exploited after the Mongol army won the battle against the Tangut at Lingwu 靈武 (near present-day Lingzhou 靈州) in 1226, where he collected rhubarb (*dahuang* 大黄). According to his biography, he later used it to cure "tens of thousands" of soldiers suffering from epidemics.[13] He served as Chinggis Khan's and Ögedei Khan's secretary later on. His influence on the Mongols' decisions might not have been as strong as historians have long believed it to be, but his proximity to the emperors, which he gained through his knowledge of various specialized arts, helped him stay visible among his peers in China.[14]

In the case of Dou Mo 竇默 (1196–1280), it was his acupuncture skills that attracted Qubilai's attention. Born into a family of humble peasants in Hebei 河北, Dou met a physician surnamed Wang 王 at the end of the Jin dynasty. After marrying Wang's daughter and moving in with her natal family, he was persuaded by Wang to take up medicine.[15] Dou later studied acupuncture with another physician, Li Hao 李浩. When the Mongols captured Kaifeng, Dou Mo fled to the Southern Song territory, only to be caught by Yang Weizhong 楊惟中 (1205–59), who was working for Ögedei Khan with Yao Shu 姚樞 (1203–80). Yang and Yao also took as captive Zhao Fu 趙復 (c. 1206–c. 1299), who would then introduce North Chinese to the commentaries of the Cheng brothers and Zhu Xi. Along with Zhao and Dou, the expeditionary army also brought 100 other Confucian scholars, as well as books, back to the north. After arriving in North China, Dou was released from captivity. Yao Shu printed the books that he had brought back and studied them with Dou Mo and Xu Heng 許衡 (1209–81) in the 1240s. Xu would later become the leader of Yuan Neo-Confucianism.[16] Their studies took Yao, Xu, and Dou far beyond Confucianism. Every day the three men sat together, discussing not just the Confucian classics but also Buddhist and Daoist texts, fortune-telling, works of various philosophers, the art of soldiery, penal codes, economy, water conservation, mathematics, and not least, medicine.[17] Xu Heng's knowledge of medicine is further evidenced by his letter to a friend, Yang Gongyi

楊恭懿 (1225–94), another politician who apparently also knew medicine. In the letter, Xu Heng reported in detail the problems that a patient had had and the therapeutic strategies that Xu and the patient had already taken. But since none of the strategies worked, they needed Yang's advice. After detailing those strategies and consequences, Xu ends the letter by comparing the strategies of two of the Four Masters of Jin-Yuan medicine—Liu Wansu 劉完素 (born between 1126 and 1132) and Zhang Zihe 張子和 (1156?–1228?)—and by saying, "If one can make use of the two masters' strengths and avoid their weaknesses, wouldn't one be close to a cure?"[18]

Dou Mo continued practicing acupuncture in the 1240s; and, because he did not discriminate between rich and poor and was good at curing illnesses, he gained high esteem.[19] Upon the recommendation of Yao Shu, who began serving Qubilai in 1251, the emperor summoned Dou in 1260. According to Xu Heng's biography, "as Dou Mo became famous for his acupuncture, he was frequently summoned by the court."[20] He eventually gained a position as a lecturer in waiting in the Hanlin Academy upon Qubilai's ascension to the throne. He wrote two books on acupuncture, *Poems on Grand Preceptor Dou's Style on Acupuncture Points* (*Dou Taishi liu zhuzhi yaofu* 竇太師流注指要賦) and *Esoteric Poems of Acupuncture Marks* (*Zhenjiu biao youfu* 鍼灸標幽賦).[21] Dou probably played the role of mentor to Luo Tianyi 羅天益, who mentioned in his book that he had intense conversations with Dou about medicine in the 1250s.[22] As we will see in Chapter 6, Luo was the last disciple of Li Gao 李杲 (1180–1251), one of the Four Masters of Jin-Yuan medicine, and later became a member of the Imperial Academy of Medicine. Luo's promotion facilitated the publication of Li's works.[23]

Dou Mo was a good example of a physician who influenced political and intellectual history, instead of just the other way around. After entering the Yuan bureaucracy in 1257, he recommended Xu Heng to the emperor, who managed to gain Xu's service in 1260. The treatise on the bureaucratic system in the *Yuan History* contends that Xu and his political patron Liu Bingzhong 劉秉忠 (1216–74) created the Yuan bureaucracy.[24] The *Yuan History* might be exaggerating Xu's role, for his political position in the early 1260s was not strong and his recommendations were not very different from his colleagues'. Even so, Xu did submit, in 1266 and 1267, two important memorials on governance, some recommendations of which Qubilai Khan later adopted. The first memorial laid out five points for Qubilai to consider: to establish the empire in a Chinese manner, to institute a proper bureaucracy, to be a righteous ruler, to promote agriculture and schools, and to pay attention to minor details. The second memorial discussed the history of the bureaucracy in previous Chinese dynasties and suggested improvements on the current system. These memorials followed a suggestion that Xu had made in person to the emperor in 1260, namely that the civil service examination was an ineffective way to recruit good government staff and that the emperor should, instead, build schools.[25]

Xu Guozhen's 許國禎 service to Qubilai (Shizu 世祖, 1214–94, r. 1260–94) was more focused on medicine than Yelü's or Dou's, although Xu used medicine to give advice on other matters. Both his grandfather and father had practiced medicine while serving, respectively, as Military Commissioner (*jiedushi* 節度使) and Assistant Military Commissioner (*jiedu panguan* 節度判官) in the Jin dynasty. Xu and his mother, Ms. Han 韓, who also excelled in medicine, had served Qubilai, even before his ascent to the throne. After Qubilai's enthronement, Xu Guozhen became Grandee of the Third Class (*ronglu dafu* 栄禄大夫, 1b) and Intendant of the Affairs of the Imperial Academy of Medicine. Subsequently Xu wrote a medical treatise, *Prescriptions for the Palace Pharmaceutical Bureau* (*Yuyaoyuan fang* 御藥院方, prefaced 1267) and would earn praise in the *Yuan History* for being not just an excellent physician but also an honest adviser to Qubilai Khan. When the emperor was procrastinating about taking a bitter medicine, and thus aggravating his illness, Xu reminded him that good medicines were bitter, just as advice from loyal subjects could be unpleasant.[26] His son, Xu Yi 許扆, would later serve not only as the Intendant of the Affairs of the Imperial Academy of Medicine but also in such non-medical positions as Minister of Rites and the Senior Vice Councilor of the Branch Central Secretariat for Shaanxi and Other Places (*Shaanxi xingsheng youcheng* 陝西行省右丞).[27]

The Mongols also recruited individuals with a good knowledge of medicine outside of China. A Nestorian Christian, ʿĪsā (Chinese name: Aixue 愛薛, 1227–1308), who was adept in various West Asian languages, calendar, and medicine, first served Chinggis Khan's grandson, Güyüg (Dingzong 定宗, 1206–48, r. 1246–48) and then his cousin Qubilai. ʿĪsā's funerary inscription suggests that he had a close relationship with the latter. It states that, when Qubilai thought of building a large Buddhist temple soon after ascending the throne, ʿĪsā persuaded the ruler to abandon the project, saying that the empire was still fighting difficult battles and should not waste money. Again indicating ʿĪsā's proximity to the ruler, the same document notes that one day, when Qubilai fell into a drunken stupor during a large party, he lay down, using ʿĪsā's lap as a pillow, and said to the imperial heir, "Having such a subject, I have no worries." In 1270, ʿĪsā recommended that the Office of Broad Grace (*Guanghui si* 廣惠司), an institution providing West Asian medical service, be established. Acting upon this recommendation, Qubilai appointed ʿĪsā head of the bureau. Subsequently ʿĪsā rose to the positions of Chancellor of the Hanlin and National History Academy (*Hanlin xueshi chengzhi jianxiu guoshi* 翰林學士承旨兼修國史, 1b), Privy Councilor (*pingzhang zhengshi* 平章政事, 1c), and Grandee of the First Class (*jinzi guanglu dafu* 金紫光録大夫, 1a). His six sons, four sons-in-law, and three grandsons all gained important government positions. One of his sons, Luqa 魯合, also became the Intendant of the Bureau of Broad Grace (*guanghui si tiju* 廣惠司提舉).[28]

Rashid-ud-Din Fazlullah (1247–1318), the author of the great world history book of this time, the *Compedium of Chronicles* (*Jāmiʿal-tawarikh*), began his service to the Il-Khans in Iran as a cook/dietician and physician. Born as a child of a Jewish apothecary, he became a Muslim at age 30 and began his official career during the reign of Geikhatu (1291–95). After he established himself as a politician and accumulated wealth, he supposedly built the Rabʾ-i Rashidi, a "clearing house" of knowledge, where scholars from all over the Eurasian continent gathered and exchanged ideas. The center included a House of Healing.

Also, he is likely to have participated in the project that translated the *Secrets of the Pulse* (*Maijue* 脉訣) into Persian.[29]

Although numerous men in Eurasia took advantage of the Mongol rulers' interest in medical art and doctors, imperial attention was not always a blessing to every physician, especially at its earlier stage. Liu Qi 劉祁, a Jin literatus who was in Kaifeng when it surrendered to the Mongols, records the suffering and fear the physicians must have felt. According to him, the leaders of the three religions, physicians, and craftsmen were forced out of the capital right before the Mongol army entered and looted the capital in 1233. The army then held the religious leaders and physicians in uncomfortable conditions near a gate of the city and plundered them of every possession before taking them to the north. Liu Qi happened to directly witness this group on their way to the north. "Alas, why am I witnessing the fall of my country directly? There were uncountable fears and pains!"[30] Elsewhere, the general of an army tried to bury religious practitioners and physicians, apparently not knowing that the emperor's expectation was to keep them alive and have them serve him.[31] These episodes remind us to see both sides. On the one hand, some physicians volunteered to work with the world conquerors and used their skills to promote themselves. On the other hand, some physicians were the Mongols' booty, forced to relocate against their wills, especially at times of turmoil.

Medical households

The Mongols began seeking systematic ways of imposing taxes on, and obtaining labor service from, the North Chinese right after they occupied Kaifeng, the capital of the Jin dynasty, in 1234. As in the *jasaq*, they bestowed privileges on physicians, although it was not until 1262 that a taxation and litigation category called "medical households" was created. While the idea of granting physicians a special status derived from the Mongols' needs as world conquerors, the concept of the household as a taxation unit originated from within Chinese society.

A glance at the history of taxation in China reveals that the dynasties before the late eighth century perceived a household merely as an assembly of taxable adults. Under the so-called Equal Field system (*juntianzhi* 均田制), established in 485 and brought to its culmination in the early Tang dynasty, the state in principle owned all land in the empire, divided it into small pieces, and distributed it equally to all adult men (and women, too, in the case of pre-Tang dynasties). In return, each person was supposed to pay equal taxes in the forms of crops, service labor, and cloth under a system known as *zuyongdiao* 租庸調. Therefore, in principle, a household's tax was determined by its number of male, and sometimes female, members.[32]

However, the household became one organic unit, so to speak, when the Tang government introduced a new taxation system called the Double-Tax System (*liangshuifa* 兩税法) in 780. Under this system, the government abandoned its former ideal of land equally distributed among people, and now determined that the tax of each household should be based on how much land it actually owned and how much its land produced. In order to implement this taxation system, the government now began to grade households according to their wealth. The Northern Song dynasty inherited the Double-Tax System and elaborated the Household Grading System. Households were categorized first into two groups, "resident household" (*zhuhu* 主戶) and "non-resident household" (*kehu* 客戶). Furthermore, the first of these was subdivided into five groups, from the "grade-one household" (*diyideng hu* 第一等戶), the richest, to the "grade-five household" (*diwudeng hu* 第五等戶), the poorest of the five.[33] The little evidence that we have regarding Jin taxation shows that Emperor Shizong 世宗 (b. 1123, r. 1161–89) of the Jin dynasty promulgated an important edict in 1180, ordering the grading of households according to their wealth. The Jin dynasty may not have graded households prior to 1180, as Yanagida Setsuko argued, but at least from this time on, the household as an integral group became an important unit of taxation.[34]

When Mongols subdued North China in 1234, the principle of taxation assumed in the *jasaq*—which took an individual man rather than a household as a unit of taxation—became a point of controversy. Qutugu, probably a Mongol politician, strongly argued that an individual man should be the unit, because that was the practice that had been used in Mongolia and the western Eurasian regions. However, Yelü Chucai, according to his biographers, convinced Ögedei Khan otherwise. He pointed out that, with households responsible for tax, if a man escaped from a village, other men in the same household would be accountable for the tax.[35] Consequently, a nationwide census was completed in 1236. Thenceforth the grain tax of a household was determined by the number of male adult members, and agricultural tools, and by the quality of its land—all data recorded in the census. Furthermore, the state silk taxes were also assessed on households based on their grades.[36]

Although the scattered records of the 1236 census do not mention tax exemptions for craftsmen, Buddhist monks, Daoist monks, or physicians, one episode indicates that physicians might have enjoyed exemptions from labor service at least some time during the reign of Möngke (Xianzong 憲宗, 1209–59, r. 1251–59). One day, this emperor granted an audience to Gao Zhiyao 高智耀, from a family that had served the Xi Xia dynasty before its surrender to the Mongols in the 1220s. Gao urged the emperor to promote Confucian scholars and grant them exemptions from labor service so that they could be educated. The emperor responded by asking, "How could Confucians be comparable to diviners and physicians?" Gao retorted, "Confucian scholars govern the people under Heaven by fulfilling moral obligations. How could these technicians be comparable [to Confucians]!" Möngke was pleased to find someone who would present his own opinion so frankly, and thus sent out an edict that no Confucians should be given labor service.[37] Of course, the overt purpose of this episode was to praise Gao's contribution to the promotion of Confucianism; but interestingly it also reveals the Mongol ruler's trust in physicians and the exemptions he had given to physicians prior to those for Confucians. In fact, this episode implies that it was Confucians who used physicians as a crutch to promote their status, rather than the other way around.

In 1262, two years after the enthronement, Qubilai Khan sent the first extant edict regarding medical households, which says:

> As to the taxes and labor service that physicians' households owe, they should pay silk, cotton, and dye taxes. Also, if they produce rice, they shall pay rice tax, and if they trade, they owe trade taxes. However, they shall be exempt from all miscellaneous service duties such as providing military supplies, raising horses and taking care of messengers in the postal relay system, and taking care of cows and personnel. When officials in appanages (*touxia* 投下, i.e., land given to imperial relatives and Chinggis Khan's important subjects) buy medicines from physicians, they should pay reasonable price and should never just take it by force. Following annual practice, households of physicians under the jurisdiction of government (*xiguan* 係官, i.e., not in appanages), should pay three *liang* of silver tax, and now they should pay with our paper money. Wang Zijun and other officials should consider a physician's wealth and status and determine their tax, and provide according to the necessities of members of Imperial Academy of Medicine who are serving in the court.[38]

This edict uses the term "physicians' households" (*yirenmei hu* 醫人每户), rather than the term "medical households" (*yihu* 醫户) that appears more often in the later sources.[39] The term *yirenmei hu* represents the hybrid nature of the origin of medical households—on the one hand, the idea of granting physicians special privileges, which came from the *jasaq*, and on the other hand the concept of the household as a unit of taxation, which had been a rule in China since the mid-Tang. Also, assuming that some appanage officials exploited physicians by commandeering their medicine for free, Qubilai Khan, as represented in this edict, attempted to play the role of guardian for the physicians—another example of closeness between Mongol emperors and physicians.

The above edict shows that Yuan medical households received discounts on the silver tax (*baoyin* 包銀), a uniquely Yuan taxation system. According to the *Yuan History*, households that did not practice medicine could owe as much as four *liang* of silver tax to the state,[40] while the above edict required medical households to pay only three *liang*. This means that being designated as a medical household was one way to pay less silver tax. The tax revenues collected from medical households, according to this edict, were to be used by members of the Imperial Academy of Medicine.

Medical households were exempted from labor service such as providing goods and services related to the military and postal system, but they were expected to give service specific to physicians. A memorial to rebuild medical schools approved by Qubilai about the same time says that professors and students of medical schools should be exempted from the labor service, such as "inspecting physicians' levy obligations" (*jianyi* 檢醫) and "temporary assignments" (*chaizhan* 差占).[41] The edict implies that medical households that did not produce medical school professors or students were obliged to engage in these services.

A regulation issued in 1298 articulated medical households' obligation to take turns to inspect and collect taxes from one another, by saying: "The prefectural and county governments should dispatch *jianyi* to count the numbers of medical households and collect levies from them."[42] No Yuan institutional texts systematically defined the "temporary service" that physicians were supposed to engage in, but we have fragmented information on the responsibilities that physicians took turns taking care of. For example, in 1263, the Department of Secretaries determined that when prisoners got sick, local physicians should take turns caring for them.[43] A Yuan gazetteer compiled in the 1320s lists "miscellaneous labor service" (*zayi* 雜役), which included, among other things, service as "chief physician" (*zhuyi* 主醫) at a Charitable Pharmacy (*Huimin yaoju* 惠民藥局), which was re-established in 1237, and "on-call physicians" (*dangzhi yigong* 當直醫工) at the circuit and prefectural offices.[44]

The Imperial Academy of Medicine

Chinese bureaucracy was never static, but the Mongol rulers, as foreign conquerors, were even less mindful of preserving rules in the Chinese bureaucracy than were the emperors of the Jin and the Song dynasties who preceded them. Thus, the Mongols were willing to ignore many of the rules of the Chinese bureaucracy in order to recruit and promote individuals whom they thought had talents that would benefit the new empire. As such, Mongols created a bureaucracy that privileged medical administrators and stratified the community of physicians according to their positions in the bureaucracy. In particular, compared to equivalent offices prior to the Yuan dynasty, the Yuan Imperial Academy of Medicine (*taiyi yuan* 太醫院) enjoyed unprecedented prestige and power.

Although sources for the period up through the Tang are scattered, we can still find evidence that Chinese dynasties maintained official positions for some physicians, even though their ranks were relatively low. Also, while they focused on serving the royal families and aristocracy in the capital in the ancient times, their responsibility increasingly included service to the people outside of the capital. The *Rites of Zhou* (*Zhou li* 周禮), an ancient text that supposedly describes the bureaucracy of an idealized Zhou dynasty, but was certainly not composed before the later Warring States period, claims that there were four kinds of doctors at that time: "physicians for internal diseases" (*jiyi* 疾醫), "physicians for nutrition" (*shiyi* 食醫), "physicians for skin problems" (*yangyi* 瘍醫), and veterinarians (*shouyi* 獸醫). According to the text, "physicians for internal diseases" were to "supervise care of the whole populace," though "the whole populace" probably was limited to the aristocracy, if not just the royal family.[45] The Qin government might have been the first to adopt the word "*taiyi* 太醫" (Imperial Physician) to refer to the doctors working in the palace. Sima Qian's 司馬遷 *The Records of the Grand Historian* (*Shiji* 史記), written in the Former Han period, said that a legendary doctor, Bianque 扁鵲, was killed by "the Qin Imperial Physician Li Xi" 秦太醫李醯.[46] This incident supposedly happened prior to the country's unification of China. Du You's 杜佑 (735–812) *Comprehensive*

Institutions (*Tong dian* 通典) said that the Qing empire called the top medical expert "Chief Imperial Physician" (*taiyi ling* 太醫令) and assigned him a role to "supervise medical matters."[47] His rank is not recorded, but because he reported to the Chamberlain for Palace Revenues (*shaofu* 少府), who was ranked in the ninth grade (*jiu deng* 九等), we can extrapolate that the Chief Imperial Physician was ranked as eighth rank or below, meaning thirteenth or lower from the top.[48] In the Former Han dynasty, the *Book of Han* (*Han Shu* 漢書) mentions two kinds of Chief Imperial Physicians, one that reported to the Chamberlain for Palace Revenues, and another who reported to the Chamberlain for Ceremonials (*taichang* 太常). Whether the two kinds of Chief Imperial Physicians had different duties or reflected temporal changes, the Chief Imperial Physician received 600 bushels (*shi* 石) as salary, ranking him ninth from the top in the sixteen ranks.[49] In the Later Han and Wei dynasties, there was only one kind of Chief Imperial Physician, who reported to the Chamberlain for Palace Revenues, and holders of this office were also granted 600 bushels.[50]

Until the Wei dynasty, the Chief Imperial Physicians supervised a large staff of doctors, semiofficially called the Imperial Physicians (*taiyi*); the organization of which he was the head, however, had no formal name. Then, in the Western Jin dynasty of the Nan-Bei chao period, a new departmental name emerged: Imperial Medical Office (*taiyi shu* 太醫署), which was led by the Chief Imperial Physician (*taiyi ling*). During the Nan-Bei chao period, the ranking of the Chief Imperial Physician varied from the seventh out of nine ranks (Northern Wei) to fourth out of nine (Northern Zhou). In the meantime, another office called the Palace Pharmaceutical Service (*shangyao ju* 尚藥局) and designated to provide medical care in the palace, emerged, while the Imperial Medical Office undertook the medical administration of the whole empire as its primary responsibility.[51] The Sui and Tang dynasties also maintained an Imperial Medical Office and Chief Imperial Physician. The ranking of the Chief Imperial Physician in the Sui bureaucracy is unknown; he ranked 7b in the Tang. As we will see later, there was a substantial effort to promote state medical education in the Tang, and the Imperial Medical Office took charge of that education.[52]

The Northern Song marked a watershed because the government gained an important means by which to codify medical knowledge and spread such codified knowledge to the regions outside the capital: printing. While the Imperial Medical Office was renamed the Imperial Medical Service (*taiyi ju* 太醫局) and continued to supervise the education of students who were later to serve in the central government, the Hanlin Medical Institute (*Hanlin yiguan yuan* 翰林醫官院) was established in 1051 and managed other features of medical administration, most importantly publishing books on pharmacology, medicine, and acupuncture. The supervisor of the Hanlin Medical Institute ranked 6b, and the number of the members of the Hanlin Medical Institute increased from 32 in 1051 to 142 in 1067, to more than 1,000 in 1114. Also, as we will later see, the Song government established a network of the Charitable Pharmacies and printed texts that determined the prescriptions to be used in these pharmacies.[53] The spread of epidemics caused by rapid urbanization motivated the government to print medical texts. Yuan Jue's teacher, Wang Yinglin, reflected on the Northern Song's printing of a medical text as follows:

> In the eighth year of the Qingli period (1048), as prescriptions and remedies were lacking for the patients afflicted by the poison of the illness (*bingdu* 病毒) in South China, the Emperor ordered the publication of a work composed of a selection of the best prescriptions from the *Taiping Era Formulary of Sagely Grace* (*Taiping shenghui fang* 太平聖惠方). This work, entitled *Prescriptions of the Qingli Period to Save People* (*Qingli shanjiu fang* 慶曆善救方) was distributed throughout the empire. The palace doctors were ordered to prepare its prescriptions and distribute them to people suffering from epidemic diseases.[54]

The Song structure of medical administration was also influenced by general politics, expanding when the so-called New Policy Faction, which in general favored state activism, was in power.[55]

The Jin dynasty carried forward the Jurchens' simple titles of officials in its early stage of rule, and then Taizong 太宗 (b. 1075, r. 1123–35) established an Imperial Academy of Medicine (*taiyi yuan*). Its chief was called the Intendant (*tidian* 提點, 5a). The functions of this office were more comprehensive than those of earlier dynasties: while the role of the Imperial Medical Service in the Song had been confined to medical education, the Jin Imperial Academy of Medicine oversaw both medical administration in general and medical education.[56]

Soon after Qubilai Khan took office in 1260, the Imperial Academy of Medicine was established as the paramount organ that oversaw medical administration. According to the *Yuan History*, it "took charge of medical matters, prepared drugs [for the imperial family] from pharmaceuticals [collected from the various regions of the empire], and presided over various medical offices."[57] It was a special agency that did not belong to any of the three major branches of the Yuan central government—the Central Secretariat (*zhongshusheng* 中書省), Bureau of Military Affairs (*shumi yuan* 樞密院), or the Censorate (*yushi tai* 御史臺).[58] It is apparent that the Imperial Academy of Medicine of the Yuan dynasty was modeled after that of the Jin dynasty because the name of the organization (*taiyi yuan*, as opposed to *taiyi ju* in the Northern and Southern Song dynasties), the name of the head of the organization (*tidian*), and the comprehensive function of this office are the same, or at least similar. One important difference, however, was the rank of the head of this Academy. The Intendant of the Imperial Academy of Medicine was ranked 5a in the Jin dynasty, but he was ranked 2a in the Yuan. This ranking fluctuated over the course of the Yuan period, but never fell lower than 4a.[59]

In the early 1260s, edicts were issued that formally established the Academy as the office responsible for monitoring physicians in the empire. In 1263, Qubilai Khan ordered that the Intendants and Commissioners of the Academy should supervise physicians and clerks in the Charity Pharmacies of the various circuits. The same edict ordered that the silver tax collected from medical households should be spent to provide for the needs of the members of the Imperial Academy of Medicine.[60] Also, in 1263, the Academy sent a request to revive local medical schools and appoint prominent physicians as instructors, and the Khan approved it.[61] In 1266, another edict was sent out to order the Imperial Academy of Medicine to govern medical households and Charitable Pharmacies.[62]

The Imperial Academy of Medicine was powerful in shaping the edicts and administrative regulations related to medicine. This should be contrasted with Song medical administrators, who were executors of governmental policies but not policy-makers.[63] To be precise, the Imperial Academy of Medicine was not the office that made final decisions. Typically, the Central Secretariat would send a matter first to a relevant ministry (e.g., the Ministry of Rites, the Ministry of Punishment, etc.), and that ministry would then consult the Imperial Academy of Medicine if the matter had to do with medicine or physicians. The Academy's proposals required the approval of the ministry and subsequently of the Central Secretariat before they became effective. Among the fourteen articles included in the "medical schools" and "medical administrators" sections in the *Sagely Administration*, however, the Academy appears in ten cases, and in all instances, the proposals submitted by the Imperial Academy of Medicine were approved.[64]

The Academy members were sometimes allowed to transfer to a governmental office that was not directly related to medicine. This is another important difference between the Yuan medical administrators and their Song counterparts. The *Yuan History* says:

> Generally, those who had been commissioned in the palace or employed by the Secretariat and Censorate were transferred into regular appointments and were able to be appointed as local administrators. Those who had been transferred from the Imperial Academy of Medicine could not follow this rule. [This was] to indicate that an official career could not be entered improperly. However, if any official of the Imperial Academy of Medicine had already received the emperor's mandate, he was transferred in accordance with [the regulations governing] the principal civil and military officials graded fifth in rank or above. As for the rest, they were promoted accordingly based upon their former ranks and positions. The employment of [their] descendants through "*yin* protection" was regulated in the same way as officials of the principal category.[65]

Officials of the first to the fifth grades received their nominations by the mandate of the emperor (*ming* 命), while officials of the sixth to ninth grades were appointed by decree (*chi* 勅) issued by the Central Secretariat.[66] Thus, the above text shows that those who received their nomination by mandate of the emperor would be treated equally, whether or not they were medical administrators.

The members of the Yuan Imperial Academy of Medicine often took advantage of this legal change. For example, Shen Jing 申敬 became a member of the Academy in 1269 and was appointed as a commissioner of the Imperial Pharmaceutical Bureau (5b), an office under the Academy's supervision (see below), in 1290. Four years later, he was appointed as a Deputy Director (5b) of the Imperial Library Directorate, which collected books, paintings, and maps from the ancient period and secret books on divination. He was then promoted to Junior Director (4b) in the same office in 1301. He ended his official career as the Lord of the Court of Imperial Sacrifices (*taichang si* 太常寺, ranked 3a at this time), which managed ceremonies and music performed at the imperial ancestral temples and the temples for Heaven, Earth, and Grain.[67]

Some members of the Imperial Academy of Medicine gained positions in local administrations. Gu Gao 谷杲, after serving as a Junior Assistant Director (4a) of the Academy, became the Director-general of Guangping circuit 廣平路.[68] Xu Yi, Xu Guozhen's son, who himself served as the Intendant of the Academy, was appointed Senior Vice Councilor of the Branch Central Secretariat for Shaanxi.[69] Yu Shizhong 俞時中, also a former Academy member, served in several posts in different local administrations.[70]

As I will show later, the methods for recruitment for the Academy evolved over time, but initially, Qubilai Khan interviewed candidates, with the help of his doctor and the first Intendant of the Academy, Xu Guozhen, or relied on his trusted subjects' recommendations. For example, in 1289, Xu invited several men reputed to be prominent physicians for such an interview. Showing a medicinal herb from West Asia, the emperor asked them to identify it. Han Gonglin 韓公麟, being the only one able to answer the question, was appointed a member of the Imperial Academy of Medicine.[71] Xu also arranged a similar interview with the emperor for another doctor, Dou Xingchong 竇行沖 (1233–1309).[72] Later, after the fall of the Southern Song, Wang Dongye 王東野, served as the Superintendent of Physicians in Yongxin prefecture 永新州 in Ji'an circuit 吉安路 and then Vice Superintendent of Physicians of the whole circuit before he was appointed to membership in the Imperial Academy of Medicine. In his case, he entered the Academy perhaps because his client, Cheng Jufu 程鉅夫 (1249–1318), was Qubilai's loyal subject.[73] As we have seen in the case of Xu Guozhen and his son Xu Yi, the Academy member's family also became Academy members. Instead of performing military service, the families of members of the Academy were required only to work for the Academy.[74]

As we have already seen in the "Medical Household" section, the Academy ordered in 1262 that the revenue collected as tax from medical households should fall under their control. In 1271, the Academicians sent a memorial to Qubilai Khan complaining that when brothers and children of the head of a medical household broke away from the household and created their own households, they would be counted as ordinary households even when the new heads practiced medicine. Arguing that such practice would not encourage the descendants to learn medicine because they would not be receiving any levy benefit of practicing medicine (such as less silver tax and the privilege to focus on medical service, not other service duties), the Academy submitted a proposal saying that it should be collecting taxes from all the descendants of medical households. The Academicians also proposed that if a descendant decided to break away from the family and the profession, the descendant's family would be treated as an ordinary household.

The Academy might indeed have been concerned about the possible decrease in the number of the doctors in the empire, and they must have been aware that the increase in the number of medical households meant increasing income for the office. The emperor approved the proposal.[75]

Under the supervision of the Imperial Academy of Medicine, many other medical administrative offices were established in and outside of the capitals. To serve the emperors and the imperial family, the Imperial Pharmaceutical Bureau (*Yuyao yuan* 御藥院, created in 1269), *Yuyao ju*, Imperial Pharmaceutical Office (*Yuyao ju* 御藥局, 1273), and Branch Imperial Pharmaceutical Office (*Xing yuyao ju* 行御藥局, 1305) were established. The Imperial Perfumes Office (*Yuxiang ju* 御香局, 1308) collected precious pharmaceuticals and perfumes from various places in and outside of the empire, compounded them, and packaged them for imperial use.[76] The Yuan government created the Office of Medicine of the Western Frontier in 1263, which was changed to the Office of Broad Grace in 1270, as detailed in Chapter 6.

The Charitable Pharmacy was also placed under the supervision of the Imperial Academy of Medicine in 1263. It was originally established in the Northern Song capital, Kaifeng, as the Medicine-Producing Bureau (*Shuyaosuo* 熟藥所) in 1076. During the Chongning 崇寧 period (1102–06), the government created the seven Charitable Bureaus of Compounding Medicine (*Heji huimin ju* 和劑惠民局), where they produced and sold medicines at discounted rates. Within a few years, during the Daguan 大觀 period (1107–10), Chen Shiwen 陳師文 and others realized that the prescription texts used by the bureaus had problems, such as missing out important ingredients, giving wrong amounts of them, or not being accurate about the efficacy of the formulae. So with permission from Emperor Huizong, they edited *Prescriptions of Great Peace for Charitable Bureau of Compounding Medicine* (*Taiping huimin hejiju fang* 太平惠民和劑局方). In the Southern Song, the book was revised several times.[77]

The Jin dynasty also built a Charitable Pharmacy, but only in the capital. Placed under the supervision of the Ministry of Rites, the office was first built in 1154. Interestingly, in 1233, when the last emperor, Aizong 哀宗, took refuge in Caizhou 蔡州, north of the Jin–Southern Song border, he created a Charitable Pharmacy there and ordered the Imperial Physicians to take turns distributing medicine to the sick. This episode not only confirms the reputed virtue of the emperor but also suggests the perceived significance of this institution in the Jin period.[78]

Soon after it defeated the Jin dynasty, the Mongol government attempted to establish Charitable Pharmacies. The Pharmacies were supposed to each be headed by a "good physician" and were built to distribute medicine to the poor. Also, as much as financially possible, a local Charitable Pharmacy was expected to provide medicine to ailing prisoners.[79] The funds came from the government, and pharmacies spent the interest on them to finance the herbs. Ögedei ordered the ten circuits in North China to establish pharmacies in 1237. Later, after Qubilai placed the Pharmacy under the supervision of the Imperial Academy of Medicine, he ordered the re-establishment of the pharmacies in Daidu 大都, Shangdu 上都, and Chengdu 成都 in 1263 and Xixia 西夏 in 1269.[80]

Medical schools

The edict to revive medical schools was sent out in 1262, two years after the enthronement of Qubilai Khan. It recognized that medical schools had existed prior to the Yuan and invoked them as precedents. The Yuan medical schools, however, were far more visible and elaborate than schools of earlier times. After giving a brief overview of medical schools prior to the Yuan, this section will examine the Yuan institution in detail.

In earliest times, medical education remained in the domain of family instruction and apprenticeship, and the state did not intervene. In 443, however, during the Liu-Song dynasty (during the Nan-Bei chao period), the emperor approved a memorial promoting a medical school; and some of the Nan-Bei chao dynasties that succeeded Liu-Song also maintained officials in charge of teaching medicine.[81]

The Sui dynasty formalized two official posts in medical education: Erudites (*boshi* 博士) and Assistant Teachers (*zhujiao* 助教). These instructors and their students were categorized by specialty: medicine (*yi* 醫), massage (*anmo* 按摩), and exorcism (*zhujin* 祝禁). A record shows that during the Sui, there were 120 medical students (*yisheng* 醫生) and 100 massage students (*anmosheng* 按摩生).[82] Elaborating on these trends, the Tang dynasty appointed Erudites and Instructors of the Imperial Medical Office in the capital, putting them in charge of educating physicians. The teachers and students had four kinds of specialties—medicine, massage, exorcism, and acupuncture. The Erudites also evaluated the performance of other physicians in the Imperial Medical Office and determined their promotions.[83] The Tang government further attempted to establish local medical schools outside the capital. To reinforce the administrative decision, in 629, to construct prefectural medical schools,[84] Emperor Xuanzong 玄宗 (r. 712–56) sent an edict in 713 emphasizing the need for reliable doctors in the countryside and ruling that one Erudite should be stationed in each prefecture.[85] The Tang bureaucracy later issued detailed rules regarding the numbers of Erudites, Assistant Teachers, and students in the prefectural schools.[86]

In the Northern Song dynasty, the faction favoring the so-called New Policies (*xinfa* 新法) promoted the government school system, which in turn stimulated an interest in medical schools. In 1044, Emperor Renzong 仁宗 (r. 1022–63) approved the suggestion of a forerunner of the New Policies, Fan Zhongyan 范仲淹 (989–1052), that the Imperial Medical Service, which focused on medical education, be established. The government also selected physicians to teach medical students in front of the Temple for King Wucheng (Wucheng wang miao 武成王廟). After setting a quota for the number of medical students, the government in 1060 distributed 120 students unequally among nine departments of medicine. During the reign of Shenzong 神宗 (r. 1067–85), several changes took place. The official post of professor (*jiaoshou* 教授) was created in the supervising agency of the Imperial Medical Service; and the quota for students was raised to 300. After being abolished briefly during the *Yuanyou* 元祐 era (1086–93), the school was revived during the reign of Huizong 徽宗 (r. 1100–25); this time, the government organized the school according to the "Three Hall System" (*sanshe fa* 三舍法), which was inspired by the government's Confucian school system: as students progressed in their studies, they were promoted from the "Outer Hall" (*waishe* 外舍) to the "Inner Hall" (*neishe* 內舍),

and then to the "Upper Hall" (*shangshe* 上舍). The Northern Song government also endeavored to build medical schools outside of the capital. During Shenzong's reign, an edict to build prefectural medical schools was issued.[87]

Continuing the Northern Song policy, the Jin dynasty had a medical school built in each of its capitals.[88] The medical school in Daxing fu 大興府 (present-day Beijing) had thirty students, and other capital schools had twenty. Outside of the capitals, various superior prefectures and defense commands (*sanfu jiezhen* 散府節鎮) had sixteen students each, and defense prefectures (*fangyu zhou* 防禦州) each had ten.[89] Another sign of imperial support for medicine is that the medical students were exempted from labor service.[90]

As the Mongols advanced in China and created the powerful Imperial Academy of Medicine, Chinese officials in the Academy and elsewhere in the bureaucracy took strong initiatives to revive medical schools. In 1262, Commissioner Wang You 王猷 and Vice Commissioner Wang Anren 王安仁 of the Imperial Academy of Medicine proposed to Qubilai Khan that medical schools be reinstated. Lamenting that medical schools had long been abandoned and that students suffered from the lack of instructors, they proposed that medical schools be built in various circuits and that locally prominent physicians be appointed as professors. Their proposal was soon approved. The memorial indicates that such schools were intended to educate sons of medical households and of merchants selling pharmaceuticals, but it also allowed that "if the educable sons of good families among commoners should wish to attend the school, they should be admitted." According to the recommendations of the memorial, professors were to be exempted from silver and silk taxes, and medical school professors and students were to be exempted from labor service such as the "inspection of physicians' levy obligations" (*jianyi*) and "temporary labor" (*chaizhan*). The circuit government was to provide the school building and the salary for a clerk (*zhushan* 主善).[91]

About the time that the 1262 edict was promulgated, the Yuan government began appointing medical school instructors. The earliest example I have found is Li Gang 李鋼 (1221–89). His funerary inscription says he was appointed as the medical school professor of Nanjing 南京 circuit in 1260, and then reappointed as the professor in Xiangyang 襄陽 in 1284.[92] Several other names show up in biographical sources. Zhao You 趙友 became the medical school professor of Jingzhao 京兆 in 1276.[93] Song Chao 宋超, after serving as the associate professor of Taiyuan 太原 medical school, was promoted in 1287 to the position of professor of the medical school in Daidu (present-day Beijing).[94]

It was probably also about this time that physician Hu Lian 胡璉 was recommended for the position of professor for the circuit medical school. This is suggested by an undated "Letter Guaranteeing Physician-Confucian Hu Lian," which was composed by a Wang Yun 王惲 (1228–1304) and reads as follows:

> In my view, Physician-Confucian Hu Lian's character is circumspect and bright. His scholarship includes *Basic Questions* (*Suwen* 素問) and all other classics. And in most cases, his medical practice has been successful. Because our circuit is lacking in medical school instructors, it would certainly be beneficial to let Lian fill the position and teach students.[95]

Given that Hu Lian was the father of Hu Zhiyu 胡祗遹 (1227–95), the letter must have been written relatively early in the Yuan period.

By promoting medical schools, the Imperial Academy of Medicine tried to eliminate "fake physicians" (*jiayi* 假醫) who were illiterate. The intention becomes clear later in 1285 when the Central Secretariat approved a regulation that specifically stated that the goal of the schools was to rectify "the problems of fake physicians."[96] However, even as early as in the late 1260s, the Imperial Academy of Medicine sent a memorial to stop the practice of "fake physicians," and Qubilai Khan approved it. The memorial lamented that some drug sellers were not fearful of "public law" and sold toxic drugs such as aconite roots (*wutou* 烏頭 or *fuzi* 附子), Purging Croton (*badou* 巴豆), and arsenic trioxide (*pishuang* 砒霜). The Academy reproached

> those who are unversed in medical texts and unfamiliar with the characteristics of drugs, and who deceive the rural and common folk, falsely claiming to be physicians, scheming for profit, and carelessly practicing acupuncture and moxibustion, thereby wrongly taking lives.

It also condemned "a certain kind of woman" who specialized in distributing medicine for abortion.[97] The Academy appears to have expected that all medical practitioners be literate—an ambitious goal, even if we take into account fairly widespread rudimentary literacy.[98] In 1269, in response to an incident in Gaotang prefecture 高唐州 around the border of the present Shandong and Hebei provinces, the Ministry of the Right confirmed:

> From now on, people of various departments [of medicine] shall each work on their specialities, and when they see a patient, [they] shall rely on medical classics to determine the symptoms, to prescribe medicine, to apply acupuncture and to burn moxa. Other than that, those who harm people's lives because they are not thoroughly familiar with the classics, do not know the properties of medicinal herbs, or indiscriminately apply acupuncture and burn moxa, shall stop practicing. If not, they shall be penalized.[99]

It is unclear whether "the classics" (*jingshu* 經書) here means the medical classics or the Confucian classics; but previous studies have suggested that it might apply to both.[100] In any case, to read either set of classics, a practitioner had to be literate.

As mentioned earlier, Xu Heng recommended Qubilai to promote schools, instead of reviving the civil service examinations. One might think that the Yuan rulers' reluctance to hold the examinations was evidence of the Mongols' suppression of Chinese culture, but Xu Heng's biography suggests that it was he and other Neo-Confucian officials who advised Qubilai in 1260 that examinations were a superficial, undesirable way of educating the people and promoting a meritocracy. To be certain, Ögedei Khan held an examination for Confucians in 1238 soon after his conquest of North China, but the primary goal was to determine which households should be considered Confucian households and be given taxation privileges as such.[101] Qubilai sent out an edict in 1261 to ban disorderly conduct in the temples dedicated to Confucius and then required Confucian school students and others interested in studying to gather in front of the temples twice every month in 1270.[102] He ordered the establishment of geomancy schools in 1262 and Mongolian schools in 1272.[103]

Out of the four different kinds of schools the Yuan established, medical and Confucian schools were most similar to one another, particularly in their relationships to medical and Confucian households (*ruhu* 儒戶). John Dardess's study has clarified that a Confucian household was "obligated to pay land tax if it owned land, and commerce tax if it engaged in commerce,"[104] but it was granted exemption from labor service. Also, a Confucian household had "automatic access to the state educational institutions,"[105] just as medical households were given admission to medical schools. Just like Confucian households that "were placed under the jurisdiction of a prefectural or county-level Confucian school (*ruxue* 儒學), or under one or another of forty-odd academies (*shuyuan* 書院),"[106] medical households were also under the jurisdiction of a medical school. As we will see in later chapters, Confucian and medical households were also treated in a special way in the law courts.[107]

Conclusion

This chapter has shown how the world looked in the eyes of Yuan Jue and his father Yuan Hong when South China became part of the Yuan dynasty. The Mongols favored and trusted physicians and politicians with medical expertise. They created medical households, a special category in the population registration system, and bestowed levy privileges. In the bureaucracy that they created in China, physicians gained positions in the Imperial Academy of Medicine and benefited from the tax that they collected from medical households. The Academy revived medical schools and hired local physicians as instructors there. It had the ambitious goal of stopping the activities of medical practitioners who were not able to read medical books. As Yuan Hong's contemporary Zheng Sixiao observed, each occupational group had its own hierarchy. We will now return to Yuan Jue's family and see how his father Yuan Hong responded to the great political changes.

Notes

1 Zheng Sixiao, "Dayi lüexu," in *Xinshi* (Beijing: Wendiange shuzhuan, preface 1905), 131.
2 Zheng Sixiao, "Dayi lüexu," 131.
3 See the entry on *jasaq* in Christopher Atwood, *Encyclopedia of Mongolia and the Mongol Empire* (New York: Facts on File, 2004), 264–65. Valentin A. Riasanovsky, *Fundamental Principles of Mongol Law* (Bloomington: Indiana University, 1965) and other earlier works assumed that a complete legal code was compiled in a relatively short period in the early twelfth century. Recent historians, however, have re-examined the assumption. For example, while accepting the existence of individual decrees, David Morgan questions the conventional assumption that the *jasaq* as a general code was ever written; see his *The Mongols* (Oxford: Basil Blackwell, 1986), 96–99. However, Igor de Rachewiltz argues, "The existence of the Jasay is well attested for the period of Činggis Qan." In his view, the "core" of the legal code was initially written soon after Chinggis Khan's election as khan; "Some Reflections on Čingis Qan's Jasay," *East Asian History* 6 (Dec. 1993): 91–104.

4 Riasanovsky, *Fundamental Principles*, 83. A similar clause can be found in Ata-Malik Juvaini, *Genghis Khan: The History of the World-Conqueror* (University of Washington Press, 1997), 599.

5 Su Tianjue, ed., *Yuan wenlei*, Guoxue jiben congshu series, 57.833. According to this document, Yelü Chucai sent a memorial to the emperor recommending him to send physicians and others to Hebei. However, this episode seems to be another example where his contributions were inflated by his biographers. On the issues of Yelü's biographies, see Sugiyama Masaaki, *Yaritsu Sozai to sono jidai* (Tokyo: Hakuteisha, 1996), in particular 26–47.

6 Song Lian et al., *Yuanshi* (Beijing: Zhonghua shuju, 1976), 158.3711 and 189.4314.

7 Song et al., *Yuanshi*, 4.70.

8 Song et al., *Yuanshi*, 209.4635.

9 Song et al., *Yuanshi*, 8.169.

10 Thomas T. Allsen, *Culture and Conquest in Mongol Eurasia* (Cambridge: Cambridge University Press, 2001), 141–42.

11 Allsen, *Culture and Conquest*, 198–202. The quotes are from 200–201.

12 Su, *Yuan wenlei*, 57.825 and 830; and Song et al., *Yuanshi*, 146.3455.

13 Su, *Yuan wenlei*, 57.831 and 838. Song et al., *Yuanshi*, 146.3455–56.

14 For careful assessments of Yelü's role and critical readings of his Chinese biographical materials, which tended to exaggerate his political influence, see Igor de Rachewiltz et al., eds., *In the Service of the Khan: Eminent Personalities of the Early Mongol-Yüan Period (1200–1300)* (Wiesbaden: Harassowitz, 1993), 136–72, and Sugiyama Massaki, *Yaritsu Sozai to sono jidai*, in particular 302–24.

15 Su Tianjue, *Yuanchao mingchen shilüe* (Beijing: Zhonghua shuju, 1996), 8.151.

16 Su, *Yuanchao mingchen shilüe*, 8.156–57 and 8.166–67. Also see the biographies of Xu Heng, Yao Shu, and Dou Mo in Song et al., *Yuanshi*, 158.3711–33; Su, *Yuanchao mingchen shilüe*, 8.151–81; and de Rachewiltz et al., *In the Service of the Khan*, 387–447. On Xu Heng's thought, see Wm. Theodore de Bary, "The Rise of Neo-Confucian Orthodoxy in Yüan China," in his *Neo-Confucian Orthodoxy in Yüan China* (New York: Columbia University Press, 1981), 1–66. On the versatility of the "*Daoxue* faction," to which Xu, Dou, and Yao belonged, see Abe Takeo, "Gensho chishikijin to kakyo," in his *Gendaishi no kenkyū* (Sōbunsha, 1972), pp. 3–53.

17 Su, *Yuanchao mingchen shilüe*, 8.166.

18 Su, *Yuan wenlei*, 37.493–94.

19 Su, *Yuanchao mingchen shilüe*, 8.152.

20 Su, *Yuanchao mingchen shilüe*, 8.166.

21 Kosoto Hiroshi, "Gendai no iyakusho, sono 3," *Gendai Tōyō igaku*, 12.1 (January 1991): 80.

22 Luo Tianyi, *Weisheng baojian*, CSJC chubian, 20.835; de Rachewiltz et al., *In the Service of the Khan*, 414.

23 Mayanagi Makoto, "*Naigaishō benwaku ron, Hi'i ron, Ranshitu hizō kaidai,*" *Myakketsu, Naigaishō benwaku ron, Hi'i ron, Ranshitu hizō, Tōeki honzō, Shiji nanchi, Kakuchi yoron, Kyokuhō hakki, Geka seigi, Ikei sokai shū*, WKIS (1989), vol. 6, kaisetsu 30–31.

24 Song et al., *Yuanshi*, 85.2119.

25 Su, *Yuanchao mingchen shilüe*, 170–71.

26 Song et al., *Yuanshi*, 168.3962–64. For *Yuyaoyuan fang*, see Kosoto Hiroshi, "Gendai no iyakusho, sono 1," *Gendai Tōyō igaku*, 11.3 (July 1990): 92–94.

27 Song et al., *Yuanshi*, 168.3964–65.

28 Song et al., *Yuanshi*, 134.3249 and 87.2220–21. Cheng Jufu, *Cheng Xuelou wenji*, Huikan, 5.243–48. See Chapter 6 for more discussions on West Asian medicine.

29 Allsen, *Culture and Conquest*, 143–45.

30 Liu Qi, *Guiqian zhi* (Beijing: Zhonghua shuju, 1983), 11.130.

31 Song et al., *Yuanshi*, 158.3711.
32 Yanagida Setsuko, "Gendai kyōson no kotōsei," *Tōyō bunka kenkyūjo kiyō*, 73 (1977): 35–36. For a comprehensive study of the Equal Field System, see Hori Toshikazu, *Kindensei no kenkyū* (1975). A succinct overview of this system is given by Hino Kaizaburō in *Ajia rekishi jiten* (1959–1962), ed. Shimonaka Kunihiko (Tokyo: Heibonsha, 1959–62), 3:30–34. For English-language literature, see Etienne Balazs, *Chinese Civilization and Bureaucracy: Variations on a Theme* (New Haven, CT: Yale University Press, 1964), especially 108–18; Denis C. Twitchett, *Financial Administration Under the T'ang Dynasty* (Cambridge: Cambridge University Press, 1970), especially 1–17; and Victor C. Xiong, "The Land Tenure System of Tang China: A Study of Equal Field System and the Turfan Documents," *T'oung Pao*, 85.4–5 (1999): 328–90.
33 For the Double-Tax System in the late Tang and Song dynasties, see Yanagida Setsuko, "Sōdai chūō shūkenteki bunshin kanryō shihai no seiritsu o megutte," *Rekishigaku kenkyū* 288 (May 1964): 4–5, and her "Sōdai kokka kenryoku to nōson chitsujo: kotōsei shihai to kyakko," in *Niida Noboru hakushi tsuitō ronbunshū*, ed. Fukushima Masao et al. (Tokyo: Keisō Shobō, 1967), 337–64. Also, see Hino Kaizaburō, "Ryōzei hō," in Shimonaka, *Ajia rekishi jiten*, 9:303–4, as well as Brian McKnight, *Village and Bureaucracy in Southern Song China* (Chicago, IL: University of Chicago Press, 1971).
34 Tuotuo et al., *Jinshi* (Beijing: Zhonghua shuju, 1975), 46.1038.
35 Su, *Yuan wenlei*, 57.834; Song et al., *Yuanshi*, 146.3459–60.
36 Su, *Yuan wenlei*, 57.835. For grain tax, see Song et al., *Yuanshi*, 93.2357; for silk tax, see Song et al., *Yuanshi*, 42.2361. For the explanation and translations of these sections of *Yuanshi*, see Herbert Franz Schurmann, *Economic Structure of the Yüan Dynasty: Translation of Chapters 93–94 of the* Yüan shih (Cambridge, MA: Harvard University Press, 1956), 65–107. Also, see Herbert Franke and Denis Twitchett, eds., *The Cambridge History of China, Volume 6: Alien Regimes and Border States, 907–1368* (Cambridge: Cambridge University Press, 1994), 375–78.
37 Song et al., *Yuanshi*, 125.3072.
38 YDZ, 32.1b. See David M. Farquhar's explanation on appanages in his *Government of China Under Mongolian Rule: A Reference Guide* (Stuttgart: Steiner, 1990), 19. For a brief overview of Japanese scholarship on appanages, see Uematsu Tadashi, "Gendai no shiden ni tsuite no ichi kōsatsu," in *Chūgoku no dentō shakai to kazoku*, ed. Yanagida setsuko sensei kokikinen ronshū henshū iinkai (Tokyo: Kyūko shoin, 1993), 231. As to *xiguan*, see usages such as *xiguan hu* (households under jurisdiction of the government) and *xiguan si* (silk yarn destined for the government) in Song et al., *Yuanshi*, 93.2361–62 and in Schurmann, *Economic Structure*, p. 99.
39 *Mei* makes a preceding noun plural in YDZ.
40 Song et al., *Yuanshi*, 93.2361–62.
41 For another example of *chaizhan*, meaning "temporary service," see YDZ, 51.4b.
42 YDZ, 9.20a.
43 YDZ, 40.10b.
44 Yu Xilu, *Zhishun Zhenjiang zhi* (Taibei: Huawen Shuju, 1968), 13.817. See below for the Charitable Pharmacies.
45 *Zhou li*, SBCK chubian, 2.1a–4b. For the historical overview of medical administration in China, see Chen Bangxian, *Zhongguo yixue shi* (Taibei: Taiwan Shangwu yishuguan, 1981; originally published in 1937); Liu Boji, *Zhongguo yixue shi* (Yangmingshan: Huagang chubanshe, 1974); Liang Jun, *Zhongguo gudai yizheng shilüe* (Hohhot: Nei Menggu renmin chubanshe, 1995); and Liao Yuqun et al., *Zhongguo kexue jishu shi: yixue juan* (Beijing: Kexue chubanshe, 1998).
46 Sima Qian, *Shiji* (Beijing: Zhonghua shuju, 1959), 105.2794.
47 Du You, *Tong Dian* (Taibei: Xinxing shuju, 1963), 25.148 *zhong*. Liang, *Zhongguo gudai*, 16. Liao et al., *Zhongguo kexue*, 136.

48 Liang, *Zhongguo gudai*, 16. In the Qin bureaucracy, the higher the number of the ranking, the higher the position. I calculated the ranking from the top so that we can compare with the cases from later periods. In the following discussion, the higher a rank is, the lower its rank number is, unless I mention otherwise.

49 Ban Gu, et al., *Hanshu* (Beijing: Zhonghua shudian, 1962), 19 *shang*.726 and 731; Liang, *Zhongguo gudai*, 16; Liao et al., *Zhongguo kexue*, 136.

50 Liang, *Zhongguo gudai*, 17; Liao et al., *Zhongguo kexue*, 184.

51 Liang, *Zhongguo gudai*, 30–32; Liao et al., *Zhongguo kexue*, 184 and 206.

52 Liang, *Zhongguo gudai*, 56–60.

53 Miyashita Saburō, "Sō-Gen no iryō," in *Sō-Gen jidai no kagaku gijutsu shi*, ed. Yabuuchi Kiyoshi (Kyoto: Kyoto daigaku jinbun kagaku kenkyūjo, 1967), 134–45; Chen Junkai, "Songdai yizheng zhi yanjiu" (Ph.D. diss., Guoli Taiwan Shifan Daxue, 1996), in particular chapters 2 and 3; Asaf Goldschmidt, "Huizong's Impact on Medicine and on Public History," in *Emperor Huizong and Late Northern Song China: The Politics of Culture and the Culture of Politics*, ed. Patricia Ebrey and Maggie Bickford (Cambridge, MA: Harvard University Asia Center, 2006), 290–91 and 304–08.

54 Wang Yinglin, *Yuhai, juan* 63, cited in Catherine Despeux, "The System of the Five Circulatory Phases and the Six Seasonal Influences (*wuyun liuqi*), a Source of Innovation in Medicine Under the Song (960–1279)," in *Innovation in Chinese Medicine*, ed. Elizabeth Hsu (Cambridge: Cambridge University Press, 2001), 145. I made minor changes to the translation. As to the relation between epidemics and the Song policy, see also Miyashita, "Sō-Gen no iryō," 123–28, and Asaf Goldschmidt, "Epidemics and Medicine During the Northern Song Dynasty: The Revival of Cold Damage Disorders (*Shanghan*)," *T'oung Pao*, 93.1–3 (2007): 53–109.

55 Chen, "Songdai yizheng," chap. 2.

56 Liang, *Zhongguo gudai*, 119; Tuotuo et al., *Jinshi*, 56.1260.

57 Song et al., *Yuanshi*, 88.2220.

58 Song et al., *Yuanshi*, 85.2119–20, and 88.2220–21. See Niwa Tomosaburō, "Genchō niokeru in, ji, kan nado no seiritsu katei nitsuite," *Mie Hōkei* 24 (Sept. 1970), for a detailed study of the fluctuations of the Yuan special agencies.

59 Song et al., *Yuanshi*, 88.2220. For a short period of time between 1283 and 1285, this agency was called *Shanyi jian*, the Directorate of Imperial Medicine, and the ranking for the chief of this office was lowered to 4a. The name was changed backed to the Imperial Academy of Medicine in 1285, and the rank of the Intendant to 2a in 1301. In the discussions to follow, I will not use the term Directorate of Imperial Medicine but instead consistently call the agency the Imperial Academy of Medicine, in order to maintain clarity.

60 YDZ, 32.1b.

61 YDZ, 32.1a.

62 Song et al., *Yuanshi*, 6.110.

63 Chen, "Songdai yizheng," p. 86.

64 YDZ, 9.18a–20a; and 32.1a–8a.

65 Song et al., *Yuanshi*, 81.2033. See Yuan-chu Lam, "The First Chapter of the 'Treatise on Selection and Recommendation' for the Civil Service in the *Yüan shih*" (Ph.D. diss., Harvard University, 1978), 133, for his translation and annotation to this text. I adopted most of it, while making some changes.

66 Paul Ratchnevsky, *Un Code des Yuan* (Paris: Libraire Ernest Leroux, 1937), 38n2. Also see Song et al., *Yuanshi*, 83.2064.

67 Wang Yun, *Qiujian xiansheng daquan wenji*, SBCK chubian, 56.1a–3b; Cheng Jufu, *Cheng Xuelou wenji*, 9.735–37; Wang Deyi, *Yuanren zhuanji*, 1.258; Song et al., *Yuanshi*, 88.2217, 88.2221, and 90.2296.

68 Liu Minzhong, *Zhong'an xiansheng Liu Wenjian gong wenj*, Beitu, 9.345–46.

69 Song et al., *Yuanshi*, 168.3964.
70 Huang Jin, *Jinhua Huang xiansheng wenji*, SBCK, 3.24a–25b.
71 Su, *Zixi wengao* (Bejing: Zhonghua shuju, 1997), 22.372.
72 Su, *Zixi wengao*, 19.310. In cases of both Han Gonling and Dou Xingchong, the initial appointments were recorded as *shangyi*. The name of this position cannot be found in either Farquhar's or Hucker's reference books on official titles and I have not seen these titles in Yuan institutional sources, either. Because the Intendant of the Imperial Academy was called *shangyi jian* for a short time in the 1280s, it seems logical to conclude that *shangyi* at this time meant a member of the Imperial Academy.
73 Cheng, *Cheng Xuelou wenji*, 13.8b and 15.15a–16a.
74 TZTG, 3.31; *Tsūsei (1)*, pp. 88–89.
75 TZTG, 3.30–31; *Tsūsei (1)*, p. 87.
76 Song et al., *Yuanshi*, 88.2221–22.
77 Miyashita, "Sō-Gen no iryō," 141–42; Chen, "Songdai yizheng," 71–77; Goldschmidt, "Huizong's Impact," 304–08. For a detailed study on the different editions of *Taiping huimin hejiju fang*, see Kosoto Hiroshi, "*Taihei keimin wazai kyoku hō* kaidai," in *Zōkō Taihei keimin wazai kyoku hō, Genshi saiseihō, Genshi seisei zokuhō*, WKIS vol. 4 (1988), kaisetsu 1–9.
78 Tuotuo et al., *Jinshi*, 5.102, 18.398, and 56.1285.
79 YDZ, 40.11a.
80 Song et al., *Yuanshi*, 96.2467–68. Also see the following: Song et al., *Yuanshi*, 4.70, 5.93, 6.119, 88.2222 and 20.425; TZTG, 21.265; and *Tsūsei (3)*, p. 16.
81 Liang, *Zhongguo gudai*, 32.
82 Wei Zheng et al., *Suishu* (Beijing: Zhonghua shuju, 1973), 22.776. Also, see Liang, *Zhongguo gudai*, 57.
83 Liu Xu et al., *Jiu Tangshu*, 44.1875–76 (Beijing: Zhonghua shuju, 1975) and Ouyang Xiu et al., *Xin Tangshu* (Beijing: Zhonghua shuju, 1975), 48.1244–45.
84 Liu et al., *Jiu Tangshu*, 2.37.
85 Song Minqiu, ed., *Tang da zhaoling ji* (Beijing: Shangwu yinshuguan, 1959), 114.595.
86 Liang, *Zhongguo gudai*, 64–67.
87 Liang, *Zhongguo gudai*, 99–100. Also see Chen Junkai, "Songdai yizheng," 56–65.
88 For a list of the Jin capitals during various periods, see Franke and Twitchett, *Cambridge History of China, Volume 6: Alien Regimes and Border States, 907–1368*, xxix.
89 Tuotuo et al., *Jinshi*, 51.1153.
90 Tuotuo et al., *Jinshi*, 47.1056.
91 YDZ, 32.1a. Also see the translation of this memorial in Yuan-chu Lam, "The First Chapter of the 'Treatise on Selection and Recommendation' for the Civil Service in the *Yüan shih*", 155–56n108.
92 Yao Sui, *Mu'an ji*, SBCK chubian, 29.11a.
93 Wei Chu, *Qingya ji*, SKQS, 5.19b–20a.
94 Cheng Jufu, *Cheng Xuelou wenji*, 8.10a.
95 Wang Yun, *Qiujian xiansheng daquan wenji*, SBCK chubian, 92.6a.
96 YDZ, 19.18a.
97 YDZ, 57.27a. Also see TZTG, 21.265–66; *Tsūsei (3)*, 17–20.
98 On the rudimentary literacy that ordinary people in the Song, Yuan, and Ming might have had, see Honda Seiichi, "*Toen saku kō: sonsho no kenkyū*," *Tōyōshi ronshū (Kyūshū daigaku)* 21 (1993): 65–101.
99 YDZ, 57.27a–b.
100 Chen Yuan-Peng cautions against assuming that the character *jing* 經 always referred to Confucian classics because the term *yijing* 醫經 was used to refer to medical classics during the Song. See his *Liang-Song de "Shangyi shiren" yu "ruyi": jianlun qizai Jin-Yuan de liubian* (Taibei: Guoli Taiwan daxue wenshi congkan, 1997), 26.

101 Ōshima Ritsuko, *Mongoru no seifuku ōchō* (Tokyo: Daitō shuppansha, 1992), 208–13. Iiyama Tomoyasu mentions the possibilities of two other examinations being held before 1276, but he presents only scanty evidence for them (*Kin-Gen jidai no Kahoku shakai to kakyo seido* [Tokyo: Waseda daigaku shuppanbu, 2011], 317–18).
102 YDZ, 31.4a–4b.
103 YDZ, 31.1a and 32.9a.
104 John W. Dardess, *Confucianism and Autocracy: Professional Elites in the Founding of the Ming Dynasty* (Berkeley: University of California Press, 1983), 16.
105 Dardess, *Confucianism and Autocracy*, 17.
106 Dardess, *Confucianism and Autocracy*, 17.
107 Dardess, *Confucianism and Autocracy*, 14–19. Also, see Ōshima Ritsuko,"Gendai no juko ni tsuite" (1981); Hsiao Ch'i-ch'ing, "Yuandai de ruhu: rushi diwei yenbian shi shang de yizhang," in his *Yuandai shi xintan* (Taibei: Xinwenfeng chuban gongsi, 1982), 1–58; and Huang Qinglian, *Yuandai huji zhidu yanjiu* (Taibei: Guoli Taiwan daxue wenxueyuan, 1977).

3 The reunification of China, 1276–1300

South Chinese elite men approached the new empire in diverse ways after the Grand Empress-Dowager Xie 謝 announced the official surrender to the Yuan army in 1276. A small number of them continued resisting the new power until 1279, while about half the men who staffed the Southern Song government chose to work for the new ruler. Yuan Jue's father Hong, an active Southern Song official until a few months before the fall of the dynasty, neither joined the resistance group nor served the Mongols, except that he received official titles from them toward the end of his life in 1298. This chapter begins by examining his political career to give a glimpse of the complex relationships that South Chinese elite men maintained with the Yuan government in the last quarter of the thirteenth century. Then I will trace how the medical institutions evolved after the Southern Song's surrender in 1276. This section will show that the medical institutions created by the Mongols, Central and West Asians, and North Chinese were slowly accepted and somewhat altered by the South Chinese during this period.

Yuan Hong's career and the Song–Yuan transition

Yuan Hong was a smart and friendly man born in a privileged family in 1245. He entered Song officialdom in the early 1260s and was then purged out of the capital in the late 1260s because of the prevailing factionalism at the time. By the time he came back to office in the early 1270s, the Song government was clearly in decline. After fighting against the Yuan army for a short period of time, he declined all the official positions and returned to his hometown.

According to Yuan Jue, Yuan Hong memorized important classics by the time he was seven *sui*. Owing to the *yin* 蔭 privilege of his grandfather, Yuan Shao, Hong gained the prestige title of Gentleman for Rendering Service (*chengwulang* 承務郎, 9b) at 17 *sui* in 1261. Yuan Shao's merit also forged a connection between Yuan Hong and his grandfather's associates, including Ma Guangzu 馬光祖 (*jinshi* 1226), the Governor of the capital at that time, who was among the first to appreciate Yuan Hong's literary talent and bureaucratic proficiency.[1]

Yuan Hong's bureaucratic career started at the beginning of the last decade of peace in the Southern Song. The Mongols had conquered North China in 1234, and in 1257, they began attacking the Southern Song (see Map 3.1). While leading an army along the Han river (*Han shui* 漢水), Qubilai heard the news that the khan of the Mongolian empire, Möngke (r. 1251–60), had died of disease while attacking Sichuan 四川. Qubilai stayed briefly in South China, performing well in the Battle of Ezhou 鄂州 (present Wuhan 武漢), but soon departed from China in 1260 to contend for the rulership of the empire, a struggle with his brother Ariq-Böke that would persist for five years. In the meantime, the Song enjoyed a respite, until the Mongols renewed their attacks in the late 1260s. Jia Sidao 賈似道 (1213–75), in charge of the Song army, took advantage of the Mongol retreat to claim "victory" in his report to the Song court. He was promoted to the position of Grand Councilor, and became the most influential figure in the last fifteen years of Southern Song politics.[2]

Yuan Hong had held several offices before receiving a demotion; Emperor Duzong 度宗 attempted to stand by him, again because of the eminence of his grandfather. According to Yuan Jue's funerary inscription for Yuan Hong, however, Jia Sidao objected, suspecting that the emperor might be giving special favors to officials from Qingyuan. Jia succeeded in purging more than sixty officials, including Hong, from their offices and forced them to return to Qingyuan. The funerary inscription specifically names seven officials who were purged

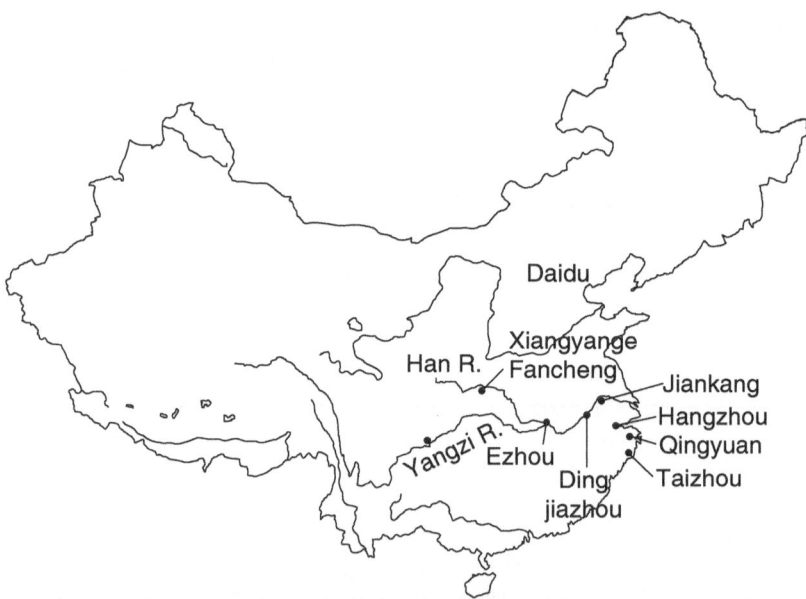

Map 3.1 Locations of Yuan Jue's and Yuan Hong's careers

(adopted from http://d-maps.com/carte.php?num_car=15277&lang=en)

with Yuan Hong.[3] Jia Sidao's antipathy toward Qingyuan was certainly not the only reason why Yuan Hong was purged. The timing of Yuan Hong's and other officials' dismissals suggests that they were closely related to conflict over Jia's controversial Public Field (*gongtian* 公田) system, innovative fiscal plans, one of which forced landlords who owned land in excess of 200 *mu* to sell a third of it to the state, to be lent directly to tenant farmers.[4] The income from state land was used to cover the increasing military costs of defending against Mongol attacks. This policy, of course, did not please many landlords, especially those rich ones in the Lower Yangzi region.[5]

Whatever the reasons for the dismissal might have been, Yuan Hong and other Qingyuan officials behaved well during their exile. According to Yuan Jue,

[They] got together once a month and discussed the words and deeds of the sages, but were not allowed to exchange opinions about current politics. My father more and more deepened his understanding of writings, took good care of himself, intentionally hid his talent, and never corresponded with people in the capital during this time.[6]

When Jia Sidao learned about Hong's "good" behavior, he nominated Yuan Hong for an honorary position to manage the Yuntai Temple (Yuntai guan 雲臺觀) in Huazhou 華州, present Shaanxi 陝西 province.[7] In 1272, Hong was appointed controller-general (*tongpan* 通判) of Jiankang super prefecture (present Nanjing).[8]

By this time, however, the Southern Song was already beginning to fall apart. Qubilai stabilized his khanship by 1264, and in 1268 he began attacking Xiangyang 襄陽 and Fancheng 樊城, two cities facing each other across the Han river, near the border of the Yuan and the Southern Song domains. As Qubilai and his strategists anticipated, it took time to defeat the Song army, but once the two cities fell in 1273, things became much easier for them. The main Yuan force went down the Han river and in 1274 subdued Ezhou, located at the intersection of the Han river and Yangzi river, without a battle. The army proceeded down the Yangzi river toward the Song capital. The news that the Yuan army would neither harm people nor steal property spread throughout Lower Yangzi region, and prompted many Song generals and people to surrender to the Yuan.[9]

It was also in late 1274 that Zhao Jin 趙溍, simultaneously the Supervisor of the Yangzi region and the Prefect of Jiankang, left the super prefecture to participate in the battles against the Yuan army along the Yangzi river. The news of his and his army's departure threw Jiankang into chaos; bandits took temporary control, and Yuan Hong campaigned against them. When Jia Sidao's army was defeated in Dingjiazhou 丁家洲 (in present-day Anhui 安徽 province), however, and Song officials including Zhao Jin surrendered to the Mongol army, Yuan Hong had no choice but to return to the Southern Song capital, Lin'an 臨安 (present Hangzhou 杭州). By the time he reached there, he already must have foreseen the fall of the dynasty. Jia Sidao's successor offered him a new position and a more prestigious title, but Hong declined all of the offers and went back to Qingyuan.[10]

In early 1276, Grand Empress-Dowager Xie announced the Song's surrender to the Yuan army. She was representing her five-year-old grandson, Zhao Xian 趙顯 (1271–1323, r. 1274–76), the last emperor of the Song dynasty. In the Song, an Empress-Dowager had the legitimate right to determine the fate of the throne, when an emperor was too young, or too ill, to do so, or if he died before naming the crown prince.[11] Thus Grand Empress-Dowager Xie's announcement marked the clear end of the dynasty in the hearts of the majority of members of the Song elite, including Yuan Hong. However, some Song men resisted her decision, and fled the capital with two brothers of the emperor and their mother, Lady Yang 楊.

Yuan Hong learned about the Grand Empress-Dowager's announcement in Qingyuan. Although his relative Yuan Yong 袁鏞 (d. 1276) and seventeen members of his family stood up for a loyalist cause, Yuan Hong was not one of them.[12] In fact, Jennifer Jay, in her detailed study of the Song loyalists, writes: "Yuan Hong (1248–98), Xie Changyuan 謝昌元 (fl. 1260–1300), and Zhao Mengchuan 趙孟傳 (fl. 1260–1300) betrayed the loyalist Yuan Yong (d. 1276) and surrendered to the Yuan general."[13] Yuan Jue's biography of Yuan Hong does not mention Yuan Yong at all, but says that Yuan Hong saved Qingyuan from a disaster by adeptly formulating a defense against the "Southern Army" (*nanjun* 南軍), the army led by the Song loyalists. Yuan Jue did not include loyalist Yuan Yong in the 1320 gazetteer for Qingyuan circuit. This compilation decision was questioned by local historians of later periods.[14] At the same time, Yuan Jue's biography mentions that Yuan Hong defended Chen Yunping 陳允平, who was to be executed because he allegedly communicated with the loyalist martyr Su Liuyi 蘇劉義 (d. 1279); Yuan Hong counseled the general of the army which had won the area that when attempting to stabilize a new country, the ruler should not summarily punish people on the basis of hearsay alone.[15]

Right after the conquest of the Southern Song, Qubilai Khan promulgated edicts encouraging Song officials to apply for positions in the new government and establishing procedures for doing so. For example, an official was supposed to bring his letter of appointment from the Song government as proof of identity, as well as two guarantors, to either central or local governments.[16] Yuan Hong was prompted to go to the new capital Daidu and saw Qubilai, who offered him positions, but he refused to take them. He demurred for the sake of his son's youth and his own "ill health," but most likely these were excuses.[17] He was perhaps testing the waters—waiting to see in which direction the new empire would go.

Qubilai Khan also engaged Jiangnan notables such as Liu Mengyan 留夢炎 (b. 1219), Wang Longze 王龍澤 (*jinshi* 1274), and Cheng Jufu to invite their associates to work for the new government. They became particularly active after 1282, when Lu Shirong 盧世榮, a North Chinese official, replaced Ahmad, a Muslim administrator, as the head of the Ministry of the Left in the Central

Secretariat. In 1282, Cheng Jufu submitted a famous memorial, "Five Points on Bureaucracy" (*Lizhi wushi* 吏治五事), advocating that they should make a list of Jiangnan literati who had served the Song government and recruit them into the new government.[18] Apparently Yuan Hong was on the recruitment list, and was offered another position in 1286, which he again declined. Cheng Jufu approached the family again in 1297, a couple of years after a new emperor, Temür (Chengzong 成宗, 1265–1307, r. 1295–1307), inherited the throne. This time, he succeeded in recruiting both father and son. Yuan Hong, however, passed away shortly after the appointment was made in 1298.

Superintendencies and judicial recognition of physicians

As the Mongol empire and South Chinese elite men such as Yuan Hong explored new relationships after 1276, the empire elaborated on the institutions that they had begun creating. One of the notable developments was the creation of the Superintendencies of Physicians (*Guanyi tiju si* 官醫提舉司, otherwise called the Directorate of Physicians, *Guanyi tilingsuo* 官醫提領所), which linked the Imperial Academy of Medicine and local medical school instructors, who directly monitored local physicians.[19] Situated in prefectural and circuit capitals, the Superintendencies of Physicians were in charge of carrying out various administrative duties, while local medical schools and the Superintendency of Medical Schools in Daidu oversaw academic aspects of doctors' activities. A Superintendent of Physicians passed a judgment on legal cases that involved physicians, in collaboration with another judge not specialized in medicine.

The Superintendency of Physicians was apparently a Yuan innovation, although we are not able to tell exactly when in the 1280s it was established. The Northern Song government began using the expression "*tiju . . . si*" as an agency name of middle rank. Charles Hucker's *A Dictionary of Official Titles in Imperial China* lists *tiju chama si* 提舉茶馬司 (Office of Horse Trading), *tiju hequ si* 提舉和渠司 (Supervisorate of Waterways), and *tiju xueshi si* 提舉學事司 (Supervisorate of Education), but neither he nor I have found any evidence for one for physicians in periods other than the Yuan.[20] The exact year when the Superintendencies of Physicians were first created, however, is unclear because of conflicting evidence. The "Annal of Qubilai Khan" (*Shizu benji* 世祖本紀) in the *Yuan History* says that the Superintendency for Physicians in Jiangnan and Other Regions was established in 1283.[21] An administrative regulation issued in 1285 and later collected in *Sagely Administration* mentions this office.[22] The "Monograph of Official Posts" (*Baiguan zhi* 百官志) in the *Yuan History* gives 1288 as the year when this office was created.[23]

A Superintendency was staffed at least by the Superintendent (*tiju* 提舉) and sometimes the Assistant Superintendent (*fu tiju* 副提舉). The Associate Superintendent (*tong tiju* 同提舉) also sometimes joined the office. These officials were assisted by clerks and escort guards.[24] Apparently some Superintendencies recruited quite a few clerks and gave them ad-hoc titles such as "Head of Medicine" (*yizheng* 醫正) and "Director of Medicine" (*yisi* 醫司). In 1298, hearing a report from a Regional Investigation Officer, the Imperial Academy of Medicine recommended to the Central Secretariat that these positions should be eliminated and the Secretariat agreed.[25]

Between the 1280s and 1304, a Superintendent's responsibilities were determined as follows. The official selected medical school instructors from within his area and with their collaboration chose students and reported the students' names, registered home addresses, and grades to the Imperial Academy of Medicine.[26] He summoned medical households to take turns in inspecting and collecting levies from other medical households.[27] When a prisoner became ill, the Superintendent was to summon a good physician to diagnose and treat him/her and write a report on the illness.[28] In the process of levying pharmaceuticals from the localities for the use of the imperial family and high officials in the central government, the Superintendent was responsible for examining the quality of herbs.[29]

Moreover, the Superintendent participated in the "mixed court" (*yuehui* 約會) when a physician was involved in a legal case. In this period, when the parties to a case came from groups that were recognized as different, a mixed court composed of judges representing each of these different groups would hear the case.[30] According to a modern Japanese historian, Iwamura Shinobu, the Yuan judicial system adopted the personal principle (*zokujin shugi* 属人主義), as opposed to the territorial principle (*zokuchi shugi* 属地主義).[31] In other words, the laws which a person in this period was to follow, and the judges to whom that person had to listen, depended on one's social group, such as ethnic, religious, and occupational groups, rather than where one lived or where the case occurred. The summary of the 1295 edict "The Litigations of Medical Households [Shall Be Held] in Mixed Courts" says: "If a physician and an ordinary person get into a fight and get involved in a lawsuit, an official governing ordinary people and a leader of the physicians shall convene a mixed court."[32]

Another edict sent in 1299 confirmed the 1295 edict that "medical household" was a category for use in determining whether a mixed court should be held. Also, in the 1299 edict, the Superintendent of Physicians was supposed not only to appear in the court but also to pass a judgment together with the officials supervising ordinary people, while the 1295 edict had said that the final decision was to be made by regular officials.[33] The 1299 edict made the mixed courts involving doctors consistent with other kinds of mixed courts, in which the leaders of two parties were supposed to pass a judgment together.[34]

Elaboration of medical schools

In 1285, around the time the Superintendency of Physicians was established, the Central Secretariat set rules for medical schools, upon the recommendations of the Ministry of Rites and the Imperial Academy of Medicine. According to the rules, students and the instructors were supposed to meet twice every month and discuss questions given by the Superintendencies of Medical Schools. This was an unfamiliar institution for the people in the Southern Song.

The Southern Song elite might have known that the supporters of the New Policies had promoted medical school systems in the Northern Song, but they were not particularly familiar with them because of the lost appeal of the New Policies and the resultant lack of governmental attention to medical schools. In the reign of Southern Song Emperor Gaozong 高宗 (1127–62), the Imperial Medical Service engaged in medical education in the capital, but the number of students enrolled in it was a third of the maximum allowed. Finally Emperor Xiaozong 孝宗 (r. 1162–89) disbanded it in 1171. Although it was revived later on and gathered students in the capital, it never recovered the vigor seen in the Northern Song period. Also, we have little evidence for prefectural medical schools.[35]

The 1285 Yuan regulation formulated a complex ranking system for medical schools. A circuit medical school should have a professor (*jiaoshou* 教授), an associate professor (*xuelu* 學録), and an assistant professor (*xuezheng* 學正). The professor was to be appointed by the emperor. Prefectural schools had either a professor or an assistant professor, depending on the prefecture's rank. They were appointed by the Intendant of the Imperial Academy of Medicine. County schools were supposed to have a lecturer (*xueyu* 學諭), to be appointed by the circuit professor. This ranking system followed the one for Confucian school instructors.[36]

Knowing that some localities had not established medical schools, the Central Secretariat clarified rules for them in 1285 as well. The regulation ordered that if a locality had not chosen a medical school instructor, the Superintendency of Physicians should have the local people recommend a doctor with broad learning and clinical excellence for the position, have him write down what kind of illnesses he had cured and three essays about therapeutic methods, and send them to the Imperial Academy of Medicine. The Superintendency and the professor collaborated to make certain each medical household and every household that sold drugs and practiced medicine would send at least one member to the school.[37]

The medical school instructors should make sure that their students learn a topic (*timu* 題目) on medical principles (*yiyi* 醫義) every month. This topic was to be chosen out of the topics on the thirteen subjects of medicine that the government, more specifically the Superintendency of Medical Schools, sent to the professors annually.[38] The Superintendency of Medical Schools (*Yixue tiju si* 醫學提舉司) was founded in 1272, abolished in 1276, and re-established in 1277. According to the *Yuan History*, the roles of this office were to supervise medical schools, to collate "works written by famous doctors," and to test drugs. The one in the capital also taught the sons of the members of the Imperial Academy of Medicine.[39] A sample topic to be discussed in medical schools read:

> Suppose a person has the following symptoms—a headache, a tight feeling in the body, a fear of cold without sweat, extreme cold without much fever, a miserable and uncomfortable look in the face, pain in the waist and back, a slight numbness in toes and fingers, not bothered by dryness, and a pulse that is floating, tight, and rough. What is the name of the syndrome, and how should one treat it?[40]

At the end of the year, the instructor was supposed to create the record of the students' achievements. In addition, he was to send the Imperial Academy of Medicine his own answers to three or four of the questions in order to prove that he was worthy of the jobs. Once a student completed study, the instructor could recommend him for governmental service to the Academy by providing information such as his name, birthplace, medical specialty, and mastery of classics.[41]

In addition to the topics on medical principles, the "students," who in the view of the regulation were all the medical practitioners in the locality, were to discuss and report on their own clinical experiences.

> Not only the medical students of various circuits, prefectures, and counties, but also the registered medical households of the jurisdiction, as well as families that just practice medicine—[in short] anyone who makes a living by practicing medicine—shall, following the above rule, report to the official of their locality on the first and fifteenth of the month, gather around the Temple of the Three Progenitors and burn incense. [There,] each shall speak about the branch of medicine he practices and the patients he has cured and shall discuss the causes of the illnesses, the circulation of *qi* according to seasons, and the adequacy of the drugs that they used.[42]

The order required that medical school students and other local medical practitioners turn in written reports of their medical practice to medical school instructors. These reports were collected every month by the prefectural and county medical school instructors and then sent to circuit medical school professors every year to be reviewed. The clinical reports were used for possible future recruitment and for the purpose of "correcting the problems of fake doctors" (*ge jiayi zhi bi* 革假醫之弊).[43]

In 1296, the system for supervising the quality of medical school instructors was revised in response to a corruption case in which a Li Kerang 李克讓 (1260–1342) had, despite his ignorance of medicine, allegedly offered bribes to become a medical school professor. The Imperial Academy of Medicine not only suggested a penalty for Li, but also expressed its concern that, although the Superintendency of Medical Schools had presumably given out 120 topics since 1285, the instructors' reports often failed to address these topics. The Imperial Academy of Medicine ruled that medical professors should submit answers to three topics on medical principles and one topic on therapeutic methods (*zhifa* 治法), and associate professors should discuss two topics on medical principles and one topic on therapeutic methods. The topics should be those that the Superintendency distributed within the previous three years, and reports on other topics would not be considered.[44]

Miaoxue

The Central Secretariat's order of 1285 determined not just the administrative and scholarly aspects of medical schools but also their religious aspects. As seen in the citation above, it mandated that medical school instructors, students, and local practitioners should assemble twice a month in front of the Temple of the Three Progenitors to worship and discuss medicine. The association between a school and a temple was important in the minds of Chinese people in the imperial period. They commonly used the term *miaoxue* 廟學 (a temple-school; temple-school complexes) to refer to this association.

Elites in imperial China valued role models in education and believed that schools should have temples in honor of Confucius and other Confucian sages. Thus, from the Han dynasty on, Confucian scholars heatedly debated which Confucian sages should be worshiped and how. According to Taga Akigorō, the most important issue up to the Tang was who should be worshiped as the Former Sage (*xiansheng* 先聖) and as the Former Teacher (*xianshi* 先師). During the time between the Han and Tang, Chinese dynasties at times treated the Duke of Zhou and Confucius as the Former Sage and Teacher, respectively; but at other times, Confucius was the Former Sage and his disciple Yanhui 顏回 was the Former Teacher. Whether to designate Confucius as the Former Sage or as the Former Teacher was an important issue because, simply put, the Former Sage was the exemplar for the students to follow and the Former Teacher merely provided assistance to that end.[45]

By the Song dynasty, Confucius's centrality was fixed, and temples dedicated to him were built in both government schools and semi-private academies (*shuyuan* 書院). Schools and academies, in addition, often had shrines dedicated to local worthies. The shrines in fact were central to the academies' physical structures, and rituals honoring these worthies were pivotal activities for the members of the academies.[46] The selection of the worthies was largely determined by the particular political and intellectual climate of any given period in the Song period; shrines to local worthies gradually became important sites where Neo-Confucian scholars promoted their own fellow scholars and ideas.[47]

During the Yuan, Temples to Confucius, officially called *Xuansheng miao* 宣聖廟, were built both in and outside the capital and were incorporated into the local academies, which by this time were under the state's close supervision, and Confucian schools. "No prefecture or county is without a school, and every school has a Temple to Confucius," says Liu Ji 劉基 (1311–75), a Yuan literatus.[48] The purpose of local Confucian schools in the Yuan dynasty was to educate, monitor, and recruit members of Confucian households into the government.[49] In 1261, Qubilai Khan ordered the Overseers (*darughachi*) and other officials to gather in front of Temples to Confucius and conduct the oblation ritual (*shidian* 釋奠) on the first day of the month.[50] In 1269, the Central Secretariat ordered that on the first and fifteenth days of the month, local officials should gather and burn incense and Confucian school instructors should lecture on classics and history to Confucian school students and "sons from ordinary families who wish to study."[51] Soon after Temür (Chengzong 成宗, 1265–1307, r. 1294–1307) ascended the throne in 1294, the government ordered that all Confucian temple-schools and local academies should conduct small rituals on every fifteenth day and large ones in spring and autumn, and should complete construction of their temple buildings.[52]

In this cultural context, we find occasional references to temples that were associated with medical education even before the Yuan period. For example, Zhang Fangyi 張方一, a Northern Song official, said that prominent doctors in 1044 began lecturing on medical classics to students in Imperial Medical Service at the Temple of King Wucheng.[53] King Wucheng was an ancient military general, Lü Shang 呂尚, who supposedly served King Wu of the Zhou dynasty and helped him defeat the Shang dynasty around the eleventh century BCE.[54] The Tang dynasty began building a temple dedicated to him and the Northern Song associated it with the governmental military school (*wuxue* 武學). They enshrined ten other historic military generals, but never doctors, implying that the temple's primary service was for the military officials and students.[55] The Song Imperial Medical Service was later relocated in the temple dedicated to a legendary physician, Bianque 扁鵲.[56] After the Song dynasty lost North China and established the temporary capital in Lin'an (present-day Hangzhou), the government built the Imperial Medical Service with a hall dedicated to Bianque, now called by his honorary title King Shenying 神應王. The building for the Service in Lin'an was built for the first time in 1156 and then renovated in the Shaoding 紹定 era (1228–33). The image of the king was accompanied by that of a legendary doctor, Qibo 岐伯.[57]

Temples of the Three Progenitors

The concept of the temple-schools culminated in the Yuan period. The primary figures worshiped in the temple associated with a medical school were the Three Progenitors (*Sanhuang* 三皇). Prior to the Yuan period, the state treated the Three Progenitors as the founders of civilization in general, while physicians privately appropriated them as their own gods. After summarizing the concept of *Sanhuang* and describing the temples dedicated to them in pre-Yuan times, this section will discuss their evolution during the Yuan period.

Extant writings from before the Tang dynasty suggest much disagreement regarding the identity of the Three Progenitors. Sima Qian of the Former Han speaks of Tianhuang 天皇, Dihuang 地皇, and Taihuang 泰皇.[58] Later texts mention Fuxi and Shennong as two of the Three Progenitors, with the third being any one of such other legendary figures as Nüwa 女媧 (also Nügua) and Suiren 燧人. Other texts counted Huangdi as one of the Five Emperors (*wudi* 五帝), another set of five legendary figures who supposedly contributed to the rise of Chinese civilization.[59]

Around the third century CE, Fuxi, Shennong, and Huangdi were grouped together as the Three Progenitors, and the Tang dynasty adopted this definition as the standard. Huangfu Mi 皇甫謐 (216–82), in his *Chronicle of the Rulers* (*Diwang shiji* 帝王世紀), treated them as the three progenitors, or "rulers." The preface to the *Book of Documents* 尚書 (*Shangshu*) also adopted this grouping.[60] Unaware that the preface was in fact a forgery, the Tang government designated the entire *Book of Documents* one of the Five Classics (*wujing* 五經), thereby securing the status of the three legendary figures as the Three Progenitors.[61]

Several Yuan inscriptions for Temples of the Three Progenitors also acknowledge Huangfu Mi's and (wrongly) Kong Anguo's 孔安國 contributions for initiating this grouping.[62]

The Three Progenitors supposedly made many contributions to Chinese civilization, including, but not limited to, the field of medicine. Fuxi, writes Huangfu Mi, taught people how to write characters and tell fortunes. He explained the principles governing how illnesses develop, and he tested hundreds of herbs to determine their medicinal values. Shennong taught people to raise crops, tested herbs, and wrote a book on pharmacology, entitled *Shennong's Materia Medica*. To continue Huangfu Mi's account, Huangdi organized an army, built ships, created drums, and ordered his subject Qibo to test herbs. *Basic Questions*, the central text of *Huangdi's Inner Classic* (*Huangdi neijing* 黃帝內經), was supposedly the record of Huangdi's conversations with Qibo.[63]

As the Tang dynasty accepted the concept of Fuxi, Shennong, and Huangdi as the Three Progenitors, they also built the first temple dedicated to them. In 747, the government "established the Temple to the Three Progenitors and the Five Emperors in the capital and conducted seasonal rituals."[64] Another source further clarifies the content of the edict:

> The Three Progenitors and the Five Emperors created things, presented rules, and provided examples. Thus, they shall be sincerely respected. . . . The five emperors are Shaohao 少昊, Zhuanxu 顓頊, Gaoxin 高辛, Tangyao 唐堯, and Yushun 虞舜. . . . Carry out regular rituals twice a year, in spring and autumn. Place both a supervisor and an assistant supervisor and order the Court of Imperial Sacrifices to monitor [them].[65]

The Tang-dynasty temple for the Three Progenitors differed from their Yuan counterparts' in three ways. First, the Tang government worshiped the Three Progenitors not because they contributed to medicine per se but because they were cultural heroes. Second, during the Tang, the Three Progenitors were worshiped along with the Five Emperors, not with the Ten Physicians. Third, only one temple in the empire was dedicated to the Three Progenitors and Five Emperors, and that was in the capital, Chang'an 長安.

During the Five Dynasties and the Song dynasty, the government sometimes built temples for an individual progenitor but not for "the Three Progenitors" as a group. However, in 1204, the Jin emperor issued an edict commanding the worship of the Three Progenitors, the Five Emperors, and the Four Kings (*Siwang* 四王, i.e., Kings Yu 禹, Tang 湯, Wen 文, and Wu 武). Even so, as was made clear in the memorial to which the edict was a response, the reason for building the temple was to revere the legendary figures for their general contributions to civilization, rather than just to medicine.[66]

Officially, the Three Progenitors were celebrated as founders of civilization. Yet, long before the Yuan dynasty, Chinese physicians had privately begun to appropriate the Three Progenitors as their role models, building on the legends that Shennong had written a book on pharmacology and that Huangdi had engaged in the first serious dialogue with physicians, as recorded in *Huangdi's Inner Classic*. This trend toward appropriating cultural heroes to legitimize medicine is evident in the case of Zhang Gao 張杲, a Southern Song physician who came from a well-established hereditary medical family. His *Essays on Medicine* (*Yishuo* 醫説) in 1189 begins with biographies of the "Three Progenitors and prominent physicians in history (*Sanhuang lidai mingyi* 三皇歷代名醫)."[67]

By the time the Mongols conquered North China, some physicians there had built their own temples to the Three Progenitors. One of the most popular poets of this period, Yuan Haowen 元好問 (1190–1257), wrote a commemorative inscription for a private temple for the Three Progenitors in 1249.[68] His inscription for the Hall of the Three Progenitors, which was built by a doctor named Zhao Guoqi 趙國器, says:

> Zhao Guoqi, a doctor in Taiyuan 太原, said, "My practice must have a foundation." He [then] constructed a large building next to his house, erected images of the three sages [i.e., Three Progenitors], and worshiped them. He also provided places for the ten prominent physicians in history, beginning with Qibo. The building has already been prepared, and the images have been arranged in a dignified manner. Introduced by Li Jinzhi 李進之 of Taigu 太谷, he asked me to write an inscription for this hall.[69]

Zhao Guoqi, who built this hall, was the head of a government-sponsored Charitable Pharmacy, but nowhere in this inscription is a government endorsement of the temple mentioned. In a significant departure from earlier government-sponsored temples for the Progenitors, this temple had the ten historic physicians accompany the Three Progenitors.

In the same inscription, Yuan Haowen expressed what I would call Daoist hesitation to the idea that he could write anything about the Three Progenitors. He started the inscription with a quotation from *The Way and Its Power* (*Daode jing* 道德經), attributed to Laozi, that said, "Of the best rulers, the people (only) know that they exist. The next best they love and praise."[70] Citing a Northern Song philosopher, Shao Yong 邵雍 (1011–77), Yuan argued that the contributions of the Progenitors were as great as that of Heaven, that none of their virtuous acts could be proven, and that their contributions could not just be reduced to benevolence. As we will see later, this inscription was in stark contrast to those written by Neo-Confucian scholars in the late thirteenth to fourteenth centuries.

Just like Yuan Haowen, an early Yuan official, Wang Yun, also attested to the existence of a temple for the Three Progenitors before it became a governmental institution. His inscription said:

> Enshrining the Three Progenitors at Wei (i.e., Weihui 衛輝 circuit, in present-day Henan 河南 province) was initiated by physicians early in the dynasty. At the altar to the right of the Temple of the City God, they set up a room and enshrined images of the Three Progenitors.[71]

Wang continued that local officials initiated the construction of a larger building than this earlier one after the central government made them an official temple.[72]

Extant legal texts acknowledged the association between the Temples of the Three Progenitors and medical schools in 1285 for the first time. This was, as we have seen, when the Central Secretariat approved the proposal sent by the Imperial Academy of Medicine that a local medical school instructor should meet with his students at the temple twice a month. Early Yuan inscriptions mentioned above suggest that the idea most likely originated in physicians' practice in North China, ruled by the Jin dynasty until 1234. This point is confirmed by the fact that the Imperial Medical Service, the only governmental office that engaged in medical education during the Southern Song period, built a temple dedicated to Bianque, not the Three Progenitors, as discussed in the last section.

Qubilai Khan's successor, Temür Khan, issued an edict recognizing the worship of the Three Progenitors as the founders of medicine in 1295. According to the *Yuan History*, the emperor

> ordered all counties to worship the Three Progenitors just as they hold rituals at the Temples to Confucius. Fuxi should be worshiped along with Goumang 勾芒, Shennong with Zhurong 祝融, and Huangdi with Fenghou 風后 and Limu 力牧. Ten people whose names appear in medical books, headed by Huangdi's subject Yu Fu 俞跗, should also be worshiped in the two hallways [flanking the main room]. Local officials should administer the rituals in two seasons, spring and autumn, and physicians should host the rituals.[73]

Since then the central government gradually elaborated on the rules for the rituals at the Temples of the Three Progenitors. In 1299, the Branch Censorate for Several Shaanxi Regions complained that although they had been told to worship the Three Progenitors and the Ten Physicians, they were given no details. This complaint led the ritual specialists in the central government to conduct research on the Tang precedent and question the authenticity of worshiping the Ten Physicians, but, in the end, they decided to keep these medical exemplars in the temple.[74] We will see more rules issued after 1300.

Local gazetteers reveal that the physical relationship between medical schools and the Temples of the Three Progenitors varied with locale. On the one hand, some localities called the entire complex a "medical school," and considered the temple to be a part of it. For example, the medical school of Qingyuan circuit consisted of the main temple (*dadian* 大殿), where the rituals for the Three Progenitors were held, and a lecture hall (*jiangtang* 講堂), where instructors and the students engaged in academic discussions. It also had a room for rituals, side rooms, hallways, and gates.[75] The circuit later added an office for officials and a room for the medical school instructor.[76] On the other hand, localities such as Zhenjiang 鎮江 circuit, simply built a Temple of the Three Progenitors and had the appointed medical school instructors meet the students at the temple.[77] The plan of Fengyuan 奉元 circuit shows no medical school but only the location of the temple.[78]

Despite the local variations, however, one point remained consistent throughout the Yuan period: the medical schools and the Temple of the Three Progenitors were treated as one institution. "Inscriptions dedicated to the Temple of the Three Progenitors" (*Sanhuang miao ji* 三皇廟記), which often appear in the collected writings (*wenji*) of Yuan literati, invariably explain the significance of medicine, praise the medical school instructors who worked hard to complete building projects, or do both; they thus remind readers that the temples were tied to medical schools. Yu Ji 虞集 (1272–1348) highlighted the close tie between the "so-called medical schools" and the Temples of the Three Progenitors when he declared, "They are actually the same."[79]

As Appendix I shows, we have evidence for about eleven medical temple-schools built before 1300. One of them was built in Yuan Jue's home circuit, Qingyuan circuit, in 1292, a year after the Assistant Regional Investigation Commissioner pointed out the lack of a medical school there. The inscription for the school was written by Yuan Jue's teacher Wang Yinglin. It started out by discussing the significance of medicine and the books attributed to two of the Three Progenitors, *Shennong's Materia Medica* and the *Huangdi's Inner Classic*. The inscription then discussed the history of medical schools and teachers in the Zhou, Tang, and Song periods and praised the Mongol ruler for creating schools in collaboration with Confucian scholars. The inscription referred to Cheng Hao 程顥 (1032–85) and Cheng Yi 程頤 (1033–1107), leading Neo-Confucian scholars in the Northern Song, who said, "Medical books say that when one's hands and legs have arthralgia (*wei* 痿) and flaccidity (*bi* 痺), they are *buren* 不仁."[80] *Buren* medically meant lacking senses, but philosophically it meant lacking benevolence. Making use of the dual meanings of this term, Cheng taught students that not being benevolent to others was like having one's hands and feet numb because if one were benevolent, he would feel others' pains as if they were his own. By citing this quotation, Wang pointed to the connection between medical theories and Neo-Confucian teachings and highlighted the significance of the new medical temple-school in Neo-Confucian terms.[81] As we will see later, such Neo-Confucian appropriation of the Temple of the Three Progenitors became more prominent after 1300.

Although the Yuan government ordered the worshipping of the Three Progenitors, they never authorized local administrations to pay for the construction and renovation of the temple buildings. These were instead funded through the private donations of local officials, physicians, and other local residents. For example, Yuan Jue's gazetteer description of Changguozhou 昌國州 prefecture in Qingyuan circuit said:

> The [medical] school is in front of the prefectural office and to the south of the Temple of Zhenwu 眞武宮. In 1292, the Superintendent of Medical Schools, Xu Ruobi 許若璧, Chen Xishou 陳錫受, and Li Jizhi 李繼之 bought a private house and built the school. In the front part of the house, the sacred images of the Three Progenitors are worshiped, and the back part is where medical school students learn and practice. In 1294, Hu Fengchen 胡逢辰,

a Confucian skilled in the art of Canggong 倉公 and Bianque 扁鵲 [i.e., medicine], arrived [here and] became the associate professor. Medical students relied on his guidance.[82]

Once the building was constructed, however, the local administration paid for the temple's ritual activities. Soon after issuing the edict of 1295, the government allowed local administrations to pay twenty-five *liang* for the temple rituals.[83]

Conclusion

This chapter has discussed the development of medical institutions from 1276 to 1300. During this time, the Superintendencies of Physicians were created, and the doctors gained the right to participate in legal trials. The rules for the medical schools for the purposes of education and government recruitment were elaborated, and the schools were associated with the Temples of the Three Progenitors, following the contemporary notion that religious activities were crucial components of proper education. While these rules all came from Daidu and were perhaps proposed by the North Chinese, the South Chinese gradually accepted them. By the 1290s, some localities, including Yuan Jue's hometown, began collecting private donations, building the temple-schools, and appointing school instructors.

Note that it was not a coincidence that Yuan Jue and his father accepted the job offers from the Yuan government in the same decade as Wang Yinglin's decision to write the inscription for the circuit medical school. Twenty years after the fall of the Southern Song, southern elites began to realize that the Mongols were going to stay in China for a long time and that it would be to their benefit to collaborate with them as much as they could.[84] When they accepted the Yuan institutions, however, they did so on their own terms. In the next chapter, we will see how medical institutions continued flourishing after 1300 and how the South Chinese elaborated on the rationale for the importance of the Three Progenitors.

Notes

1 *Qingrong*, 33.6a.
2 Miyazaki Ichisada, "Gakushū no eki zengo," in his *Ajiashi kenkyū*, vol. 1 (Kyoto: Tōyōshi kenkyū kai, 1957); Miyazaki Ichisada, "Nan-Sō matsu no saishō Ka Jidō," in his *Ajiashi kenkyū*, vol. 2 (Kyoto: Tōyōshi kenkyū kai, 1959); and Sugiyama Masaaki and Kitagawa Seiichi, *Sekai no rekishi: Dai Mongoru no jidai* (Tokyo: Chūō kōronsha, 1997), 132–34. As to Jia Sidao, see also Herbert Franke, "Chia Ssu-tao (1213–1275): A 'Bad Last Minister'?", in Arthur. F Wright and Denis Twitchett, eds., *Confucian Personalities* (Stanford, CA: Stanford University Press, 1962), 146–61.
3 *Qingrong*, 33.7b.
4 C. Bradford Langley, "Wang Ying-lin (1223–1296): A Study in the Political and Intellectual History of the Demise of the Sung" (Ph.D. diss., Indiana University, 1980), 277–294.
5 Miyazaki, "Nan-Sō matsu no saishō Ka Jidō" (1959), 208–10.
6 *Qingrong*, 33.8a.
7 Yuntai is listed as one of the major Daoist temples supervised by the Song government in Tuotuo, *Songshi* (Beijing: Zhonghua shuju, 1977), 170.4681, but the position of

temple manager was apparently nominal in the Southern Song since it was under Jin rule and later under Mongol rule.

8 *Qingrong*, 33.8a.
9 Sugiyama and Kitagawa, *Sekai no rekishi*, 152–56.
10 *Qingrong*, 33.8b–9b.
11 See Reiko Shinno, "Sōdai no kō to teishi ketteiken," in *Chūgoku no dentō shakai to kazoku*, ed. Yanagida setsuko sensei kokikinen ronshū henshū iinkai (Tokyo: Kyūko shoin, 1993), 51–70.
12 Chang Bide et al., eds., *Songren zhuanji ziliao suoyin* (Taibei: Dingwen shuju (1974–1984), 3.1865.
13 Jennifer W. Jay, *A Change in Dynasties: Loyalism in Thirteenth-Century China* (Bellingham: Western Washington University, 1991), 173.
14 Xu Shidong, *Song-Yuan Siming liuzhi jiaokan ji*, ZGFZCS (vol. 580), 6.6a–17b.
15 *Qingrong*, 33.11a.
16 Uematsu Tadashi, *Gendai Kōnan seiji shakai shi kenkyū* (Tokyo: Kyūko shoin, 1997), 227–231.
17 *Qingrong*, 33.11b.
18 Uematsu, *Gendai Kōnan seiji shakai shi kenkyū*, 230–31.
19 David M. Farquhar translated *Guanyi tijusi* as "Superintendency of Medical Households" in his *The Government of China Under Mongolian Rule: A Reference Guide*, but I am translating it as "Superintendency of Physicians" because some documents call this position *Guan yiren tijusi*, indicating that the office supervises *yiren* (physicians), not just *yihu* (medical households). David M. Farquhar, *The Government of China Under Mongolian Rule: A Reference Guide* (Stuttgart: Seiner, 1990), 135; YDZ, 9.18a–18b.
20 Charles O. Hucker, *A Dictionary of Official Titles in Imperial China* (Taibei: Nantian shuju, 1988), 493–95.
21 Song Lian et al., eds., *Yuanshi* (Reprint, Beijing: Zhonghua shuju, 1976), 12.251.
22 YDZ, 32.2a–2b and 4.18a–19b.
23 Song et al., *Yuanshi*, 88.2222.
24 Song et al., *Yuanshi*, 88.2222.
25 YDZ, 9.19b–20a.
26 YDZ, 9.18a–19b and 32.2a–2b.
27 YDZ, 9.19b–20a.
28 YDZ, 40.10b–11a.
29 YDZ, 32.6a.
30 Iwamura Shinobu, "*Gen tenshō* keibu no kenkyū: keibatsu tetsuzuki," *Tōhō gakuhō (Kyoto)*, 24 (1954): 82–96.
31 Iwamura, "*Gen tenshō* keibu," 63–82.
32 YDZ, 53.21b.
33 YDZ, 32.2a.
34 Iwamura, "*Gen tenshō* keibu," 82–96. Also, the 1295 edict in the Yuan edition of *Sagely Administration* looks as if it was originally left blank and then someone later copied from other versions to fill that in—a sign of possible manipulation or mistakes.
35 Chen Junkai, "Songdai yizheng zhi yanjiu" (Ph.D. diss., Guoli Taiwan Shifan Daxue, 1996), 33–37 and 65–67.
36 YDZ, 9.18b.
37 YDZ, 9.19a.
38 YDZ, 32.2a and 9.18a.
39 Song et al., *Yuanshi*, 88.2222.
40 YDZ, 9.18a. The text says, "not bothered by dryness" (*bu fanzao* 不煩燥) but might have meant "not easily agitated" (*bu fanzao* 不煩躁). The latter is a medical term listed in Li Jingwei et al. eds., *Zhongyi da cidian* (Beijing: Renmin weisheng chubanshe, 1995), 1292.

41 YDZ, 32.2a–2b and 9.18a–18b.

42 YDZ, 32.2b and 9.18b. The same passage shows up in both the places, differing in one character only.

43 YDZ, 9.18b.

44 YDZ, 32.2b and 9.19b. Li Kerang's funerary inscription, written half a century later, is found in Xu Youren, *Zhizheng ji*, YRCK, 58.10a–11a. The funerary inscription does not refer to this scandal.

45 Taga Akigorō, *Tōdai kyōiku shi no kenkyū: Nihon gakkō kyōiku no genryū* (Fumaido, 1953), 84–92.

46 For temples dedicated to Confucius in Song government schools, see Ma Duanlin, *Wenxian tongkao*, Guoxue jiben congshu ed. (Taibei: Xinxing shuju, 1962), 43.409 and 44.413–15. Also, *Qinding xu wenxian tongkao*, commissioned by the Qianlong Emperor, Guoxue jiben congshu ed., 48.3221–22. For temples dedicated to Confucius and local worthies in academies, see Linda Walton, "Southern Song Academies as Sacred Places," in *Religion and Society in T'ang and Sung China*, ed. Patricia Buckley Ebrey and Peter N. Gregory (Honolulu: University of Hawai'i Press, 1993).

47 Ellen Neskar, *The Politics of Prayer: Shrines to Local Former Worthies in Sung China* (forthcoming). Also see her "The Cult of Worthies: A Study of Shrines Honoring Local Confucian Worthies in the Sung Dynasty (960–1279)" (Ph.D. diss., Columbia University, 1993).

48 Liu Ji, *Chengyibo wenji*, *juan* 6, cited in Chen Gaohua, "Yuandai de difang guanxue," *Yuanshi luncong* 5 (1993): 160–89.

49 John W. Dardess, *Confucianism and Autocracy: Professional Elites in the Founding of the Ming Dynasty* (Berkeley: University of California Press, 1983), 17. Also see Morita Kenji's review of studies on the relationship between Confucian households and Confucian schools, in his *Gendai chishikijin to chiiki shakai* (Kyūko shoin, 2004), Chapter 1.

50 YDZ, 31.4a.

51 YDZ, 32.4b.

52 YDZ, 31.4b–5a; Song et al., *Yuanshi*, 76.1901.

53 Chen, "Songdai yizheng zhi yanjiu," 57.

54 Sima Qian, *Shiji* (Beijing: Zhonghua shudian, 1959), 32.1479–80.

55 Tuotuo et al., *Songshi*, 105.2555–58.

56 Chen, "Songdai yizheng zhi yanjiu," 15.

57 Jian Shuoyou, *Xianchun Lin'an zhi*, 12.18b–19a.

58 Sima Qian, *Shiji*, 6.236.

59 Gu Jiegang and Yang Xiangkui, "Sanhuang kao," in *Gushi bian*, 7.*zhong*, ed. Lü Simian and Tong Shuye (Shanghai: Kaiming shudian, 1941).

60 See Gu and Yang, "Sanhuang kao."

61 For centuries, scholars considered Kong Anguo, of the Former Han dynasty, to have been the author of the preface; but Qing-dynasty scholars demonstrated that it was the forgery of an unknown author of the Wei-Jin period (third to fifth centuries CE). For an English-language overview of the history of the preface to *The Book of Documents*, see Benjamin Elman, *From Philosophy to Philology: Intellectual and Social Aspects of Change in Late Imperial China* (Cambridge, MA: Council on East Asian Studies, Harvard University, 1984), 177–80, 200–02, and 207–12.

62 For example, Liu Shen, *Guiyin wenji*, YRCK, 1.20b–21a, and *Qingrong*, 25.2b–3a.

63 Huangfu Mi, *Diwang shiji*, CSJC chubian, 2–5.

64 Liu Xu et al., comp., *Jiu Tangshu* (Beijing: Zhonghua shuju, 1975), 9.221 and 24.915.

65 Wang Pu, *Tang Huiyao*, CSJC, 22.430.

66 *Qinding xu wenxian tongkao*, 3548.

67 Zhang Gao, *Yishuo*, SKQS, *juan* 1.

68 Yuan Haowen, *Yishanji*, SKQS, 32.22a–23b. The inscription simply says it was written in *jiyou* 己酉 year. The only *jiyou* year in Yuan Haowen's life was 1249.

69 Yuan, *Yishan ji*, SKQS, 32.22a–23b. See also *Quan Yuanwen*, 1:22.358.
70 *The Wisdom of Laotse*, trans., ed., and with an introduction and notes by Lin Yutang (New York: Modern Library, 1976), chap. 17, p. 114. Also, see *Rōshi*, translated and annotated by Hachiya Kunio (Tokyo: Iwanami Shoten, 2011), 17.
71 Wang Yun, *Qiujian ji*, SKQS, 59.1a.
72 Wang, *Qiujian ji*, 59.1a.
73 Song et al., *Yuanshi*, 76.1902.
74 YDZ, 30.14a–b.
75 Yuan Jue, *Yanyou Siming zhi*, ZGFZCS (vol. 578), 14.16a–b.
76 Wang Yuangong, *Zhizheng Siming xuzhi*, 8.1b–2a.
77 Yu Xilu, *Zhishun Zhenjiang zhi* (Taibei, Huawen shuju, 1968), 8.483, 11.656, and 17.915–16.
78 Li Haowen, *Chang'an zhitu*, SKQS, *shang*.11b–12a.
79 Yu Ji, *Daoyuan leigao*, YRCK, 23.30b.
80 Cheng Hao and Cheng Yi, *Henan Chengshi yishu*, 2 *shang*.15, in their *Er-Cheng ji* (Beijing: Zhonghua shuju, 1981), vol. 1. They also refer to medical and philosophical meanings of *buren* in *Henan Chengshi yishu*, 2 *shang*.33. The *Huangdi's Inner Classic* has a chapter on the *bi* syndrome and another on *wei* conditions, and in both the chapters, *buren* is listed as one of the major symptoms. See Maoshing Ni, trans. *The Yellow Emperor's Classic of Medicine: A New Translation of the Neijing Suwen with Commentary* (Boston, MA: Shambhala, 1995), chaps. 43–44; and Ishida Hidemi, Katsuta Masayasu, Suzuki Hiroshi, and Hyōdō Akira, trans., *Gendaigo yaku Kōtei daikei somon (chū)* (Chiba: Tōyō gakujutsu shuppansha, 1992), 157–81.
81 Yuan Jue, *Yanyou Siming zhi*, 14.13b–14a.
82 Yuan Jue, *Yanyou Siming zhi*, 14.19b.
83 YDZ, 30.14b–15a.
84 Langley, "Wang Ying-lin," 471–72; Morita Kenji, *Gendai chishikijin to chiiki shakai*, 213–32.

4 South Chinese participation in the imperial politics, 1300–68

Only 7 *sui* when the Southern Song surrendered to the Mongol army, Yuan Jue had a political career dramatically different from his father Yuan Hong's. Accepting positions in the Yuan central government, Yuan Jue spent time in both the capitals, Daidu and Shangdu, and was in close contact with Mongol rulers and their Central and West Asian advisers. The difference in the father's and the son's careers reflected larger social changes occurring in South China in the second half of the 1290s. Twenty years had passed since the Mongols took over South China, and the generation that had been active adults at the time of conquest was retiring or passing away. Moreover, the relatively peaceful imperial succession from Qubilai to Temür in 1294 and Temür's conservation of Qubilai's policies appeared to promise political stability.[1] Jennifer Jay's study of Song loyalism concludes with 1300 because "[b]y then, many loyalists had died, or their loyalism had in most cases become insignificant or transformed into a more accommodating acceptance of the new dynasty."[2] This chapter will first follow Yuan Jue's career path and views on education as a window onto the ways the South Chinese participated in Yuan politics. I will then show that the medical bureaucracy in the fourteenth century retained the form set in the late thirteenth century but that the South Chinese changed its focus in subtle ways.

Yuan Jue's career and the mid-Yuan politics

The Yuan government offered Yuan Jue the first governmental position as headmaster of Lize 麗澤 Academy in Wuzhou circuit 婺州路 around 1295 when he was in his twenties.[3] Although he did not take this position, he soon took office in the imperial capital, Daidu, as a Collector of the Hanlin and National History Academy (*Hanlin guoshi yuan jianyue* 翰林國史院檢閱, 8a). He was promoted gradually within this academy to the post of a Compiler of the First Class (*Hanlin daizhi* 翰林待制, 5a). He was then transferred to the Academy of Scholarly Worthies, and became an Auxiliary Academician (*Jixianyuan zhixueshi* 集賢院直學士, 3a). Because of illness, he took leave of office and went home to Qingyuan for a while, but eventually returned to the same position. He finally became a Hanlin Expositor (*shijiang xueshi* 侍講學士, 2b) in 1321, resigned from that office in 1324, and passed away in 1327 at age 61.[4]

To appreciate the official posts that Yuan Jue achieved, we must first understand the significance of the Hanlin Academy in Yuan politics and culture. In the early Tang, it was the emperor's private cultural salon; but in 738, Emperor Xuanzong 玄宗 (r. 712–56) permitted its members to draft edicts. At this time Hanlin scholars held positions elsewhere, but their power gradually began to compete with and to supersede that of the Central Secretariat (*zhongshu* 中書), which had drafted edicts and shaped the policy-making process since the Nan-Bei chao period. In the Song dynasty, the Hanlin scholars, who advised and lectured to the emperor and drafted edicts, were better respected than the members of the Secretariat. By the Yuan dynasty, the Academy was a regular government agency, also charged with compiling official historiography, as its title, the Hanlin and National History Academy, indicates. It continued enjoying political power, and its members sometimes even appropriated positions in the Secretariat.[5] Yuan Jue was cognizant and proud of that power, once commenting that "The [most] desired [position] in the court is [one in] the Hanlin."[6]

The Hanlin Academy was also one of the major literary centers in the Yuan dynasty. Yuan Jue and other poets in Daidu gathered around the Academy, sought to realize the old Chinese literary ideal in which close subordinates of the emperor occupied the center of the empire's literary circle and in which political engagement and literary activity went hand in hand. Yuan Jue's poetic style was conservative and followed Tang conventions, but the content of his poems showed curiosity and openness toward new things and toward the realities of Yuan life. For example, Yuan Jue often depicted characteristic Yuan images, such as white grass used for fuel in Daidu, or the palace, houses, and desert landscape in Shangdu, where he often accompanied Mongol emperors summering in the north. According to a modern scholar, Yoshikawa Kōjirō, Yuan Jue and his friends formed a new trend, as poets who lived in pre-1300 South China often expressed implicit or explicit resistance to the new regime.[7]

Yuan Jue also worked for the Academy of Scholarly Worthies (*Jixian yuan* 集賢院), which supervised schools and oversaw Daoist clergy and fortunetellers.[8] This Academy and the Hanlin Academy were merged for at least two years in the 1280s, and some of their personnel, Cheng Jufu for example, continued to be affiliated with both the offices even after they separated.[9] This explains why Yuan Jue went back and forth between the two academies.

Early in 1314, Ayurbarwada Khan sent an edict to determine the content of the civil service examinations, which were to be revived half a year later, citing the memorial sent by both the Hanlin Academy and the Academy of Scholarly Worthies.[10] The revival of the examinations is usually attributed to the fact that Mongol rulers in the early thirteenth century, Emperors Temür (r. 1294–1307) and Ayurbarwada, were sympathetic to Chinese culture and valued officials with Chinese learning. The emperor who occupied the imperial throne between the reigns of these two emperors, Haishan (Wuzong 武宗, 1281–1311, r. 1307–11), is generally characterized as an emperor little affected by or interested in Chinese culture, but his disposition appears to have had not much negative effect on the school system; after all, his reign lasted only three and a half years.[11]

Another, and perhaps more important, reason for the revival of the examination was a large number of vacancies caused by death, retirement, and arrest in the 1300s. Before 1314, government officials were recruited through recommendations, and many of them were officials of the former dynasties. A modern historian, Uematsu Tadashi, estimates that more than half of the Southern Song government officials remained in the bureaucracy after the Mongol occupation. This first generation of local officials, however, died or retired around the turn of the century, while the central government had increasingly become suspicious of "local bullies" occupying local and provincial administrations, to the extent that a large number of suspected local elites were arrested in the early 1300s.[12] They added the civil service examinations as another way to recruit scholars to fill the vacancies.

Yuan Jue, as a member of the Hanlin Academy and the Academy of Scholarly Worthies, was involved in the process that eventually led to the revival. He was initially opposed to it because he thought the examinations had led to the demise of the Southern Song. In an undated memorial on national schools, he criticized the civil service examinations as they were held toward the end of that dynasty. He cited Yang Wan 楊綰 (d. 777), an official in the Tang dynasty, who said:

> Those taking examinations on poetry (*jinshi*) are reciting the contemporary literature and not familiar with the Classics and history. Those taking examinations on the Classics (*mingjing* 明經) are just memorizing difficult words and submitting their own writings to promote themselves. There is no sense of "giving up one's own seat to welcome the wise."[13]

Yuan Jue then added, "The end of the Song was not far from this." He continued:

> The civil service examinations are now abolished, and our dynasty established a national school system in order to give deep education to the children of the elite. It is like the Tang dynasty, which established erudites for each of the Five Classics, charging each erudite to professionally master one Classic. They asked one another difficult questions to fathom the meaning of each classic thoroughly.[14]

He believed that a scholar-official should have a specialty, which he should understand in depth.

Hu Yuan 胡瑗 (993–1059) and Zhu Xi, in his view, valued expertise on in-depth knowledge in the Song dynasty:

> As to the essentials of current affairs, Hu Yuan of the Song dynasty established methods of teaching at his school in Huzhou 湖州, and lectured on rituals, administration of justice, mobilization for defense and agriculture, grain tribute, and river management. Morning and night, practical matters of statecraft were expounded and studied. Zhu Xi also discussed the examination system; he gathered various commentaries to the Classics, among them, those by Zheng [Xuan] 鄭玄 (127–200), Ouyang [Xiu] 歐陽脩 (1007–1072), Wang

[Anshi] 王安石 (1021–1086), and Lü [Zuqian] for the *Book of Odes*;[15] Kong [Anguo] 孔安國, Su [Shi] 蘇軾 (1036–1101), Wu Yu 吳[棫] (*jinshi* 1124), and Ye [Mengde] 葉夢得 (1077–1148) for the *Book of Documents*.[16] These former Confucians used their minds-and-hearts to truly understand this and administer things (*xingshi* 行事).[17]

In other words, although Zhu Xi compiled the Four Books to show his students the essence of the Way, it was not his intention to let students take short-cuts, said Yuan Jue.

To continue his argument, however, the elite by the end of the Southern Song abused Zhu Xi's legacy. They studied the Four Books only as a convenient summary and did not pay attention to the details presented in other Confucian classics.

> At the end of the Song, the learning of Zhu Xi came to be respected, and [the people repeated his texts over and over] to the extent that their lips were rotten and their tongues were exhausted. They now stop [their scholarly pursuit once they studied] Zhu Xi's commentaries to the Four Books. The minutiae of judicial courts, accounting, tax collection, and the census were all considered vulgar. Governmental clerks competed to abandon them and engaged in empty talks and just sat straight. That was why the dynasty collapsed and nobody could save it.[18]

In Chapter 1, we learned that he had his personal reasons—the deaths of his mother, father, and wife—why practical matters and specialized knowledge to get them done were important. That was why he thought medicine was particularly important. We now know that he had public concerns. He thought the indifference to in-depth knowledge of the Southern Song elite was a cause of the fall of the dynasty.

The Hanlin Academy and the Academy of Scholarly Worthies agreed with Yuan Jue that the examination on poetry was not necessary but recommended to the emperor that the Four Books and the Five Classics should be tested and that Zhu Xi's interpretations of the books should be central.[19] Yuan Jue contributed to the examinations after the revival, despite his past opposition. He wrote questions for the provincial examination in Daidu in 1317, for the metropolitan examination in 1321, and for the provincial examination in Jiangzhe 江浙 in 1326.[20] His local gazetteer for Qingyuan said, "The former emperor (i.e., Ayurbarwada) respected literary tradition and Confucians, and he forcefully re-established the civil service examination, encouraging students to work even harder."[21]

The "medical service examinations"

As the revival of the civil service examinations became a topic of heated debates in the early fourteenth century, the privileges of medical administrators, and the methods used to recruit them, came under scrutiny as well. The fact that some of the members of the Imperial Academy of Medicine managed to have their sons and nephews appointed as Academy members became controversial. Some people argued that medical schools should teach and test on the Neo-Confucian Four Books, not just on medical classics. A year after he ordered the establishment of the civil service examination, Ayurbarwada ordered the establishment of what I call the "medical service examination."

The first complaint regarding the privileges of the Imperial Academy of Medicine came unexpectedly from the Bureau of Military Affairs. They argued in 1303 that the Academicians stretched the definition of a "family" or a "household" so that their male members would not have to serve in the Yuan military. The Bureau was referring to Mongolian families, many of which had been placed under the category of "military households" (*junhu* 軍戶) after having settled down in China. Sons of military households were usually conscripted into the Yuan military, although parents were allowed to keep at least one son at home. The members of the Imperial Academy of Medicine could serve in the Academy, instead of the military. Responding to the Bureau's concern that the number of soldiers would diminish if the practice continued, the emperor sent an edict saying that only the children and wives of the Academicians should be allowed to leave military households but that their brothers and other male relatives must serve in the military.[22]

Should the medical school instructors be found not to be fulfilling their responsibilities, they were penalized, according to a regulation sent by the Central Secretariat in 1305. It was issued in response to a memorial sent by an official, Li Fengxun 李奉訓, who lamented that even though there were already excellent regulations about how medical school instructors should guide their students, they were not properly implemented. The new regulation ordered that the first time a professor allowed students to neglect their studies, a month's salary would be withheld; an associate professor or a lecturer would be penalized seven *liang* 兩; and their supervisors (*tidiaoguan* 提調官) half a month's salary. Medical school professors received a salary of ten to twelve *liang*, almost as much as professors at the Confucian school, by the 1320s, when *Sagely Administration* was published. For the second offense, a professor would forfeit two months' salary; an associate professor or a lecturer fourteen *liang*; and the supervisors one month's salary. An instructor who disobeyed the rule for a third time would be interrogated (*quzhao* 取招), and, although the penalty would be deliberated on a case-by-case basis, each incident would be publicized. The regulations outlined similar but somewhat lighter penalties for instructors and supervisors who delivered lectures of low quality at the medical schools.[23]

In the same year, a debate on the subjects of study at medical school took place. It started out with a memorial sent by Wang You 王祐, the Prefect of Zezhou 澤州 in present Shanxi 山西 province, which argued that physicians must learn Confucian classics to improve the quality of their practice. The members of the Academy of Worthies and the Hanlin Academy agreed with Wang You and recommended:

> As for the medical teachers, we should order a good physician who knows the classics to take up the job and to gather junior medical students, and lecture on *Basic Questions*, *The Classic of Difficult Problems*, [Zhang] Zhongjing 張仲景 ['s *Treatise on Cold Damage*], [Wang] Shuhe 王叔和 ['s *Classic of the Pulse*], Secrets of Pulse (*Maijue* 脉訣), etc. Also, they have to be familiar with the Four Books (i.e., *Analects*, *Mencius*, the *Great Learning*, and the *Doctrine of the Mean*) and thoroughly understand them. If one does not thoroughly understand [those books], he should be prohibited from healing activities and should not be allowed to practice medicine.[24]

Receiving this memorial which proposed that physicians should not only read medical books but also the Four Books, the Ministry of Rites in turn asked the Imperial Academy of Medicine for its opinion. Through the Academy and the Superintendency of Medical Schools, the professor of the medical school in Daidu was asked to respond to this proposal. He expressed fierce opposition. In his memorial, he first politely acknowledged the significance of Confucian learning for everyone and then established the authority of the medical profession by arguing that good physicians were learned.

> The Four Books are in fact the basis of [all] learning and the gate to the promotion of morality. Whether a literatus, military man, physician, or fortuneteller, all should learn [those books]. [But then] why should it be only physicians? Physicians should thoroughly understand the circulatory phases and seasonal influences of Heaven and Earth, and the pharmaceutical nature of herbs. In order to understand the circulatory phases and seasonal influences, [one should] have a deep insight into the subtlety of the Way in the *Book of Changes*, and in order to know the pharmaceutical natures, one should be widely familiar with the names of things in the *Books of Odes* and the *Literary Expositor* (*Erya* 爾雅). Also, to be able to discuss illnesses, to examine, and to know symptoms, [physicians should] of course master the *Book of Documents*, *Spring and Autumn Annals*, and the *Three Rites* [i.e., *Book of Rites*, *Rites of Zhou*, and *Etiquettes and Rites*]. Then why should they study only the Four Books?[25]

The Daidu professor said, however, that the fact that physicians needed to be learned did not mean that they should be given examinations on every book.

> Examining the students on the books of various philosophers and histories is a method to examine Confucians. In order to take the examination of "Erudite in [Confucian] Classics," one should specialize in one major Classic, and also study each commentary to the *Analects* and the *Mencius*, but we cannot ask them to be accountable for other books and examine them on those books.[26]

Finally, he argued that it was important for physicians to be specialized in medicine and thus be primarily tested on their knowledge of medicine.

Moreover, for those practicing medicine, if their skill is not sophisticated, they cannot become top-level experts, and if they do not focus on their specialty, they cannot excel. Therefore, we suggest that we follow the examination method that we have already established, and if one does not master the classics in our subjects, he shall be prohibited from healing and shall not practice medicine.[27]

The Daidu medical school professor's memorial was approved by the Superintendency of Medical Schools, the Imperial Academy of Medicine, the Ministry of Rites, and the Central Secretariat.

At this time the Central Secretariat approved of a list of the "thirteen subjects" (*shisan ke* 十三科) of medical study: internal and miscellaneous medicine (*dafangmai zayi ke* 大方脉雜醫科), pediatrics (*xiaofang mai ke* 小方脈科), wind medicine (*fengke* 風科), childbirth medicine and medicine for women's miscellaneous illnesses (*chanke jian furen zabing ke* 產科兼婦人雜病科), ophthalmology (*yanke* 眼科), medicine for the mouth and teeth as well as for the throat (*kouchi jian yanhou ke* 口齒兼咽喉科), medicine for bones and for war injuries (*zhenggu jian jinzu ke* 正骨兼金鏃科), dermatology (*chuangzhong ke* 瘡腫科), acupuncture (*zhenjiu ke* 鍼灸科), and charms and spells (*zhuyou shujin ke* 祝由書禁科).[28] They called this list "thirteen subjects" obviously because they counted the ones connected by the word *jian* 兼 (as well as, e.g., *chanke jian furen zabing ke*) as two subjects, not one. Moreover, the regulation of 1305 listed the medical classics to be studied for each subject. For internal and miscellaneous medicine, a student had to study *Basic Questions*, *Classic of Difficult Problems* (*Nanjing* 難經), *Shennong's Materia Medica* (*Shennong bencao* 神農本草), Zhang Zhongjing's 張仲景 *Treatise on Cold Damage Disorders* (*Shanghan lun* 傷寒論), and selected *juan* of the *Comprehensive Record of Sagely Benefaction* (*Shengji zonglu* 聖濟總錄). *Basic Questions*, the *Classic of Difficult Problems*, *Shennong's Materia Medica* and different portions of the *Comprehensive Record of Sagely Benefaction* were assigned for pediatrics, wind medicine, childbirth medicine, medicine for women's miscellaneous illnesses, ophthalmology, medicine for the mouth and teeth as well as for the throat, medicine for bones and for war injuries, dermatology, and acupuncture. For charms and spells, *Basic Questions* and Sun Simiao 孫思邈's *Supplementary Prescriptions Worth a Thousand Golds* (*Qianjin yifang* 千金翼方) were assigned.[29] The lists of subjects and textbooks were similar to the ones in the Northern and Southern Song, with one important exception—the Yuan adoption of the *Comprehensive Record of Sagely Benefaction*.[30] We will discuss the historical significance of this book later.

The Ministry of Punishments communicated with the Central Secretariat regarding physicians' malpractice in the 1310s. First, in 1311, they complained generally about "fake physicians" (*yongyi* 庸醫) who prescribed wrong drugs or applied acupuncture in a wrong way. One of the victims of the malpractices that they mentioned was a daughter of a military general Sudai'er 速歹兒, presumably a *Semu*. They proposed that all the sons of medical households and other households who wished to study medicine be required to attend a medical school twice a month and pass the examinations given by the instructors. The Central Secretariat approved the proposal. Second, in 1313, the ministry questioned the quality of physicians' services for prisoners. They recommended that the Superintendent of Physicians test a doctor's ability before he let him take care of a prisoner. If the prisoner died and malpractice was proven, not just the physician but also the Superintendent faced punishment.[31] Again the ministry's recommendation was approved.

Half a year after the details of the civil service examination were determined in 1314, the Investigating Officers at the Office of Surveillance sent to the Censorate a report that recommended the establishment of an examination system to recruit medical administrators, or the medical service examination. It started out by questioning the occupation of the Academy positions by the relatives of the existing members:

> As to medical practice, if doctors have learned and understood [medicine], they can prescribe drugs [and cure illnesses]. If they prescribed medicine despite having a low level of medical understanding, they would harm people's lives. Some members of the Imperial Academy of Medicine at the court have acquired high levels of learning. Other members may or may not have understood medicine because they are young, have inherited their fathers' or brothers' positions, or have relied on their relatives' support. Some medical school instructors and Superintendents of Medical Households in various localities have not understood medicine. Now we are recruiting Confucians through the civil service examinations. We should have the Academy establish the examination format, have them test doctors' understanding, and assign jobs to those who have mastered medicine.[32]

Agreeing with the Office of Surveillance, the Censorate sent the report to Ayurbarwada Khan (Emperor Renzong) with their comments, and he sent an edict approving their recommendation to establish the medical service examinations.

The Imperial Academy of Medicine responded to the edict a year and a few months later by submitting a memorial to the Ministry of Rites, which in turn sent it to the Central Secretariat. The memorial detailed the concrete plans for the examination system to recruit new medical administrators in such a way that incumbents would not lose their positions. It argued that the Academy had collaborated with two Investigation Officers at the Office of Surveillance to test all the Academicians. The memorial also pointed out that the emperor had permitted them to exempt medical school instructors from the examinations and instead to rely on Regional Investigation Officers to monitor their services because they had been tested as they were promoted. At the same time, the Academicians recommended that Superintendents or Directorates of Physicians should take the exam, and if they failed they should quit medical practice although they could still continue doing managerial work. Finally, the memorial suggested examinations for those who had not yet held any positions in the Yuan medical bureaucracy. Modeled after the civil service examination, a provincial examination (*xiangshi* 鄉試)

for the doctors should be held in the autumn every three years, followed by a metropolitan examination (*huishi* 會試) a year later. Members of medical households and other households were eligible to apply, according to the suggestion, as long as they could find a guarantor for their character and learning. The candidates would be tested on the meanings of the Classics, therapeutic methods, and herbal qualities. Out of the thirty successful candidates, the first class would become members of the Imperial Academy of Medicine, the second class the assistant superintendents of physicians, and the third class medical school professors.[33] The Central Secretariat approved the proposal.

The establishment of the medical service examination system was important because it meant that the Yuan government recognized the significance of a rigorous recruitment system and merit-based hierarchy for doctors, not just regular government officials. However, I have not seen any biographies of medical administrators that mention the examinations. This reminds us that the civil service examination was an *additional* method of governmental recruitment in the Yuan period. In other words, the Yuan elite took the examination as a speedy way to climb up the ladder of official success, not the only way.[34] The medical service examination at most complemented, but did not replace, the existing recruitment system.

Medical administrators and buildings

Whatever the recruitment method for medical administrators might have been, the Yuan central and local administrations created and filled a large number of positions for them. They also encouraged local elites to construct and renovate relevant medical temple-schools. Local gazetteers, biographical materials, and medical texts attest to these points.

Of the men who staffed the Imperial Academy of Medicine in the Yuan period, fifty-five are easily identifiable. Of these, twenty-three are listed in Wang Deyi's *Index to Biographical Materials of Yuan Figures* (Appendix II). When the Academy approved Wei Yilin's 危亦林 *Effective Pharmaceutical Recipes by a Hereditary Physician* (*Shiyi dexiao fang* 世醫得效方) in 1339, twenty-three members of the Academy signed to acknowledge the greatness of this book. Only one man, Zhang Yuangui 張元桂, is listed in both lists. Interestingly, six out of the twenty-three members listed in Wei Yilin's book had names that were not Chinese (Appendix III). Also, a prominent politician Yol-Temür 月魯帖木兒 (d. 1352), was appointed as the Director of the Academy in 1348, even though neither his relatively long biography in the *Yuan History* nor a funerary inscription written by Wei Su 危素 mentions his skills as a physician.[35] Apparently, high positions in the Imperial Academy of Medicine became so prestigious that its posts were given to some politicians as honorary titles.

We have substantial evidence for the Superintendencies of Physicians at various levels of the local administrations. The *Yuan History* names seventeen circuits in North China and five Branch Central Secretariats (*xing zhongshusheng* 行中書省, hereafter BCS) as the localities that established the superintendencies (See Table 4.1). The list of medical administrators based on Wang Deyi's *Index*

Table 4.1 Superintendencies of Physicians listed in *Yuan History*

Place name	Rank	Associated position(s)		
		Superintendent	Associate superintendent	Assistant superintendent
Metropolitan Area (Zhongshu sheng 中書省)				
Daidulu 大都路	5b	×	×	×
Baodinglu 保定路	5b	×	×	×
Zhangdelu 彰德路	5b	×	×	×
Dongpinglu 東平路	5b	×	×	×
Hejianlu 河間路	5b	×		×
Daminglu 大名路	5b	×		×
Jinninglu 晉寧路	5b	×		×
Datonglu 大同路	5b	×		×
Ji'ninglu 濟寧路	5b	×		×
Guangpinglu 廣平路	5b	×		×
Ji'ninglu 冀寧路	5b	×		×
Ji'nanlu 濟南路	5b	×		×
Xinghelu 興和路	5b	×		×
Weihuilu 衛輝路	5b	×		
Huaiqinglu 懷慶路	5b	×		
Liaoyang 遼陽 Branch Central Secretariat (BCS)				
Liaoyanglu 遼陽路	5b	×		×
Da'ninglu 大寧路	5b	×		
Henan 河南 BCS	6b	×	×	×
Jiangzhe 江浙 BCS	6b	×	×	×
Jiangxi 江西 BCS	6b	×	×	×
Huguang 湖廣 BCS	6b	×	×	×
Shaanxi 陝西 BCS	6b	×	×	×

Source: Song Lian et al., *Yuanshi* (Beijing: Zhonghua shuju, 1976), 88: 2222 and 91: 2312.

gives names of superintendents and associate superintendents of physicians in Jiangzhe 江浙 BCS, Jiangxi 江西 BCS, and Pingjiang circuit 平江路 (present-day Suzhou 蘇州).[36] The biographical materials not cited in the *Index* further reveal that appointments were made at levels below the circuits in North China and the Branch Central Secretariats in South China. For example, Wang Cheng was named as the Superintendent of Physicians of Cangzhou 滄州 prefecture (in Hejian circuit 河間路).[37] The Imperial Academy of Medicine appointed You Laiweng 游萊翁 as the Superintendent of Physicians of Jianchang circuit 建昌路 in the Jiangxi 江西 BCS.[38] Wei Yilin was the Assistant Superintendent of Physicians in Nanfeng 南豐 prefecture in the same BCS.[39]

In contrast, the evidence for buildings for the Superintendencies of Physicians is almost non-existent. A gazetteer for Qingyuan circuit, compiled in 1342, says:

Superintendency of Physicians. [It was] established in 1288. The Imperial Academy of Medicine ordered that the Superintendency should be headed by a Superintendent, Associate Intendant, and Assistant Intendant . . . . [In Qingyuan circuit,] it does not have a building [of its own]. Thus, [it] oversees various matters at the Charitable Pharmacy.[40]

No other Yuan local gazetteer mentions buildings for the Superintendencies. One suspects that local administrations did not feel the need or justification to construct a building for them, given the relatively small number of appointments per Superintendency to be made.

Local physicians, local elites, and government officials collaborated to construct and renovate medical temple-schools in their localities. Local gazetteers and commemorative inscriptions dedicated to the temple-school complexes identify when and where the temple-schools were built and enable us to explore what motivated local residents to implement the laws. We have evidence for about fifty-five temple-schools in the Metropolitan Area (Zhongshusheng 中書省), Henan-Jiangbei 河南江北 BCS, Jiangzhe 江浙 BCS, Jiangxi 江西 BCS, Huguang 湖廣 BCS, and Shaanxi 陝西 BCS combined (See Appendix I). The appendix provides evidence from Yuan primary sources only. I have excluded information available in Ming gazetteers because the gap between when the temples wereconstructed or renovated in the Yuan and when the Ming gazetteers were compiled is too great, and because the Ming gazetteers do not necessarily provide the original construction dates. It is the case, however, that some Ming gazetteers and an early Ming map give thorough information about the prefecture's Yuan-period medical temple-schools.[41] In other words, Ming sources make it clear that more medical temple-schools were built than those I have listed in the appendix.

The construction of local medical temple-schools was not only widespread but also highly concentrated, from the circuit level on down to the prefectural and county levels. Nine circuits (Daidu, Xingyuan 興元, Pingjiang, Zhenjiang 鎮江, Qingyuan, Jiankang 建康, Ji'an 吉安, and Fuzhou 撫州 circuits) had more than one complex each. In Qingyuan circuit, almost every prefecture and county built its own complex. According to the "Geography Section" (Dili zhi 地理志) of the *Yuan History*, Qingyuan circuit supervised two prefectures (Changuo 昌國 and Fenghua 奉化) and four counties (Yin 鄞, Xiangshan 象山, Cixi 慈溪, and Dinghai 定海).[42] As the appendix indicates, both the prefectures and two out of the four counties (Cixi and Dinghai) built either a medical school or a temple. Only two administrative units lacked the complex: Xiangshan county, which was the most remote county from the circuit capital; and Yin county, where the circuit capital was, and which already had a circuit medical school. Zhenjiang circuit also built temples for the circuit and two out of its three prefectures, leaving out only Dantu county 丹徒縣, probably for the same reason that Yin county had no temple.

We have ample evidence for medical instructors. The *Index to Biographical Materials of Yuan Figures* [hereafter *Yuan Index*], shows that seventy-seven out of the 16,000 Yuan men listed were medical administrators, and forty of these were instructors at local medical schools (Appendix II). This is significantly different from the *Index to Biographical Materials of Song Figures*, which was compiled primarily by the same group of modern historians using roughly the same criteria as the *Yuan Index*. Of the nearly 15,000 entries in the *Index to Biographical Materials of Song Figures*, twenty-eight identify medical administrators who worked in the central government, but the *Index* offers no indication that they held positions in local administrations or local medical schools.[43] Chen Yuan-Peng's list of writings dedicated to physicians further shows that medical administrators listed in the *Yuan Index* were only the tip of the iceberg.[44] According to my own close reading of primary sources mentioned in the *Yuan Index* and Chen Yuan-Peng's list, some of those physicians and medical administrators had family members who were physicians, medical school instructors, and medical administrators. Thus one can identify a few hundred names of Yuan-dynasty medical administrators.

Direct evidence is available for educational activities in medical schools. The funerary inscription dedicated to Yan Shouyi 嚴壽逸 (1278–1348) offers one glimpse:

> Our [Yuan] dynasty established medical schools, and admitted students. You [i.e., Yan Shouyi], as a son of a Confucian family, were admitted to the school. The school official named Zeng 曾 (*zi* Zhaoxian 昭先) from Luling taught *Huangdi's Inner Classic* but [your] classmates were unable to understand [his lectures]. You alone understood the real meaning [of the *Inner Classic*] thoroughly. When [you were] older, you, through your ability, became known in your hometown as a physician, and were eventually chosen as the associate professor of Nanfeng prefecture medical school.[45]

Educational activities are also mentioned in reference to Ge Yinglei 葛應雷 (1264–1323), who was professor at Pingjiang circuit. One eulogy of Ge states:

> In the tenth year of the Dade 大德 era (1306), upon being recommended, [Ge Yinglei] filled the position of the medical school professor. He built the Temple, reclaimed arable land [to support the school], and educated many disciples, many of whom later became good physicians.[46]

Ge is also mentioned in an inscription commemorating the renovation of the Pingjiang circuit medical school, by Mou Yan 牟巘 (1227–1311):

> Ge Yinglei has succeeded in his responsibilities [as head of the medical school]. Previously he had, as an Intendant, daily followed the Prefect's order and collaborated with him to encourage physicians to establish the [school] field. Now, having taken responsibility at the [medical] school, he has supervised its construction . . . He encourages the students and tells them that physicians' moral duty is to aid the people.[47]

Certainly, we do not have as much information about the actual educational and academic activities as we have about the buildings and instructors themselves. This is probably because during the Yuan times, students at the medical schools continued to receive day-to-day instruction from family members or through apprenticeship. However, as seen in the funerary inscription for Yan Shouyi, the gatherings at the medical schools still provided opportunities for young practitioners to interact with senior physicians; and such opportunities must have been important to those whom I would call "first-generation medical students," who were not born into families that had produced generations of physicians. Moreover, because the law required that students be able to read medical texts and write medical essays, participation in the gathering gave them prestige as educated physicians, making the occupation more appealing to elite families.

Praying to the Three Progenitors

In the fourteenth century, the Yuan government and elites elaborated on not just the educational and administrative aspects but also the religious aspects of medical temple-schools. The inscriptions dedicated to the Temples of the Three Progenitors reveal the intentions behind their construction and renovation, as we have begun to see in the last chapter. The construction and renovation projects also fulfilled the political, social, and spiritual needs of various constituencies. In particular, elites in South China were eager to define the Temples for the Three Progenitors in Neo-Confucian terms.

In 1305, the Central Secretariat established that the circuits (*lu* 路) should pay one *ding* 錠 each for spring and autumn rituals at the Temple for the Three Progenitors, and superior prefectures (*snafu* 散府) and other prefectures should pay twenty-five *liang*. In 1317, in response to inflation, the Secretariat ordered these payments to be doubled. The amount that the government paid reflected its priorities. Both in 1305 and 1317, the Temples of the Three Progenitors, along with the Temple to Confucius, were awarded the largest amount of ritual fees. The government ordered local administrations to pay less for rituals for the God of the Soil and Grain (*sheji* 社稷) and the Masters of Wind, Rain, and Thunder (*fengyu leishi* 風雨雷師).[48]

In 1308, the Branch Central Secretariat for Huguang and Other Places raised questions about the order in which the images of Goumang, Zhurong, Fenghou, and Limu were arranged and the colors of their clothes. Upon the Central Secretariat's request, the Ministry of Rites, citing the *Book of Rites* (*Li Ji* 禮記) and *Records of the Grand Historian* (*Shiji*) and assuming that the Three Progenitors should face south, suggested that Goumang and Zhurong should be on the left side of the Progenitors and face Fenghou and Limu sitting on the right side. At the same time, the ministry insisted that, since the appearance and dress of the four companions were no longer known, localities should not create images for them but should instead make wooden tablets with characters identifying each figure, as in "Goumang's Spirit (*shen* 神)."[49]

Roughly twenty authors dedicated the extant inscriptions for the medical temple-schools throughout the Yuan period. Most of them were politically and intellectually prominent figures at the time. At least twelve of them served as members of the Hanlin and National History Academy or the Academy of Scholarly Worthies, whose members generally enjoyed high cultural prestige and great political power during this period; some were considered pre-eminent Neo-Confucian thinkers.[50] In other words, these authors were not poor literati writing with the goal of receiving gifts. Rather, aware that the temples had an empire-wide cultural significance, they lent their prominence to the temples in localities where they had personal ties; they expected that their sponsorship of the construction or renovation of temples would, in return, enhance their status and power.

The inscriptions dedicated to the Yuan medical temple-schools promoted various political and ethico-religious beliefs and thus functioned like inscriptions dedicated to Confucian schools, local academies, temples, and shrines in the late Southern Song. In the Yuan period, authors used inscriptions for the medical temple-schools to achieve three goals: to network, to legitimate imperial power, and to conceptualize medical practice as a means to achieving the Way. Many inscriptions provide information regarding how and by whom the construction or renovations were initiated and completed. The authors often had important personal connections with the people who participated in the construction or renovations. For example, when Cheng Jufu 程鉅夫 (1249–1318), who served as an important bridge between Chinese literati society and Mongol rulers, wrote an inscription for the land endowment for the medical school of Yongxin prefecture 永新州, he focused on the donor Wang Dongye, a member of the Imperial Academy of Medicine.[51] Before he wrote the inscription, Cheng had penned an essay expressing his gratitude to Wang for having saved his life and submitted it to the imperial court to support its decision to promote Wang as a member of the Imperial Academy of Medicine.[52] The inscription for the medical school land endowment gave Cheng an opportunity to reinforce his personal and political network.

While advancing their own interests, Cheng Jufu and others used the inscriptions to legitimize the Mongol emperors as proper rulers for the Chinese people. In particular, they stressed that the rulers had created medical schools to promote the people's welfare. Cheng wrote:

> The Three Progenitors not only contributed to medicine, but are worshiped by all those who study medicine. Is this not because, in dealing with people, the Sages are concerned first about what might make people sick and only later about [curing] the sickness itself? I understand that after [our] sacred dynasty was successfully established, it asked [all] counties and prefectures to build schools and teach medicine. This is truly wonderful. Is this not just like the mind-and-heart of the ancient sages who were always concerned about the people?[53]

Yu Ji 虞集, a mid-Yuan Hanlin academician, similarly enhanced the legitimacy of the Mongol emperors by praising the policy that every prefecture and county should establish Temples of the Three Progenitors and have physicians lead rituals. Yu Ji interpreted such acts as "the supreme indication that [Yuan rulers] were trying to let people live their lives and to fulfill their own fate."[54]

The interest in strengthening the legitimacy of the Yuan ruler suggests why, in some cases, Mongol rulers, imperial family members, and non-Chinese official initiated and contributed to the construction or renovations. Qubilai Khan had a sculptor Liu Yuan 劉元, whose family was from Baodi 寶坻 (in present-day Tianjin 天津), carve the statues of the Three Progenitors in Shangdu. He had mastered the sculpturing technique of western India by studying with Aniga 阿尼哥 (1245–1306), a man from present Nepal. Liu won praise in the *Yuan History*: "His Three Progenitors in Shangdu were extremely ancient and pure. Those who had eyes to recognize thought he was able to express the subtlety of the Three Sages." Qubilai Khan gave one of the palace women in marriage to Liu Yuan and ordered him to supervise artisans. Eventually the sculptor became a high official.[55] In Quanning circuit 全寧路, it was a Mongol imperial grand princess who proposed and financed the temple construction.[56] In Jiankang circuit 建康路, it was Temüke 帖木歌 who, along with Zhao Jian 趙簡, made financial contributions to renovate the Temple so as to welcome Bayan 伯顏 on his visit from the capital; their initiative greatly encouraged the officials, physicians, and local elites in the prefectures and counties to make contributions.[57]

Finally, and most importantly, the inscriptions for the Temples of the Three Progenitors were where authors used Neo-Confucian terms to conceptualize the temples' place in society. As we saw in the last chapter, Yuan Jue's teacher Wang Yinglin began justifying medical temple-schools by citing Cheng Hao's words. Wu Cheng 吳澄 (1249–1333), who was a prolific writer, important Neo-Confucian thinker, and popular teacher, articulated this point even more sharply than Wang did. In Wu Cheng's view, which is revealed in his inscription commemorating the 1331 renovation of the temple in Fuzhou circuit 撫州路, the throne's decision had two important implications. First, Wu Cheng stated, "By building the Temples of the Three Progenitors at medical schools, [the government] made clear who the founders of the Way of Physicians (*yidao zhi zu* 醫道之祖) were," whereas the Temples to Confucius were the government's endorsement for "what the Way of Confucians respects" (*rudao zhi suo zong* 儒道之所宗).[58] Differentiating the Way of Physicians from that of Confucians, Wu Cheng wrote:

> The Way of Confucians embodies the totality of the Way, thus enabling the society to enjoy the happiness of peace, so that people can live their lives. The Way of Physicians employs an aspect of the Way, thus enabling the world to avoid calamities such as injury, illness, and early death, so that people can live their lives.[59]

According to Wu Cheng, it was only by focusing on their own specialty that physicians could fulfill their role in society—to prevent people from the tragedy of early death.

Wu Cheng's argument reveals that the Yuan government's decision to let the Three Progenitors represent the Way of Physicians had a second, more important, implication. By worshiping both the Three Progenitors at medical schools and Confucius in the Confucian schools, the Yuan government was paying respect to the set of sages he called "the Fourteen Sages" (*Shisi sheng* 十四聖) and the values they represented. The fourteen sages were the Three Progenitors, the legendary Five Emperors (*Wu di* 五帝, i.e., Shaohao 少昊, Zhuanxu 顓頊, Gaoxing 高辛, Yao 堯, and Shun 舜), the ancient Four Kings (*Si wang* 四王, i.e., Kings Yu 禹, Tang 湯, Wen 文, and Wu 武), the Duke of Zhou, and Confucius.[60] Wu wrote:

> The Three Progenitors were the first [three] of the Fourteen Sages, and Confucius was the last of them. Confucian schools worship the last [sage] in order to honor his contribution to assemble the sages' achievements. Medical schools worship the first [three sages] in order to honor their contributions to blaze the path for the sages.[61]

In his view, although the social statuses of the fourteen sages differed, their "Way" (*dao* 道) was the same because "they all appropriated Heavenly Virtue as their own virtues, Heavenly Mind-and-Heart as their own minds-and-hearts, and lived the mandate of the Heavenly people."[62]

Wu Cheng also wrote:

> Whether we call it the Way of Confucians or of Physicians, it is still the Way of the Sages. Although there is difference between [employing] an aspect [of the Way] and [embodying] the totality [of the Way], in terms of enabling people to live their lives, there is no distinction.[63]

In other words, a physician could aspire to become a sage, not by imitating a Confucian (*ru* 儒), but simply by focusing on his own expertise. For this reason, Wu Cheng insisted that the government's decision to choose the first three of the fourteen sages as the physicians' role models was proper.

When writing the inscription commemorating the renovation of the Fuzhou temple, Wu Cheng was in tune with other Yuan-period Neo-Confucians who had expanded the concept of the Lineage of the Way (*Daotong* 道統) back to the ancient period and had placed physicians' role models, the Three Progenitors, at its beginning. *Daotong* was a fictive master–disciple lineage through which the proper Way was supposed to have been transmitted since ancient times. Han Yu 韓愈 (768–824) initially conceived of the Lineage in his "Origin of the Way" (*Yuandao* 原道), but he did not refer to the Three Progenitors. Instead he started out with Yao: "Yao transmitted this [Way] to Shun. Shun transmitted this to Yu."[64] Several centuries later, when Li Youwu 李幼武 (fl. 1261) augmented Zhu Xi's *Words and Deeds of Celebrated Statesmen* (*Mingchen Yanxing lu* 名臣言行錄) and drew the "Diagram of Transmission of the Lineage of the Way" (*Daotong chuanshou zhi tu* 道統傳授之圖), he also started the Lineage from Yao.[65] The *Yuan History* credits Zhao Fu 趙復, an early Yuan scholar, for establishing the Three Progenitors' places in the Lineage.[66] In drawing his "Diagram of the transmission of the Way" (*Chuandao tu* 傳道圖), he inserted the Three Progenitors at the top of the Lineage.[67] Xu Heng 許衡 also begins with his discussion of the Way with the Three Progenitors.[68] An early Yuan official, Hu Zhiyu 胡祗遹, states:

> If one did not read the *Book of Changes*, *Book of Odes*, *Book of Documents*, *Analects*, or *Mencius*, one would not be able to see the sages' contributions, and the sages one would know would be Mencius and those who followed him. Only Han Yu wrote the *Origin of the Way* and discussed this matter thoroughly. Before the Duke of Zhou and Confucius were King Wen and King Wu, before King Wen and King Wu were King Yu, King Tang, King Yao, and King Shun. The Three Progenitors were the teachers of King Yao and King Shun.[69]

Obviously, Hu Zhiyu had the concept of *Daotong* on his mind when he wrote this passage, which was part of his inscription commemorating the construction of the Temple of the Three Progenitors for Zhangde circuit 彰德路.

By the late Southern Song, many Neo-Confucians were creating shrines and temples dedicated to men whom they considered to have been transmitters of the Way. Historians call these structures "Transmission shrines."[70] After Zhao Fu incorporated the Three Progenitors into *Daotong* in the early Yuan, many Yuan-period followers of the Learning of the Way perceived the Temple of the Three Progenitors as a Transmission shrine and therefore were motivated to collaborate with local physicians to build one in their own locality.[71]

The newly established civil service examinations reflected Wu Cheng's and others' argument that the Three Progenitors were the founders of the Way. A question that Wu Cheng's disciple Yu Ji drafted for the palace examination said: "Had it not been for Fuxi, Shennong, and Huangdi, the Way would not have existed." The examinees were then asked to discuss the contributions of each of the Three Progenitors and other members in the Lineage of the Way.[72]

Whatever the reasons might be, being involved in the construction and renovation of the Temple of the Three Progenitors was considered so important that it compelled authors of funerary inscriptions to cite it among the good deeds of the deceased. For example, Li Fang 李芳, a medical school professor, worked so hard to construct the Temple of the Three Progenitors in his locality that his illness was exacerbated and his demise hastened, said Huang Jin 黃溍 (1227–1357).[73] We also have a funerary inscription for a man surnamed Gong 龔, a Confucian school professor, who wrote a draft inscription for a Temple of the Three Progenitors as his last piece of writing before his death.[74]

The practice of worshiping the Three Progenitors in the governmental temples culminated in 1349, when the Yuan government determined the exact procedure and created music for the spring and autumn rituals at the Temple of the Three Progenitors in the capital. Responding to a memorial sent by an Investigation Commissioner of Jiangxi and Hudong 湖東 Regions, Wenshune 文殊訥, the Central Secretariat instructed the Ministry of Rites to deliberate this matter. As a result of the deliberations, responsibilities for the rituals were divided as follows: the Court of Imperial Sacrifices would establish the ritual procedure, the Ministry of Works would manufacture ritual utensils, Jiangzhe 江浙 BCS would make the musical instruments, Erudites in the Court of Imperial Sacrifices would select the music, and the Hanlin and National History Academy would write the lyrics. Other offices provided sacrificial objects, ritual money, and grain. One hundred and forty-eight "medical households" (i.e., physicians) were selected to participate in the ritual as "temple households and the students of the rituals and music" (*miaohu liyue sheng* 廟戶禮樂生) and were probably taught to perform dances at the ceremony. The head of the Imperial Pharmaceutical Bureau learned the music and had forty-two musicians play various instruments.[75]

According to the 1349 regulations, preparation for the ceremony would begin on the eighth day of the ninth month of the following year. On the next day (the ninth day of the ninth month), when all the civil and military officials in the central government "assisted" at the ceremony by observing the process respectfully, and when musicians played the music with lyrics lauding the Three Progenitors, the Officiant of the Three Libations (*sanxian guan* 三獻官), representing the emperor, would offer wine. Ritual and music (*liyue* 禮樂) were, according to Confucian thought, integral components of governance and thus lent respectability to the Temple of the Three Progenitors. The lyrics were written by Huang Jin, born in Yiwu 義烏 in present-day Zhejiang 浙江 province.[76]

Charitable Pharmacies: development and criticism

In addition to adopting medical temple-schools in ways that suited their own religious convictions, the South Chinese elites also maintained and possibly expanded the Charitable Pharmacy system that they inherited from the Southern Song period. In contrast to the Jin domain, in which the evidence for the Charitable Pharmacy branches outside of the capital cities is relatively scanty, the Pharmacy offices were built all over the Southern Song territory. The Yuan government began building the system before 1276, but it apparently did not fare well until South China joined the empire and strengthened it. By the end of the Yuan period, a large amount of money was invested in the Pharmacy system, while some physicians influenced by North Chinese medical theories began expressing severe criticism of the therapeutic assumptions behind the system.

We have a fair amount of evidence for branch offices of the Pharmacy in the Southern Song outside of the capital. For example, the three Southern Song gazetteers for Lin'an 臨安, the capital at that time, allow us to trace the development of the Pharmacies there. The *Records of Lin'an in the Chunyou Era* (*Chunyou Lin'an zhi* 淳祐臨安志), compiled in 1152, records an office called the "Medicine-Providing Bureau" (*Shiyaoju* 施藥局).[77] The *Records of Lin'an in the Qiandao Era* (*Qiandao Lin'an zhi* 乾道臨安志), compiled in 1169, indicates the locations of one office that produced medicine and four offices that sold medicine.[78] The *Records of Lin'an in the Xuanchun Era* (*Xianchun Lin'an zhi* 咸淳臨安志), compiled in 1268, states that one more office to sell medicine was established.[79] The *Records of Siming in the Kaiqing Era* (*Kaiqing Siming xu zhi* 開慶四明續志), compiled in 1259, shows that in the area almost equivalent of the Yuan-period Qingyuan circuit, there were thirteen branch stores under the supervision of the Charitable Pharmacy.[80]

Certainly some people in the Southern Song were critical of the Pharmacy, but at that time, the issues were about corrupt officials. For example, Yu Wenbao 俞文豹 said in a book printed in 1250 that "*Huimin ju* 惠民局 (The Bureau to benefit people; the Charitable Pharmacy) is actually *huiguan ju* 惠官局 (The Bureau to benefit officials); *heji ju* 和劑局 (The Bureau to combine medicine) is actually *heli ju* 和吏局 (The Bureau to appease the clerks)."[81] Zhou Mi (1232–98) wrote:

> When the [Song] dynastic founder started this institution, we can say [the Pharmacies were the product of] benevolence. However, problems were showing up everywhere [by the Southern Song]. The clerks and pharmacists stole [the medicines to be sold at the Pharmacies].

Moreover, he said, they intentionally mislabeled cheap medicines as expensive ones to make profits. He lamented, "Although [the name of the bureau] is *huimin* (benefiting people), none of the drugs benefit the ordinary people even a little." According to him, the government officials and the powerful instead acquired all of them.[82]

Although the Yuan government was not so successful at building Charitable Pharmacy branches in the thirteenth century, they ended up investing a lot of money in the system in the fourteenth century. According to the *Yuan History*, the Pharmacy system lost the monetary principal (*guanben* 官本) in 1288 and thus its entire operation was shut down until its revival in 1298. While the early Yuan system uniformly provided 100 *liang* to its few branches, the new system took the number of the ordinary households (*minhu* 民戶) in each locality into account and gave more funding to the branches in more populated areas.[83] Two doctors were placed in every office in a larger circuit, and one in a smaller circuit and a prefecture. The *Yuan History* has a table of government funds used for the Pharmacies (see Table 4.2). In the Yuan-dynasty plan of the Fengyuan circuit 奉元路 capital, we can find the Pharmacy there also (Figure 4.1). All three counties in Zhenjiang circuit had Pharmacy branches.[84] The branches for Qingyuan circuit and Fenghua prefecture 奉化州 are mentioned in the *Continued Records of Siming in the Zhizheng Era* (*Zhizheng Siming xuzhi* 至正四明續志) as well as one in Jiqing circuit 集慶路 in the *New Records of Jingling in the Zhizheng Era* (*Zhizhen Jinling xinzhi* 至正金陵新志).[85] In Guangzhou circuit 廣州路, there was a Charitable Pharmacy for Soldiers and People (*huiji junmin yaoju* 惠濟軍民藥局).[86]

At the same time, some Yuan doctors influenced by the medical theories developed in the Jin domain became critical of the therapeutic assumptions behind the system of the Pharmacy, not just the officials who did not follow the rules. Zhu Zhenheng 朱震亨 wrote in *Expounding the Bureau Prescriptions* (*Jufang fahui* 局方發揮):

Table 4.2 Government funds for Charitable Pharmacies

Region	Funds
Metropolitan Area (*Fuli* 腹裏, *Zhongshu sheng* 中書省)	3,780 *ding* 錠
Henan Branch Central Secretariat (BCS) 河南行省	270 *ding*
Huguang BCS湖廣行省	1,150 *ding*
Liaoyang BCS遼陽行省`	240 *ding*
Sichuan BCS 四川行省	240 *ding*
Shaanxi BCS 陝西行省	240 *ding*
Jiangxi BCS 江西行省	300 *ding*
Jiangzhe BCS 江浙行省	2,615 *ding*
Yunnan BCS 雲南行省	*zhenba* 眞趴 11,500 suo 索
Gansu BCS 甘肅行省	100 *ding*

Notes:
Ding: a unit of the currency in the Yuan.
Ba: the name of a shell fish, the shells of which were used as currency in Yunnan.

Source: Song Lian et al., *Yuanshi* (Beijing: Zhonghua shuju, 1976), 96: 2468.

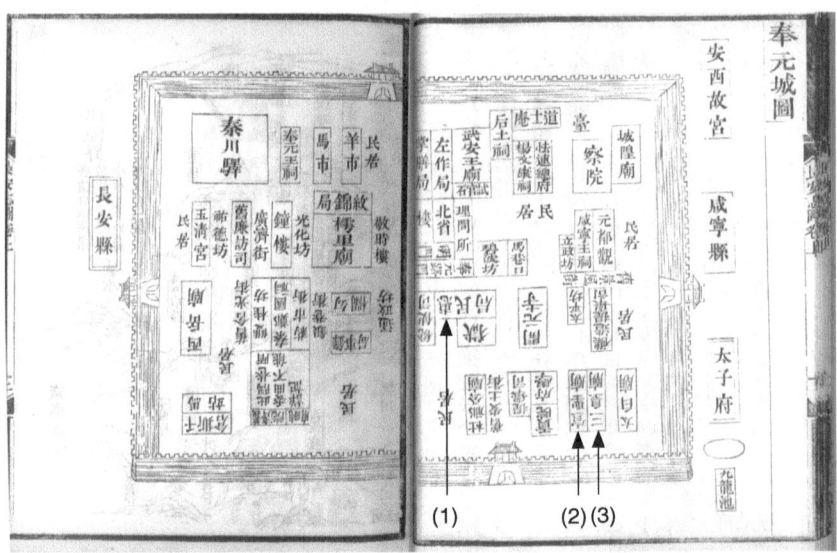

Figure 4.1 A Yuan-dynasty plan of Fengyuan circuit capital (present-day Xi'an 西安 city). (1) Charitable Pharmacy; (2) Temple to Confucius; (3) Temple of the Three Progenitors.

Source: Li Haowen 李好文, *Chang'an zhitu* 長安志圖, 1784 edition in Jingxuntang congshu 經訓堂 叢書, *shang*.11b–12a. Courtesy of Library of Congress.

In the book called *Prescriptions of the Medicine-Combining Bureau* (*Hejiju fang* 和劑局方), one can look up the prescription based on one's symptoms and take medicine. One does not need physicians. One does not need to study.

As soon as one buys the pills, the pain of illnesses gets healed. What can be more benevolent than this! From the Song until now, the government has maintained [the prescriptions in the book] as the law. Physicians use [the book as the basis of their] practice. Patients rely on it to survive. People have learned it, and it has become a custom. However, I doubt it. Why? Ancient people considered medical practice something sacred and subtle. Also, the meaning of medical understanding can be transmitted, and a physician's knowledge might be deep. But [a physician] has to make decisions case by case. It is like a general facing his enemy or a sailor sailing a boat.[87]

Note that Zhu Zhenheng's criticism was of the theoretical assumption behind the Pharmacy system. He argued that medicine should only be prescribed by an experienced physician with the ability to make case-by-case judgments based on a firm theoretical foundation. He was different from Southern Song critics who complained about the clerks not following the rules. As we will see later, Zhu Zhenheng, born in Yiwu 義烏 in present-day Zhejiang, went out of his way to learn theories developed by doctors in the former Jin domain.

Nominalization of medical households?

The local gazetteers written in the Song and Yuan show that the laws regarding medical households were fairly well implemented across the empire. The term "medical households" also appeared in documents not directly relevant to the registration system. However, this system was apparently not as reflective of reality in the fourteenth century as it might have been in the thirteenth century because the central government had not surveyed the occupations of the heads of households since 1290.

No extant gazetteers from the Song mention anything about medical households, while the term "medical households," as one of many household categories, appears in three Yuan local gazetteers. These Yuan gazetteers also discuss the Song household system, but again they do not mention occupational categories for the Song. For example, the Yuan gazetteer for Changguo prefecture 昌國州 indicates only two household categories for the Song—resident households (*zhuhu* 主户) and non-resident households (*kehu* 客户)—but seven for the Yuan—ordinary households (*minhu* 民户), Confucian households (*ruhu* 儒户), medical households (*yihu* 醫户), salt-making households (*zaohu* 竈户), crafts households (*jianghu* 匠户), military households (*junhu* 軍户), and constabulary households (*dabuhu* 打捕户).[88] The gazetteer for Jiqing circuit also records only the distinction between resident and non-resident households for the Song, but gives thorough lists of occupational categories, including medical households, for the Yuan households.[89] The last of the three, the gazetteer for Zhenjiang circuit, also shows that the local administration categorized households partially according to occupations and that "medical households" was one category.[90]

Fifteen Yuan gazetteers are extant, so one might wonder why twelve of them did not mention the "medical households." Of the fifteen, eight (*Yuan Henan zhi* 元河南志, *Chang'an zhitu* 長安志圖, *Qisheng* 齊乘, *Zhizheng Kunshan junzhi*

至正崑山郡志, *Yanyou Siming zhi* 延祐四明志, *Zhizheng Siming xuzhi, Leibian Chang'an zhi* 類編長安志, and *Xijin zhi* 析津志) did not have a "households and population" section either because it was never written or because it was lost in later centuries. Apparently the Yuan local gazetteers were less standardized than those compiled in the later periods, so the compilers of the Yuan gazetteers apparently were creative in determining what kinds of sections to include in a local gazetteer. For example, the compilers of the gazetteer for present-day Luoyang 洛陽 (*Yuan Henan zhi*) chose to focus on historical remains of this city, which had been the capital of many dynasties prior to the Yuan and one of the major cultural centers in North China, rather than discussing more economic and practical matters.[91]

Also, three out of the remaining seven gazetteers have a "households and population" section but do not mention medical households for obvious historiographical reasons. The *Records of Qinchuan* (*Qinchuan zhi* 琴川志) focuses on pre-Yuan matters.[92] The *Records of Wuxi* (*Wuxi zhi* 無錫志) gives only the total number of the households, mentioning no household categories.[93] The *Records of Nanhai in the Dade Era* (*Dade Nanhai zhi* 大德南海志) adopts only rough categorization—whether a household is originally from the north (*beiren* 北人) or from south (*nanren* 南人).[94]

The only gazetteer that has a relatively long list of household categories but does not mention medical households is *Records of Jiahe in the Zhiyuan Era* (*Zhiyuan Jiahe zhi* 至元嘉禾志). I cannot deny the possibility that this locality in fact did not adopt the category of medical household. There is, however, also a possibility that the category was "hidden" in the six categories mentioned in this gazetteer—Confucian households, Buddhist monks (*seng* 僧), Buddist nuns (*ni* 尼), Daoists (*dao* 道), postal households, and ordinary households.[95] As I will show below, some local administrations treated medical households as a subcategory of ordinary households. A medical-households category might have also existed in this locality, subsumed within ordinary households, and thus did not show up in the statistics in the gazetteer.

The three Yuan gazetteers that list medical households in their "households and population" section show that medical households constituted around 0.5 percent of the entire households in a locality (See Table 4.3). In the three counties and two prefectures in Jiqing circuit (present-day Nanjing), medical households constituted between 0.2 and 0.4 percent of the households. Medical households also made up 0.2 percent of the registered households in Changguo prefecture of Qingyuan circuit. Medical households were 0.2 or 0.3 percent of the native households (*tuzhu* 土著) in the three counties of Zhenjiang circuit (present-day Zhenjiang), except for the area under the administration of the Municipal Affairs Office (*lushi si* 錄事司) of Zhenjiang circuit, in which 0.7 percent of native households were medical households. According to Farquhar, a Municipal Affairs Office was established in the major city of each of 100 of the 184 circuits in the Yuan dynasty.[96] As Table 4.3 shows, these percentages are usually similar to the percentages of Confucian households, another important parallel between medical households and Confucian households.

Table 4.3 Numbers and percentages of medical households and Confucian households

	Medical households number (%)	Confucian households number (%)	Total registered households number
Jiqing Circuit 集慶路			
Municipal Affairs (*lushisi* 録事司)	–	–	18,205
Jiangning county 江寧縣	75(.3)	75(.3)	22,705
Shangyuan county 上元縣 (Southerner *nanren* 南人)	94(.3)	74(.3)	29,277
Jurong county 句容縣 (Southerner)	137(.4)	116(.3)	34,801
Lishui prefecture 溧水縣 (Southerner)	121(.2)	337(.6)	57,896
Liyang prefecture 溧陽縣 (Southerner)	108(.2)	137(.2)	63,482
Zhenjiang Circuit 鎮江路 (Natives, *tuzhe* 土著)			
Municipal Affairs	69(.7)	254(2.7)	9,469
Dantu 丹徒縣	66(.2)	32(.1)	28,462
Danyang 丹陽縣	77(.3)	72(.2)	29,024
Jintan 金壇縣	88(.3)	379(1.2)	32,516
Changguo Prefecture 昌國州	43(.2)	58(.3)	22,649

Sources: Zhang Xuan, *Zhizheng Jinling xinzhi*, Sanshiqi, 8.5a–12b. Yu Xilu, *Zhishun Zhenjiang zhi* (Taibei: Huawen Shuju, 1968), 3.157–180. Feng Fujing et al., *Dade Changguozhou tuzhi*, ZGFZCS, 3.1a–2a.

Although the category of medical households was fairly universally implemented, the patterns of implementation varied. In particular, there were inconsistencies among different localities regarding the relation between medical household and *minhu* (ordinary households). In some cases medical household was a subcategory of ordinary household, and in other cases it was a category of equal ranking. For example, the *Records of Changguo Prefecture in the Dade Era* (*Dade Changguo zhou tuzhi* 大德昌國州圖志) indicates that both medical households and ordinary households were among the seven subcategories of *gaiguan hu* 槩管戶 (registered households) in Changguo prefecture.[97] This is also the case in Zhenjiang circuit.[98] However, the *New Records of Jiqing Circuit in the Zhizheng Era* shows that in Jiangning county 江寧縣, a medical household was a subcategory of ordinary households.[99] Furthermore, the last gazetteer shows us that such inconsistency existed even among counties and prefectures within the same circuit, recorded in the same gazetteer. While Jiangning county and Lishui county 溧水縣 of Jiqing circuit treated medical households as a subcategory of ordinary households, Shangyuan county 上元縣, Jurong county 句容縣, and Liyang county 溧陽縣 in the same circuit considered medical households independent from ordinary households.[100]

Unfortunately, the total numbers and percentages of medical households are not so reliable, especially in the fourteenth century. In the thirteenth century when the Yuan government was actively expanding their own area of rule, nationwide censuses were held several times to record households in each locality and to determine their levy obligations.[101] After the census in 1290, however, the Yuan government stopped re-evaluating the labels on households. In 1301, Huguang Branch Secretariat received a communiqué from the Secretariat for State Affairs, saying:

> As to the household registry for physicians, report them as medical households if they were already registered as medical households and still serve the government as medical households. Those who were included in the registry every year after that should be reported to the Branch Central Secretariat as ordinary households. As to Confucian and medical households established as such by 1290, they will be, following the edict, exempted from miscellaneous labor service. However, those registered later [as ordinary households] shall not get consideration separately. Instruct your subordinate departments to implement this.[102]

This administrative order stated that the label of "medical household" should remain within the group of physicians who started practice before 1290. The same went for the label of "Confucian household." Jiqing circuit apparently followed this administrative order and thus titled a subsection of the "Households and Population" (*hukou* 戶口) section as "Households and Population Determined in 1290" (*Dayuan Zhiyuan ershiqi nian benlu chaoji hukou* 大元至元二十七年本路抄籍戶口), before giving numbers of various kinds of households.[103] In other words, the households of physicians who began medical practice after 1290 were not categorized as medical households, even though the numbers of physicians increased.

Despite uneven implementation and increasing numbers of physicians whose households were not labeled as medical households, the institution of "medical households" was far more than just a paper category. To say the least, "medical households" became a common term beyond documents directly related to a levy system. For example, Yuan Jue did not create a section devoted to recording numbers of households and population in his gazetteer, *Records of Siming in the Yanyou Era*, but he mentioned that a Prefect "encouraged the medical households in the neighborhood to contribute [to construction of a medical school]."[104] For another example, an inscription for the Temple of the Three Progenitors in Haining prefecture 海寧州 uses the expression "thirty households registered as physicians" (*qiji yu yizhe* 其籍於醫者) along with "other households gathered money to buy farming land to finance a Temple for the Three Progenitors."[105] These examples suggest that Yuan people generally knew that physicians enjoyed some privileges and carried obligations different from other occupational groups. Also, the fact that the term "medical households" appear in eulogistic writings, as in these examples, suggests that the term "medical households" did not have a negative connotation.

Conclusion

This chapter has discussed the post-1300 development of medical institutions, after some descendants of the former Southern Song subjects, like Yuan Jue, began serving the Mongol empire. Soon after the revival of the civil service examinations in 1314, the government established an examination system to select medical administrators. At the same time, local government officials and elites continued constructing and renovating medical temple-schools. While giving Mongol emperors and their collaborators credits for creating the system, the authors of the inscriptions dedicated to the Temples of the Three Progenitors made sure to incorporate the buildings in their own Neo-Confucian landscape. The Yuan government also let the Charitable Pharmacies flourish, just as the Southern Song government did. At the same time, the Yuan government was flexible as to how the occupation-based house registration system was implemented in each locality. Such flexibility was probably necessary as Mongol emperors, their Central and West Asian advisers, and North Chinese elites sought ways to collaborate with the South Chinese.

I have pointed out how the rationales for the Temples of the Three Progenitors changed over time. While Yuan Haowen's inscription, as discussed in Chapter 3, cited the book attributed to Laozi, the legendary founder of Daoism, Wu Cheng's inscription discussed the Lineage of the Way as Neo-Confucians developed it. We will now look at the two authors' and other literati's discussions of their experiences with illness and doctors to see if we can identify a similar trend.

Notes

1 Herbert Franke and Denis Twitchett, eds., *Cambridge History of China, Vol. 6: Alien Regimes and Border States, 907–1368* (1994), 490–560. The discussion of Temür's conservation of Qubilai's policies can be found in pp. 496–98.
2 Jennifer W. Jay, *A Change in Dynasties: Loyalism in Thirteenth-Century China* (Bellingham: Western Washington University, 1991), 11.
3 Dai Biaoyuan's farewell essay on the occasion of Jue's departure to Lize Academy is dated in 1295, and thus I assume that the appointment was made sometime shortly before that (Dai Biaoyuan, *Shanyuan wenji*, SKQS, 12.18a–20a.). Apparently Yuan Jue declined the offer after the essay was written.
4 Song Lian et al., eds., *Yuanshi* (Beijing: Zhonghua shuju, 1976), 172.4025–26; Su Tianjue, *Zixi wengao*, SKQS, 9.9a–9b.
5 Charles O. Hucker, *A Dictionary of Official Titles in Imperial China* (Stanford, CA: Stanford University Press, 1985), 223; Umehara Kaoru, *Sōdai kanryō seido kenkyū* (Kyoto: Dōhōsha, 1985), 68–70; David M. Farquhar, *The Government of China Under Mongolian Rule: A Reference Guide* (Stuttgart: Steiner, 1990), 127–28; and Yamamoto Takayoshi, "Gendai ni okeru kanrin gakushiin ni tsuite," *Tōhōgaku*, vol. 12 (1955).
6 *Qingrong*, 24.9a.
7 Yoshikawa Kōjirō, *Sō-Min shi gaisetsu* (Tokyo: Iwanami Shoten, 1963), 110–14. Also see Abe Takeo, "Gensho chishikijin to kakyo," in his *Gendaishi no kenkyū* (Tokyo: Sōbunsha, 1972).
8 Song et al., *Yuanshi*, 87.2192.
9 Song et al., *Yuanshi*, 172.401–18.
10 YDZ, 32.8b.
11 Franke and Twitchett, eds., *Cambridge History of China vol. 6: Alien Regimes and Border States*, 907–1368, chap. 6, passim.
12 Uematsu Tadashi, "Gendai Kōnan no chihōkan nin'yō ni tsuite," in his *Gendai kōnan seiji shakaishi kenkyū* (Tokyo: Kyūko shoin, 1997), 222–70.

13 *Qingrong*, 41.28b. Yang Wan's quote is found in Ouyang Xiu et al., *Xin Tangshu* (Beijing: Zhonghua shuju, 1975), 44.1166.
14 *Qingrong*, 41.28b.
15 *Zhuzi yulei*, a collection of dialogues between Zhu Xi and his disciples, gathers some of Zhu's critiques of various commentaries to *Odes* (Shu Jingde, comp., *Zhuzi Yulei*, [Reprinted in 1872, Yingyuan shuyuan] 80.24b–28b). This section shows that Zhu in fact studied commentaries written by various authors. Zheng Xuan was a Han-dynasty scholar who annotated *Odes*. Ouyang Xiu wrote *Maoshi benyi* 毛詩本義, Wang Anshi *Shizhu* 詩註, and Lü Zuqian *Lüshi jiashu du shi ji* 呂氏家塾讀詩記 (Chang Bide et al., *Songren zhuanji ziliao suoyin*, 5:3748, 1:277, and 2:1212).
16 Zhu's knowledge of various commentaries to *Documents* can be seen in Shu Jingde comp., *Zhuzi Yulei, juan* 78. Su Shi wrote *Shuzhuan* 書傳, Wu Yu *Shu bizhuan* 書裨傳 and Ye Mengde *Shuzhuan* 書傳 (Chang Bide et al., *Songren zhuanji ziliao suoyin* [Taibei: Dingwen shuju, 1974–84], 5:4313 and 2:1112; Tuotuo, *Songshi* [Beijing: Zhonghuan shuju, 1977], 202.5042–43).
17 *Qingrong*, 41.29a.
18 *Qingrong*, 41.29a.
19 YDZ, 30.9a.
20 *Qingrong*, 42.1a–4b. He also wrote two "questions to test *jinshi*" (*shi jinshi cewen* 試進士策問)" in1318 and 1324 (*Qingrong*, 35.4a–6a).
21 Yuan Jue, *Yanyou Siming zhi*, ZGFZCS (vol. 578), 13.1a.
22 TZTG, 3.31; *Tsūsei (1)*, 88–89; Hsiao Ch'i-ch'ing, *The Military Establishment of the Yuan Dynasty* (Cambridge, MA: Council on East Asian Studies, Harvard University, 1978), 17–18 and 23.
23 YDZ, 32.5a–6a. Also see TZTG, 21.260, and *Tsūsei (3)*, 2–3. For another use of *quzhao* that means "interrogate," see *Tsūsei (1)*, 177. A medical school professor's and a Confucian school professor's salaries are shown in YDZ, 15.2b.
24 YDZ, 32.3a.
25 YDZ, 32.3b.
26 YDZ, 32.3b.
27 YDZ, 32.3b.
28 YDZ, 32.4a. Note that in some cases, two subjects were combined into one and thus there were altogether ten subjects, instead of thirteen.
29 YDZ, 32.4a.
30 For the lists of subjects and textbooks studied toward the end of the Northern Song, see Xu Song, ed. *Song huiyao jigao* (Beijing: Zhonghua shuju, 1957), *ce* 55, *chongru* 3.2213, and Asaf Goldschmidt, *The Evolution of Chinese Medicine: Song Dynasty, 960–1200* (London: Routledge, 2009), 53. For Southern Song, see Chen Junkai, "Songdai yizheng zhi yanjiu" (Ph.D. diss., Guoli Taiwan Shifan Daxue, 1996), 33 and 35.
31 YDZ, 32.7a.
32 TZTG, 21.264–65; *Tsūsei (3)*,14–16.
33 YDZ, 32.7a.
34 Iiyama Tomoyasu, *Kin-Gendai no Kahoku shakai to kakyo seido: Mōhitotsu no "shijin" sō* (Tokyo: Waseda daigaku shuppanbu, 2011), 292.
35 Song et al., *Yuanshi*, 144.3433–35: *Quan Yuanwen*, 48: 1477.413.
36 Nie Jujing 倪居敬, Zhang Yuanshan 張元善, and Ge Yinglei 葛應雷 served in the Superintendency of Physicians in Jiangzhe BCS; Chen Geng 陳庚 in Jiangxi BCS; and Ge Yingze 葛應澤 in Pingjiang circuit. See Appendix II.
37 Su Tianjue, *Zixi wengao*, SKQS, 19.312.
38 Yu Ji, *Yu Ji Quanji* (Tianjin: Tianjin guji chubanshe, 2007), *xia:* 953.
39 Wei Yilin, *Shiyi dexiao fang* (Beijing: Renmin weisheng chubanshe, 1990), p. 12.
40 Wang Yuangong, *Zhizheng Siming xuzhi*, ZGFZCS, 3.7a.
41 See, for example, *Zhengde Songjiang fu zhi*, TYG Xubian, 11.19a–22b. Citing the early Ming map of Taiyuan prefecture, Ikeuchi Isao argues in "Genchō no gunken saishi ni tsuite" that almost all the counties and prefectures in the Yuan built a

Temple. Ikeuchi's chapter is in *Chūgoku ni okeru oshie to kokka*, ed. Noguchi Tetsurō (Tokyo: Yūzankaku shuppan, 1994).

42 Song et al., *Yuanshi*, 62.1496–97.

43 Chang Bide et al., *Songren zhuanji ziliao suoyin*. Medical administrators listed in this index are Wang Keming 王克明 (1:293), Wang Jixian 王繼先 (1:374), Kong Shiqing 孔世卿 (1:391), Zhu Gong 朱肱 (1:571), Song Daofang 宋道方 (1:779), Du Riqian 杜日遷 (2:809), Du Risi 杜日思 (2:809), Li Gun 李袞 (2:863), Li Xun 李詢 (2:890), Li Duan 李端 (2:898), Li Shouwen 李守文 (2:968), Li Zhongzhang 李仲章 (2:972), Li Zongyuan 李宗元 (2:985), Li Shilao 李師老 (2:1020), Li Shizu 李師祖 (2:1021), Zhuo Zunguo 卓遵國 (2:1410), Xia Rixuan 夏日宣 (3:1811), Xia Rihua 夏日華 (3:1811), Qin Jie 秦玠 (3:1866), Ban Hanqing 班漢卿 (3:1879), Xu Xi 許希 (3:2155), Chen Gao 陳高 (3:2461), Chen Yijian 陳易簡 (3:2591), Chen Zhaoyu 陳昭遇 (3:2599), Feng Wenzhi 馮文智 (4:2750), Zhao Jiuling 趙九齡 (4:3378), Zhao Zihua 趙自化 (4:3459), and Liu Han 劉翰 (5:3903).

44 Chen Yuan-Peng, *Liang-Song de "shangyi shiren" yu "ruyi": jianlun qizai Jin-Yuan de liubian*, 241–48.

45 Wei Su, *Wei Taipu wen xuji*, YRCK, 6.12b.

46 Huang Jin, *Jinhua Huang xiansheng wenji*, SBCK chubian, 38.8a.

47 Qian Gu, ed., *Wudu wencui xuji*, SKQS, 38.8b.

48 YDZ, 30.15b–16b.

49 YDZ, 30.15a.

50 For the Hanlin and National History Academy, see Yamamoto, "Gendai ni okeru kanrin gakushiin ni tsuite," 81–99. The members of this academy who authored inscriptions to the Temples of the Three Progenitors and references to their biographies in *Yuanshi* are as follows: Hu Zhiyu (170.3992–93), Wang Yun 王惲 (167.3932–35), Wei Chu 魏初 (164.3857–59), Wu Cheng 吳澄 (171.4011–14), Cheng Jufu 程鉅夫 (172.4015–33), Liu Guan 柳貫 (181.4189), Yu Ji 虞集 (181.4174–182), Jie Xisi 揭傒斯 (181.4184–87), Huang Jin 黃溍 (181.4186), Xu Youren 許有壬 (182.4199–4203), and Su Tianjue 蘇天爵 (183.4224–27). Liu Guan, Yu Ji, Jie Xisi, and Huang Jin were called by their contemporaries, the "Four Great Confucians" (*rulin sijie* 儒林四傑).

51 Cheng Jufu, *Cheng Xuelou wenji*, Huikan, 13.8b–9a. Cheng had been taken as a hostage by the Mongols, but was later chosen as a close adviser to Qubilai Khan. He recruited many Chinese elites into the new government. See Song et al., *Yuanshi*, 172.4015–18. On his political role, see Uematsu, *Gendai Kōnan seiji shakaishi kenkyū*, 229–31.

52 Cheng Jufu, *Cheng Xuelou wenji*, 15.15a–16a.

53 Cheng Jufu, *Cheng Xuelou wenji*, 12.1a.

54 Yu Ji, *Daoyuan leigao*, YRCK, 23.28a.

55 Song et al., *Yuanshi*, 203.4546. Also, see Yu Ji, *Daoyuan xuegu lu*, SKQS, 7.24a–26b. On Aniga, see Christopher Atwood, *Encyclopedia of Mongolia and the Mongol Empire* (New York: Facts on File, 2004), 52, 345, 540, and 609.

56 Liu Guan, *Daizhi ji*, SKQS, 14.4b.

57 Wu Cheng, *Wu Wenzheng gong ji*, YRCK, 21.2a.

58 Wu Cheng, *Wu Wenzheng gong ji*, 21.3a.

59 Wu Cheng, *Wu Wenzheng gong ji*, 21.3b–4a. To translate this passage, I referred to Hymes, "Not Quite Gentlemen? Doctors in Sung and Yuan," *Chinese Science* 8 (1988): 52.

60 Wu Cheng, *Wu Wenzheng gong ji*, 21.3b.

61 Wu Cheng, *Wu Wenzheng gong ji*, 21.4a.

62 Wu Cheng, *Wu Wenzheng gong ji*, 21.3b.

63 Wu Cheng, *Wu Wenzheng gong ji*, 21.4a.

64 Han Yu, *Hanyu quanji jiaozhu* (Chengdu: Sichuan daxue, 1996), 5:2665. To translate this passage, I referred to Thomas A. Wilson, *Genealogy of the Way: The Construction and Uses of the Confucian Tradition in Late Imperial China* (Stanford, CA: Stanford University Press, 1995), 78–79.

65 Zhu Xi and Li Youwu, *Song Mingchen yanxing lu wuji* (Taibei: Wenhai chubanshe, 1967), 3:1731.
66 Song et al., *Yuanshi*, 189.4314. See section 2 on the circumstances that brought Zhao Fu to North China and spread the Cheng brothers' and Zhu Xi's commentaries.
67 Zhao Fu, *Xianru Zhaozi yangxing lu*, comp. Chen Tingjun, 1856, *shang*.8a–b.
68 Xu Heng, *Luzhai yishu*, SKQS, 10.6a–b.
69 Hu Zhiyu, *Chaishan daquanji*, SKQS, 10.3a.
70 See Ellen Neskar, "The Cult of Worthies: A Study of Shrines Honoring Local Confucian Worthies in the Sung Dynasty (960–1279)" (Ph.D. diss., Columbia University, 1993), Part II.
71 To the best of my knowledge, no concrete evidence suggests that the Temple of the Three Progenitors was built as a Transmission shrine prior to the Yuan. None of the Song gazetteers mentions anything about the Temples of the Three Progenitors. Also, I searched the word "Sanhuang" on the Siku Quanshu database, but it did not lead me to any such evidence.
72 *Quan Yuanwen*, 26:815.25.
73 Huang Jin, *Wenxian ji*, SKQS, 8 *shang*.48b.
74 Deng Wenyuan, *Baxi ji*, SKQS, *shang*.48b.
75 Song et al., *Yuanshi*, 77.1915.
76 Song et al., *Yuanshi*, 77.1915–20. Also, see Huang Jin, *Huang Wenxian gong ji*, CSJC chubian, 115–18. For compact overviews of rituals and music in Confucian thought, see, for example, Mizoguchi Yūzō et al., eds., *Chūgoku shisō bunka jiten* (Tokyo: Tokyo daigaku shuppankai, 2001), 230–38, and 445–51. See Song et al., *Yuanshi*, 181.4187–89, for Huang Jin's biography.
77 Shi E, *Chunyou Lin'an zhi*, Sanshiqi, 7.21b–22a.
78 Zhou Cong, *Qiandao Lin'an zhi*, Sanshiqi, 1.9a.
79 Jian Shuoyou, *Xianchun Lin'an zhi*, Sanshiqi, 9.9a–b.
80 Mei Yingfa, *Kaiching Siming xuzhi*, Sanshiqi, 2.19a–20b.
81 Yu Wenmao, *Chuijian silu*, cited in Chen, "Songdai yizheng," 76.
82 Zhou Mi, *Guixin zashi*, cited in Chen, "Songdai yizheng," 76.
83 Song et al., *Yuanshi*, 96.2467.
84 Yu Xilu, *Zhishun Zhenjiang zhi* (Taibei: Huawen Shuju, 1968), 13.798. This text gives detailed location for *Huimin yaoju* for Dantu county 丹徒縣 of this circuit, but ones for Danyang 丹陽 and Jintan 金壇 counties are followed by the word "missing" (*que* 缺). This means that the Pharmacies existed but the information regarding their exact locations had become unclear by the time the extant version of this book was printed. The book uses the word, "has not been built" (*weijian* 未建) or "do not have" (*wu* 無) when an institution or property did not exist at the time of the compilation (e.g., 11.657).
85 Wang Yuangong, *Zhizhing Siming xuzhi*, ZGFZCS, 3.7a and 16a. Zhang Xuan, *Zhizheng Jinling xinzhi*, Song-Yuan fangzhi congkan, 6 *shang*.26a.
86 Chen Dazhen, *Dade Nanhai zhi*, SYD Xubian, 10.10b.
87 Zhu Zhenheng, *Jufang fahui*, his own preface, cited in Tanba Mototane, *Chūgoku iseki kō* (reprint, Bejing: Remin weisheng chubanshe, 1956), 594.
88 Feng Fujing et al., *Dade Changguo zhou tuzhi*, 3.1a–2a.
89 Zhang Xuan, *Zhizheng Jinling xinzhi*, Sanshiqi, 8.1a–12b.
90 Yu Xilu, *Zhishun Zhenjiang zhi*, 3.157–180.
91 *Yuan Henan zhi*, Sanshiqi. Li Haowen, *Chang'an zhitu*, ZGFZCS. Yu Qin, *Qisheng*, Sanshiqi. Yang Hui, *Zhizheng Kunshan zhi*, Sanshiqi. Yuan Jue, *Yanyou Siming zhi*, ZGFZCS (vol. 578). Wang Yuangong, *Zhizheng Siming xuzhi*, ZGFZCS. Luo Tianxiang, *Leibian Chang'an zhi*, SYD Xubian. Xiong Mengxiang, *Xijin zhi jiyi* (Bejing guji chubanshe, 1983).
92 Sun Yingshi, *Chongxiu Qinchuan zhi*, Sanshiqi (titled *Qinchuan zhi*).

93 *Wuxi zhi*, SYD Xubian, 1.10b.
94 Chen Dazhen, *Dade Nanhai zhi*, 6.2b.
95 Xu Suo, *Zhiyuan Jiahe zhi*, Sanshiqi, 6.7419–20.
96 Farquhar, *The Government of China Under Mongolian Rule*, 416.
97 Feng Fujing et al., *Dade Changguo zhou tuzhi*, 3.1b–2a.
98 Yu, *Zhishun Zhenjiang zhi*, 3.162–164.
99 Zhang, *Zhizheng Jinling xinxhi*, Sanshiqi, 8.6a–7a.
100 Zhang, *Zhizheng Jinling xinzhi*, Sanshiqi, 8.2a–12b.
101 Otagi Matsuo, "Mōkojin seiken chika no kannchi ni okeru hanseki no mondai," in *Haneda Hakase shōju kinen Tōyōshi ronsō*, by Haneda hakase kanreki kinenkai et al. (Kyoto: Tōyōshi kenkyūkai, 1950), and Herbert Franz Schurmann, *Economic Structure of the Yüan Dynasty: Translation of Chapters 93–94 of the* Yuan shih (Cambridge, MA: Harvard University Press, 1956).
102 YDZ, 17.9b.
103 Zhang, *Zhizheng Jinling xinzhi*, Sanshiqi, 8.5a.
104 Yuan Jue, *Yanyou Siming zhi*, 14.17b.
105 Huang Jin, *Jinhua Huang xiansheng wenji*, 47.5b.

5 Illnesses and doctors in patients' eyes

In addition to inscriptions dedicated to medical temple-school complexes, Yuan Jue wrote prose and poetry about doctors. He wrote, for example, a preface to a medical text written by Gao Yiqing, his friend from his hometown, and a postscript to Gao's grandfather's *Diagram of Channels* (*Maitu* 脉圖).[1] Yuan's writings mentioned that Gao's family had been respected since the Song period and that he and the grandson visited each other frequently in their childhood. In another instance, Yuan dedicated a seven-character regulated verse (*lüshi* 律詩) to the Hall of Rescuing Lives (Jisheng tang 濟生堂) built by a doctor named Liang 梁 in Luling 廬陵 in present-day Jiangxi province. This verse praised the doctor for having talent similar to a legendary doctor, Liu 劉, who supposedly had performed a charm therapy (*jinjia shu* 禁架術).[2] Furthermore, Yuan wrote a seven-character ancient-style poem (*gushi* 古詩) about this legendary doctor and compared him to another legendary figure, Zhao Bing 趙炳, from the Later Han period, who was said to have cured diseases simply by paying respect to spirits with river water and dried mulberry skin.[3]

A modern historian, Chen Yuan-Peng, has identified roughly 400 pieces of writing dedicated to doctors written by sixty-six literati from the late Jin through the early Ming period. My follow-up study shows that Chen's list is fairly thorough, except that I have found even more. These writings were farewell poems, prefaces to farewell poems, poems dedicated to doctors' offices, prefaces to medical texts, funerary inscriptions, biographical tales (*zhuan* 傳), and short essays (*shuo* 説). We cannot find such a large number of writings for doctors in Song literary collections (*wenji*).[4] This increase in writings dedicated to physicians was partly due to the development of printing and to the literary networking that Yuan elites were passionately engaged in.[5] It was also due to the higher status that elite physicians enjoyed in Yuan politics and culture. Because of their higher status, they had better connections with elite society and, more importantly, higher self-esteem with which to prevail upon (sometimes quite adamantly) their literati friends and clients to write for them and their families.

Analyzing prose, poetry, and medical records, written by five literati from the late Jin to Yuan, this chapter will describe the illness experiences from the elite clients' point of view and the close relations that elite doctors forged with their clients.[6] I will also show that the discourses about the doctors reflected the complex philosophical and religious situations of the time. Because the "Iron Curtain," or political and cultural barriers, separated the discursive practices of the Jin and the Southern Song territories, the ways in which the literati eulogized doctors were different in North and South China.[7] The late Jin and early Yuan literati focused on the doctor's membership in what we would call the elite society and his ability to participate in China's literary tradition (*wen*). In contrast, Southern Song literati had been increasingly converted to the Learning of the Way (*Daoxue*), which emphasized the significance of the values and behaviors proper to "Confucians" (*ru*), and thus sought out "Confucian doctors" (*ruyi*) or doctors who continued their study and practice as Confucian scholars. At the same time, literati continued paying attention to the fact that medical art required specific skills not necessarily possessed by all Confucian scholars.

Yuan Haowen (1190–1257) and Yan Jian (1212–89)

A late Jin-dynasty scholar-official and poet, Yuan Haowen, was himself knowledgeable about medicine and was a good friend of an eminent physician, Li Gao, and other doctors. When the Jin dynasty fell in 1234, Yuan Haowen was in the capital, Kaifeng, and was captured by the Mongols. After he was released in 1235, his friend helped him build a new house in Guanshi 冠氏 (in present-day Shandong 山東 province).[8] At the same time, he actively traveled to other places including Dongping 東平 (also in present-day Shandong province), a cultural center of this period, and befriended the area's hereditary lord, Yan Shi 嚴實. Li Gao accompanied Yuan Haowen from Kaifeng and eventually to Dongping in 1238. Li afterwards went back to his hometown Zhending 眞定 (in present-day Hebei province), and Yuan visited there several times.[9] Yuan expressed great admiration for Li and other educated doctors, but it did not matter to him whether or not they were Confucians. His writings on doctors were in sharp contrast with those of Yan Jian 硯堅 (1212–89), who depicted Li Gao as a Confucian doctor.

Yuan Haowen learned medicine in adulthood and practiced it sometimes. After describing a formula for skin tumors (*ju* 疽) in his collection of essays, he said:

> [When my father got a tumor on his temple], I was stupid and young. I was always preparing for the civil service examination, and I did not know anything about medicine or drugs . . . My father hired [a quack] and passed away. Later I came back to the hometown, learned the prescription in the family study, and cured other people. I discovered that it had a variety of effects. . . . If a son does not know medicine, the calamity can be as serious as this.[10]

He said elsewhere that his family used to own a large number of medical texts before they were lost during the Mongol conquest of North China. In 1242, he collected dozens of prescriptions that he knew were effective and compiled a book titled *The Yuan Family's Collection of Verified Prescriptions* (*Yuanshi jiyan fang* 元氏集驗方).[11]

His knowledge of medicine helped him select a good doctor for himself in 1248. According to the medical case record written by Yuan and later incorporated into Li's *Dongyuan's Experimental Formulas*, Yuan had just arrived at the house of his first daughter's marital family in Zhending when he found a small abscess (*xiao chuang* 小瘡) at the upper back of his neck.[12] Because it did not hurt or feel itchy, he paid no attention to it for the first two days. Even when he saw Li Gao on the third day, Yuan did not say anything about the abscess because the pain was still subtle. A few days later, however, it became severe, and he heard a rumor that a Mr. Liu in town had died of a tumor on the head. Yuan asked his family to invite a doctor, who prescribed him a medicine. On the following day, the doctor returned with another doctor, and they together told Yuan that it would take eighteen days for the pus to come out and three months to heal. Yuan panicked because he thought he had read in a medical classic that an abscess with pus was almost always fatal. The fact that his father had died of a skin tumor might have aggravated the anxiety. He begged a friend to bring Li Gao. After examining the abscess, Li told him that it was serious enough that Yuan was correct to have invited Li, but that it would heal soon.

In the medical case record, Yuan was frank about his anxiety and the emotional and practical support that he gained from his doctor-friend. Yuan specifically noted, "Li talked and smiled as usual after examining the abscess." Li then applied moxibustion, prescribed medicine different from the one the other two doctors had used, and explained to Yuan in detail which channel needed care and how various ingredients should work together. After taking the medicine, Yuan slept well, and when he woke up, the abscess was substantially smaller than the night before. Being afraid that the abscess might have gone through the neck to the throat, however, he invited Li back. Li came in to tell him happily, "The abscess has flattened. In several days, the scab will be formed and you will be able to go outside." A few days later, it was a nocturnal emission that alarmed Yuan again. Thinking that it was a sign that he would die soon, he was horrified but not able to tell that to anyone, until Li came back.

> [Li] asked me jokingly, "After you took the medicine, you experienced three effects, but you have not told me. Why?" He then asked me in rapid succession, "In the past few days, you have more appetite, right?" I said, "Yes." [He] asked [me] again, "Your legs were weak before, but when you walk now, you feel strong, right?" I said, "Yes." Then he said, "In your last night's dream, there was a 'change in the snowy sleep' (*xiaomei zhi bian* 霄寐之變). Why are you not volunteering the information to me?" [The last question] made me laugh because I would never have told him that![13]

Using a literary term, "the change in the snowy sleep," to refer to the emission, the literati doctor elegantly communicated to his patient that it was a sign that Yuan was recovering, just like his improved appetite and ability to walk. Only six days after Li Gao began taking care of him, Yuan had recovered completely. Li, according to Yuan, saved other patients with the same illness all in fourteen days.

Toward the end of the record, Yuan praised Li Gao for being able to understand the "unspoken secrets" (*buyan zhi mi* 不言之密)" in the human body. He said:

> Medicine is not easy, and curing the head and back abscess is particularly hard. Hereditary doctors (*shiyi* 世醫) would apply their [practical] skills (*ji* 技) in hopes of getting results. The only person in my life who can get the results and calculate the unspoken secrets in the body is Li Gao.[14]

"Hereditary doctors" was a common term used to refer to doctors coming from families that produced generations of doctors. Li did not come from such a family, and he was better than them, Yuan says.

A year later in 1249, Yuan wrote a preface to Li's *Treatise on the Spleen and Stomach*. To highlight the significance of Li's book, he disparaged hereditary doctors more than he did in the medical case record discussed above. He said:

> I think for a long time, hereditary doctors did not differentiate "excess" (*youyu* 有余) and "depletion" (*buzu* 不足). When the Incident of 1232 (i.e., the fall of Kaifeng) occurred, a million people died because eating, drinking, and fatigue damaged them. Everyone said that Cold Damage caused the deaths. However when I read Li's *Distinguishing Inner and Outer Damages* and *On Damages Caused by Eating, Drinking, and Fatigue*, I learned the mistakes of hereditary doctors. Isn't it very sad that one would make mistakes on people when his scholarship is not brilliant (*xueshu buming* 學術不明)?[15]

In other words, in Yuan's mind, a typical hereditary doctor was shallow and did not understand the complex mechanisms that caused illnesses.

Certainly, he was not critical of all the doctors who came from a family that had practiced medicine for generations. His funerary inscription for Lu Chang 盧昶, his relative by marriage, said that Lu's family had been famous north of the Yellow River for their craft (*fangji* 方伎). The inscription praised Lu for diligently studying the family scholarship (*jiaxue* 家學) since he had been young and asserted that he was not tired of it even at an old age. According to Yuan, Lu had read an enormous number of medical texts written by doctors since the ancient times. He had served in the Jin dynasty's Palace Pharmaceutical Bureau (*Shangyao ju*) and authored medical texts himself. The poem attached to the inscription started by saying, "The sacred learning of Qibo and Huangdi (*Qi-Huang shengxue* 岐黃聖學) is shining like the sun and stars." The sacred learning of Qibo 岐伯 and Huangdi 黃帝 referred to the *Inner Classic* which, in Yuan's view, Lu Chang had mastered.[16] Despite Lu's family background, Yuan never used the term hereditary doctor, perhaps because of its negative connotation.

If Li was not a hereditary doctor, what kind of doctor did Yuan think Li was? Yuan instead used the term "doctor of the realm" (*guoyi* 國醫) to praise Li. Yuan's preface to Li's unpublished book, *The Records of Cold Damage* (*Shanghan huiyao* 傷寒會要), said, "In the past when I was living in the capital (i.e., Kaifeng), I heard that the resident Li Gao was considered a doctor of the realm but I had not met him yet."[17] Yuan also used the term "doctor of the realm" for other excellent doctors. He once wrote a seven-word regulated verse for "Doctor of the Realm Wang Zeming" (*guoyi Wang Zeming* 國醫王澤明).[18] Yuan's funerary inscription for a literatus mentions books written by "Doctor of the Realm Zhang Zihe [i.e., Zhang Congzheng 張從政] from Wanqiu" (*guoyi Wanqiu Zhang Zihe* 國醫宛丘張子和).[19]

Yuan's preface to Li Gao's *The Records of Cold Damage* made an interesting distinction between a doctor of the realm and a doctor. It said:

> [Li's] family was wealthy, so he did not live on his craft. [His] behavior was more than prudent, so people dared not call him a doctor. When an elite man with a lot of money became ill, [Li] would be straightforward and rarely bend down. Unless someone had a critical illness that could not be cured, he could not see Li.[20]

This passage illuminates the complex class relations that affected doctor–client relations at the time. Elites in the Jin capital felt uncomfortable calling him a doctor because the term implied someone working for money. They expressed their respect for Li's profound knowledge of medicine by calling him a doctor of the realm.

Whether for Li or other doctors, Yuan never used the term "Confucian physcian" (*ruyi*), which had been coined at latest by 1113, right before North China was occupied by the Jurchens.[21] Apparently, it mattered to him more whether a doctor came from the elite class that participated in the civil service examination than whether he was a Confucian. In a preface to a medical text written by Zhou Mengqing 周夢卿, for example, Yuan said:

> [Zhou], however, had the *qi* of studying as a civil service examination candidate (*juzi xiqi* 舉子習氣). After reaching middle age, he studied medicine and fortunetelling. . . . Even though he had courage to eliminate a thousand troops by himself, he did not enjoy fighting and taking human lives lightly.[22]

By saying, "Zhou had the *qi* of studying as an examination candidate," he was referring to the fact that the doctor was preparing for the Jin dynasty's examination before he joined the Mongols' army.[23] In Yuan's view, Zhou understood medicine and the value of human lives, despite his military career, thanks to his early education as an examination candidate. In the Jin period, a Chinese candidate chose between the poetry track (*shifu* 詩賦) and "the meaning of the Classics" (*jingyi* 經義). The former was more popular than the latter, and the texts for the "meaning of the Classics" were mostly the so-called old annotations (*guzhushu* 古注疏) completed in the Tang period.[24]

Yuan Haowen cited books other than Confucian classics to justify choices that doctors made. For example, to justify the physician Wu Bianfu's 吳辨夫 decision to build his own gravesite before passing, Yuan cited a phrase from one of the poems written by Tao Yuanming 陶淵明 (326–427): "Why was it necessarily

bad to be buried naked? One must loosen [and understand beyond] the surface"
(裸葬何必惡, 人當解其表).[25] This poem was titled "Drinking No.11," and made
fun of Yan Hui 顏回, Confucius's disciple who died destitute at age thirty. The
poem's overall theme was that no matter how famous one might become posthumously, it would be meaningless if one did not enjoy life now.[26] The phrase
cited above referred to Yang Wangsun 楊王孫 in the Former Han period, a Daoist
who ordered his son to bury him without coffin or clothes upon his death so that
he would be close to the earth.[27] Citing this phrase and the deeds and words of
several other poets and artists, Yuan assured readers that as someone who had
engaged in medical art (*fangji* 方伎) for many years and had seen changes in the
world, Wu was making a decision in accordance with his predecessors.[28]

Yuan's discussions about elite doctors provide a sharp contrast with Yan
Jian's 硯堅 (1212–89) biography of Li Gao, written in 1267, which painted Li
as an ideal Confucian. The biography started out with two episodes in which Li's
friends attempted to change his seriousness. Once at a party, the story goes, they
had a courtesan lean against him and pull on his clothes. Li became so angry
that he removed his clothes and burned them. In another occasion, said Yan, a
courtesan forced him to drink a little bit of alcohol, only to see him spit it out. He
was taught Confucian classics like the *Analects*, *Mencius*, and the *Chronicle of
the Spring and Autumn Period* by prominent scholar-officials and later built an
academy on his estate to which he invited Confucian scholars. To continue with
Yan's description, Li was a filial son who regretted not having been able to choose
the right doctor for his dying mother. Li asked his disciple Luo Tianyi whether he
was studying medicine to make money or to spread the Way (*chuandao* 傳道). Li
was satisfied when Luo's answer was, "Only to spread the Way."[29]

The difference between Yuan's and Yan's representations of Li reflected the
difference in the authors' cultural orientations. Yuan was typical of the Jin literati,
among whom the Learning of Su Shi 蘇軾 (1037–1101; *Suxue* 蘇學), a great
poet from the Northern Song, gained enormous popularity.[30] Yuan's loyalty was
to *wen*, defined as "the cumulative tradition of writings (the classics, histories,
philosophers, and belles lettres) as the legacy of civilization" and "individual cultural accomplishments: literary prose and poetry, calligraphy, and (sometimes)
painting."[31] Even when, for example, he wrote a funerary inscription for Zhao
Bingwen 趙秉文 (1159–1232), one of the small group of scholars who valued the
legacy of the Cheng brothers, Yuan started out with a discussion of the history of
wen, continued on to Zhao's political career, and then praised the excellence of his
prose, poetry, and calligraphy. Only toward the end of this relatively long inscription did Yuan comment on Zhao's revival of the Way (*dao* 道).[32] When Yuan
eulogized doctors, he paid little attention to the question of whether or not they
were Confucians. Rather, he focused on proving that a doctor was part of the class
that participated in the great tradition of writing. Note that Yuan Haowen lived
during the period when the Complete Reality Sect (*Quanzhen zong*), a Daoist sect
founded by Wang Zhe 王嚞 (1113–70), had converted twenty percent of the population in the areas north of the Yellow River. Although Yuan was ambivalent about
the sect's power as a group, he was respectful of some of the leaders of the sect.[33]

In contrast, Yan was raised as a serious follower of the Learning of the Way movement in the Southern Song. He was a great-grandson of Zhu Xi and a grandson of Zhu's close disciple, Huang Gan 黃榦 (1152–1221). He had been a student at the Huang family school since childhood. In 1235, Yan was captured and brought from South to North China by the Mongol army. In 1252, he gained Confucian-household status in Zhending. He was appointed as the professor of Zhending Confucian school and eventually as the Director of Studies at the National Institute (*guozi jianxue siye* 國子監學司業) that oversaw the National University. A *Daoxue* scholar, Su Tianjue 蘇天爵 (1294–1352), later praised Yan for working hard to clarify the art of the Way (*daoshu* 道術).[34] It is thus understandable that Yan paid attention to Li's behaviors that matched *Daoxue* values.

Wang Yun (1227–1304)

Born in Weizhou in present-day Henan province, Wang Yun was only eight *sui* when the Jin dynasty fell. Unlike Yuan Haowen, who never served the Yuan government, Wang was recruited into it when Qubilai Khan ascended to the throne in 1260.[35] Active throughout his life until he retired as an Academician at the Hanlin and National History Academy at age seventy-four, he nonetheless suffered from several health issues, such as broken teeth, visual difficulties, and frequent stomach aches, and extensively wrote poems and essays about them. Although he appears to have been familiar with both the Complete Reality Sect and the *Daoxue* Learning, he tended to eulogize his doctors as good Confucians, not good Daoists.

Wang was shocked when his tooth broke for the first time when he was reaching forty *sui*. His five-character ancient-style poem titled "A Song of a Broken Tooth" (*Zhechi yin* 折齒吟) started by boasting that his teeth had been strong even though his hair had been "whiter than snow," his vision blurred, and his hearing weak. Then suddenly, he said, one of his teeth broke one morning while he was eating breakfast. The incident made "little children so sad that they stopped playing and the ailing wife so shocked that she almost expired" (群稚慘不嬉, 病妻驚欲絕).[36] He also wrote a seven-character regulated verse titled, "A Song of a Broken Tooth for Self-Consolation" (*Zhechi yin zi wei* 折齒吟自慰). It started with a phrase, "In the morning, a tooth broke, making the Five Deities shocked" (朝來齒折五神驚). He ended this poem with a sense of acceptance: "In this world, is there anything that does not wax and wane (世間何物不虧盈)?"[37]

Wang also lamented eye problems, probably toward the end of his life. His seven-character regulated verse titled, "Writing Thoughts with Ailing Eyes" (*Bingmu shuhuai* 病目書懷), started with a phrase, "With ailing eyes, [I get] confused when looking at things at ordinary times" (病眼平時視物疑). Perhaps seeing flashing lights in his eyes, he then said, "Moreover, [I am] prohibiting wind and fire from chasing after each other inside" (更禁風火內交馳). He then compared himself to frogs, whose eyes stick out, and sharks, whose tears fall all day, and bemoaned his pain and unclear vision. At the end, the poem says, "Putting my face on a pillow continuously, [I] suffered for a month

(悠悠伏枕三旬苦). How can [I] find a golden spatula to scrape the surface [of my eyes] (安得黃金刮膜鎞)?"[38]

Using a golden spatula to cure one's blindness had been a well-known metaphor, if not a well-known practice. The first known reference was in *Mahāparinirvāṇa Sūtra* (*Daban niepan jing* 大般涅槃経), a Buddhist text translated into Chinese in the fifth century. It compared followers of Buddhism to the blind gathered around a good doctor who would use a golden spatula to cut the surface of his patient's eye to help them see.[39] Another reference to a golden spatula is found in a biography of a filial son in the sixth century, which says that after he prayed for seven days, he dreamed of an old man using a golden spatula to cure his blind grandfather's vision.[40] Du Fu 杜甫 (712–70), in yet another instance, used the metaphor in a poem that he wrote toward the end of his life in 766.[41] "If traditional Chinese medicine is known for its hesitation to develop surgical interventions to treat illness, this is certainly not true in traditional Chinese ophthalmology," write the modern translators of a fifteenth-century ophthalmological text, *Essential Subtleties on the Silver Sea* (*Yinhai jingwei* 銀海精微).[42] Although it is unclear whether Wang Yun pursued surgery as a realistic option, he certainly used the metaphor to express his strong desire for a cure. He also mentioned this metaphor in a poem dedicated to an ophthalmologist, Du Jinshan 杜金山.[43]

Wang Yun suffered from recurring stomach problems for twenty years before he saw a doctor named Hu Qizhi 胡器之 in the 1280s. By that time, he had seen doctors in various places in North China, where he worked as an official. When he first had the stomach problem in Daidu 大都 in the 1260s, he saw a doctor who prescribed him a black drug from West or Central Asia (*xuan huji* 玄胡劑). Between 1272 and 1276, when he was serving as the Supervisor in the directorate-general (*zongguanfu pan'guan* 總管府判官) of Pingyang circuit 平陽路, he saw another doctor who prescribed a medicine named Divine Treasure (*shenbao* 神寶) to "attack" his abdomen. It caused great pain and severe bowel movements. After being prescribed another drastic medicine by a Mr. Chen, he finally met Hu in the 1280s in his hometown. Hu gave Wang a small tablet containing *zhusha* 朱砂 (cinnabar). Seeing Wang wondering if such a small tablet could be efficacious, Hu assured him that once he swallowed the medicine, he would feel mild bowel movements and that the pain would stop after he had passed some stools. After seeing Wang's body react to the drug in the way he had predicted, Hu prescribed soup containing *houpu* 厚朴 to condition it.[44] Wang later wrote a medical essay detailing his experience and presented it to Hu as a token of gratitude.[45] Wang also wrote a seven-character regulated verse to celebrate Hu's longevity.[46]

Wang promoted Confucian learning as an official. When he submitted a document titled *Summary of Matters Concerning the Crown Prince* (*Chenghua shilüe* 承華事略), to Qubilai's first son and crown prince at the time, Zhenjin 眞金 (1243–85), he listed "Respecting Confucian Scholars" (*chongru* 崇儒) as one of the twenty actions that he thought the prince, as the future ruler, should take.[47] He also wrote an essay titled, "The Use of Confucians" (*Ruyong pian* 儒用篇), in which he argued that benevolence, righteousness, rites, and music that "scholars" (*shi* 士) had mastered were the most important tools with which a country could maintain peace and order.[48]

At the same time, he was close to the Daoist sects and was among the scholar-officials at the time who believed that there were common grounds for the Confucian and Daoist teachings. His paternal grandmother, Ms. Han 韓, was an active member of the Taiyi 太一 sect, founded in his hometown in the late 1130s. Her uncle Han Ju 韓矩, for whom Wang wrote a funerary inscription, was the second leader of this sect.[49] Wang wrote another inscription for the third leader of the sect, Wang Shouqian 王守謙, because he was Yun's distant paternal relative.[50] Wang Yun dedicated an inscription to Li Zhiyuan 李志遠 (1169–1254), who became the leader of the Complete Reality Sect in 1238. Wang eulogized him for being effective in making its members preserve the order by turning some of the sect's rough followers, those who had been as cruel as "tigers" and "wolves," into gentle and considerate people.[51] Wang's preface for the *Extended Meanings of Laozi* (*Laozi yanyi* 老子衍義), written by a Daoist monk, praised the book for pointing out that a lot of words in the *Laozi* were rooted in the ideas of "governance and pacification" (*zhiping* 治平).[52]

Wang was close to doctors as well and dedicated numerous writings to them. His wife's father, Tui De 推德, was a doctor and served the Jin dynasty as a medical administrator. He had learned the craft from his stepfather, Mr. Du 杜, whom his mother had married after his father's passing. Wang's funerary inscription praised Tui for benevolent actions that he took in the 1230s at the time of the Mongols' conquest of North China. According to the inscription, he made a large quantity of medicinal soup and offered it to people who were suffering from illnesses at the same time that he offered rice to the hungry.[53]

Wang used the term "doctor of the realm" (*guoyi*), but he also used the terms "Confucian-doctor" (*ruyi*) and "doctor-Confucian" (*yiru* 醫儒) to praise elite doctors. He called his own doctor, Hu Qizhi, who solved his stomach problems, a *guoyi*.[54] In the meantime, he presented a seven-character verse to a *ruyi*, Xu Dengsun 徐登孫.[55] When he recommended Hu Lian 胡璉 as the medical school professor in Weihui circuit, he referred to him as *yiru*.[56] Wang thought a Jin-dynasty doctor, Li Mi 李泌 (*hao* Daoyuan 道源), was a "Confucian and doctor" (*ru er yi zhe* 儒而醫者).[57]

Wang explained the reasons why a doctor could be called a Confucian. Citing Han Yu 韓愈 (768–824) and Fan Zhongyan 范仲淹 (989–1052), both of whom had compared doctors to ministers, Wang said, "If one compares doctors with ministers, the essence (*ti* 體) and manifestations (*yong* 用) [of the two] are different, but they are the same with regards to the fact that they save people."[58] In his preface to Luo Tianyi's *The Treasuries of Life Protection* (*Weisheng baojian* 衛生寶鑒), he argued that medical learning was part of the *Daoxue* project of "investigating things and extending knowledge" (*gewu zhizhi* 格物致知). Given the tens of thousands of words written about medicine since the ancient times, he said, someone must investigate these words and must share the results of the research, drugs, with people.[59] In his preface to Zhang Yuansu's 張元素 annotations to the *Classic of Difficult Questions* (*Nanjing* 難經), he said that medical classics like *Difficult Questions* and *Basic Questions* were like the *Chronicle of the Spring and Autumn Period* and the *Classic of Changes*. Despite the large number of words contained in these books, they had not captured the true meanings of the ancient sages' teachings. Thus, Wang argued that Zhang's annotation to *Difficult Questions* was equivalent to the *Great Learning* (*Daxue* 大學), a book that *Daoxue* scholars thought summarized the essence of their learning.[60] Growing up mostly after the fall of the Jin dynasty, Wang was among the new generation of scholar-officials in North China promoting the Learning of the Way, thus praising elite physicians as Confucian doctors.

Wu Cheng (1249–1333)

Wu Cheng 吳澄, a leading *Daoxue* theoretician, was born twenty-seven years before the fall of the Southern Song dynasty into a scholarly family in Fuzhou 撫州 in present-day Jiangxi province. His grandfather held a *jinshi* degree and excelled in poetry, prose, astronomy, and calendar studies. Wu Cheng was most likely quite healthy throughout his life and lived to the age of eighty-five *sui*. A funerary inscription for him said that he had no serious eye or ear problems even toward the end of his life.[61] We have very few extant sources in which he complained about his own illnesses. However, he dedicated at least fifty-one writings to a variety of doctors, far more than any other literatus in the Jin and Yuan periods did.[62] The writings reveal the significance of medicine to his life and philosophy. They also show that he was aware of medical innovations that originated in the north but that he believed in the quality of doctors in the south.

As a *Daoxue* philosopher, Wu Cheng belonged to Zhu Xi's academic lineage but was sympathetic to Lu Jiuyuan's philosophy as well. As David Gedalecia summarizes, Zhu and Lu emphasized "the moral attainment through the spiritual awakening of the inner self," but they had differed as to the extent that book learning could contribute to the awakening process. Zhu considered most important "an awakening through the objective truths, or principles (*li* 理), especially as conveyed in classics," while Lu thought that one should "recover the universal cosmic comprehension inherent in one's nature and transcend book learning."[63] Wu Cheng began reading Zhu Xi's commentaries on the Four Books by the time he was ten *sui* and began studying with Cheng Ruoyong 程若庸 (fl. 1260s) around the time he was fifteen *sui*. Cheng had been a student of Shen Guiyao 沈貴瑤 and Rao Lu 饒魯 (fl. *c.* 1256), both of whom belonged to the "branch" of Huang Gan 黃榦, Zhu's son-in-law and favorite disciple.[64] At the same time, Wu Cheng was influenced by Cheng Shaokai 程紹開 (1219?–80), who attempted to synthesize Zhu's and Lu's teachings.[65]

Wu Cheng was open not only to the two different trends within the Learning of the Way but also to Daoism. He fled to a Daoist monastery during the period of the Song–Yuan transition. In the monastery, he met Lei Siqi 雷思齊, who later became the Lecturer of the Daoist School (*xuanxue jiangshi* 玄學講師) of the Celestial Master Way (*Tianshi dao* 天師道) sect. Wu later wrote a commentary to the *Laozi*, in which he tackled the question of commonalities and differences between the two teachings.[66]

Spending his first twenty-seven years under the Southern Song regime and the next fifty-eight years under the Mongols, Wu Cheng's relationships with both governments were mixed. He never gained a *jinshi* degree nor served in the Southern Song government. Even though he had an excellent political connection—his classmate Cheng Jufu, in charge of recruiting South Chinese elite to the Yuan government—Wu did not serve the new government until he accepted a position as the Deputy Director of the Institute (*guozi jian cheng* 國子監丞) in 1308. He was later promoted to a Director of Studies (*siye* 司業) in 1311, but he suddenly departed from the position in 1312, just before the civil service examination was revived by the Yuan government. This fact, along with the passages cited below, make us suspect that Wu was opposed to the revival.[67]

Just like many members of other Fuzhou elite families, some of Wu Cheng's relatives had practiced medicine since around the time of the Mongol occupation.[68] The little information we have about Wu Cheng's father, Shu 樞, does not say he was a doctor but that he was "good at making medical formulae" (*shan weifang* 善爲方). The father was remembered for his benevolent act of boiling medicine for tens of families when the doctors in town were too afraid to provide care for the victims of an epidemic (*dazha* 大札).[69] Wu Cheng's half-brother Wu Rui 吳瑞 was a doctor.[70] Wu Yifeng 吳一鳳, a grandson of Wu's "clansman" (*zongren* 宗人), was another doctor and was the assistant professor of the medical school in Jianchang 建昌 prefecture in present-day Jiangxi.[71] A daughter of Wu's younger sister was married to a doctor, who served as the medical school professor of Yugan 餘干 prefecture, also in present-day Jiangxi.[72]

Under these circumstances, Wu Cheng also had read medical books since he was young and applied his knowledge to make certain that his family members were provided with proper care. In his preface to his good friend Li Ji'an's 李季安 *Summary of the Inner Classic* (*Neijing zhiyao* 內經指要), he wrote, "Since I was young, I have liked this classic and always wanted to discuss it with others."[73] His preface to a book on the pulse written by Yao Yizhong 姚宜仲 says, "I never mastered medicine, but I like the writings [on it],"[74] and then critiqued Yao's theory in detail. Such an expression of modesty and interest can also be seen in his essay dedicated to a doctor, Dong Qiqian 董起潛: "I never studied medicine but enjoy reading books like the *Inner Classic*, the *Classic of Difficult Questions*, and the *Classic of Pulses* (*Maijing* 脉經)."[75] When his grandfather was gravely ill, Wu Cheng stayed up for over ten nights to make certain that the grandfather was given proper medicine and food.[76] Many years later, when his grand-nephew was ill, Wu felt the child's pulse and discussed it with a doctor.[77]

Wu Cheng asserted that all Confucians must know medicine. His essay dedicated to a medical school teacher said that the Way of medicine (*yi zhi dao* 醫之道) and the Way of Confucians (*ru zhi dao* 儒之道) were close for the following reason:

> The Way of Confucians is benevolence. Love is the function of benevolence (*ren zhi yong*). Love's top priority is for one's parents and for one's own body. They are the greatest love. [As the *Book of Rites* says,] "One's parents are the roots of one's body." So not remembering to love one's parents means that

one has forgotten one's own roots. [The *Records* also says,] "One's own body is his parents' branch." So not loving one's own body means that one is hurting [the parents'] branch. If a person is not a doctor, who can love his parents and his own body and make sure that [his parents and he] live long and are healthy? Therefore, Confucians must know medicine. The Way of medicine is profound.[78]

In other words, in Wu Cheng's view, medicine was an integral component of the central value in Confucian teaching: filial piety. His belief that a good Confucian should be familiar with medicine was reflected in his "Lineage of Learning" (*xuetong* 學統), the list of readings that he thought Confucians should master. Three out of the twenty-eight books in his list were medical books: the *Inner Classic*, the *Treatise on Cold Damage*, and the *Classic of Eighty-One Difficult Questions* (*Bashiyi nanjing* 八十一難經).[79]

Just like Wang Yun, Wu Cheng acknowledged that a Confucian could and should make use of his reading skills to understand the principles in the difficult ancient medical classics. For example, his preface to a Yuan medical book, *Critiquing the Book of Vitalizing Humans* (*Huoren shu bian* 活人書辯) compared its author, Dai Qizong 戴啓宗, to the Cheng brothers, who saw the significance of the *Great Learning* and the *Doctrine of the Mean*, which used to be chapters buried in the messy *Book of Rites*. Wu argued that Dai made a great contribution in clarifying the meaning of the *Treatise* by critiquing Zhu Gong's 朱肱 (*jinshi* 1088) popular book on the *Treatise on Cold Damage Disorder*.[80]

Wu Cheng did not, however, think book learning and understanding of medical principles were sufficient to make a good doctor. He argued that a good doctor should most importantly have sincerity (*cheng* 誠), or a sincere wish to cure his patients' illnesses. In his inscriptions for pediatrician Zeng Zhongqian's 曾仲謙 hall named "The Hall of Sincere Quest" (*Chengqiu tang* 誠求堂), he compared a good doctor to a loving mother. He said a child's illness was hard to treat because his pulses were hard to feel and he could not explain what he liked to eat. To continue Wu's words, a mother would, however, understand what was happening inside of the child's body because she loved him so much and because she sincerely wanted to understand why he was suffering.[81] He said, "Sincerity could feel spirits (*shenming* 神明) and penetrate through gold and stones." In the same inscription, he cited a clause from the *Great Learning*, which said "[One should serve the parents, elder brother, and the country] as if one would care for a baby." As many, if not all, the South Chinese literati must have known by this time, this phrase is followed by sentences that said, "So [their actions] may not be exactly right but not wrong. No woman has learned how to raise a baby before she gets married."[82] In other words, a sincere wish to have perfect knowledge was not as important as sincerely wishing to serve one's family (in the case of a Confucian) or patients (in the case of a doctor).

Interestingly, Wu sometimes expressed his great disappointment in self-styled Confucians in his essays for doctors. For example, in his farewell essay for Fang Shiweng 方實翁, he said that although Confucians might not sound bad when they talked about politics and social issues, their actions did not match their words. "What they say are empty words (*xuyan* 虛言)!" deplored Wu. In contrast, in his view, Fang was talented in doing substantial things (*shi* 實). He asked, "Did they not used to say that Confucians' emptiness does not level with doctors' substance?" In other words, Wu admired Fang's substance and resented Confucians' emptiness.[83]

Wu's farewell essay to a doctor, He Qingchang 何慶長, revealed specifically what kind of "Confucians" Wu despised:

> Whenever I think of the culture at the end of the period, I repeatedly feel sad and sigh. At the end of the Song period, when children became a little older and learned to write essays for the civil service examinations, they claimed in small voices that they were better than their contemporaries. Then they became shallow and arrogant, and said that they were better than eight or nine out of ten people. They would most likely not wait until they passed the exam and had become an official to become arrogant. When occasionally they passed the provincial examination, they would be even more arrogant. When they occasionally even went to the National University, they would become even more arrogant. Their proud words and thriving energy were enough to move the prefectures and shake the hometown. What they thought from the morning to the evening, and what they did from the first till the end, all came from their own selfish human desire. They had no intention to save the world or aid people whatsoever.

In other words, Wu thought that the civil service examinations had caused young men to be arrogant and thus moved them away from attaining Confucian sagehood.

To continue with the farewell essay for He Qingchang, Wu stated that He Qingchang's great-uncle He Boyu 何伯玉 was an exception because he was modest even though he had passed the provincial examination at the end of the Southern Song period. Wu praised He Boyu's nephew He Jixin 何季新 and great-nephew He Qingchang for practicing medicine. Wu said:

> If you set your mind and manage your behavior (*lixin zhixing* 立心制行) as Great-Uncle Boyu did and use [your mind and behavior] to save the world and aid the people, the effect should be more than what Confucians can accomplish. As I part with Qingchang, how can I not expect a lot from him?[84]

Wu was suggesting here that a young man was more likely to realize true Confucian sagehood by becoming a doctor than by passing an examination. The followers of the Learning of the Way in the Southern Song had certainly been critical of the examinations and of their own contemporaries who had been concerned only about passing them. Wu Cheng's argument, however, was more powerful than his Southern Song counterpart's because he had seen the demise of the Southern Song dynasty.

Wu's mixed feelings toward contemporary Confucians seem to have made him egalitarian when comparing a Confucian doctor and a hereditary doctor. Wu said in his essay for a member of the Imperial Academy of Medicine, Wang Yuanzhi 王元直, "If one is not a hereditary [doctor], there are some skills he may not have learned. If one is not a Confucian [doctor], there are some principles which he may not know with much sophistication."[85] In other words, Wu thought both kinds of doctors had strengths and weaknesses, and a truly good doctor should have the strength of a Confucian doctor and that of a hereditary doctor.

In a poem dedicated to a hereditary doctor, Fan Wenru 范文孺, who specialized in curing hemorrhoids, Wu said, "Ancient people praised a doctor from a family that has produced three generations of doctors (*sanshi zhi yi* 三世之醫)." Fan's mother was a daughter of a man who was the seventh-generation doctor in his family. Fan's father learned his medical skills from the father-in-law and passed them down to Fan, making him the ninth-generation doctor. Note that the phrase in the *Book of Rites* that Wu had on his mind (*yi bu sanshi, bu fu qiyao* 醫不三世, 不服其藥) had allowed two interpretations. *Bu sanshi* could be interpreted as "not having been learned in three medical classics" as well as "not having come from a family that has produced three generations of doctors." Although the former would have favored Confucian scholars, Wu adopted the latter interpretation and used it as a way to eulogize Fan and his ancestors' medical skills and secret prescriptions.[86]

At the same time, Wu sometimes pointed to the weakness of hereditary doctors. For example, in a "presentation preface (*zengxu* 贈序)," dedicated to a physician, Chen Yudao 陳與道, Wu said that people sought out a hereditary doctor, as well as an older doctor, because they wrongly thought his prescriptions and skills had stood the test of time. Wu argued, "Some hereditary doctors have messed up their ancestors' achievements; some old doctors have grown stupid and cannot be compared to young bright doctors."[87] In other words, he thought hereditary doctors might have had access to treatments kept secret in their families, but they would not be able to apply them well if they were not good doctors themselves.

Wu Cheng acknowledged that a Daoist monk could be an excellent doctor. When he dedicated a preface to a monk, Deng Ziran 鄧自然, for example, Wu said:

> His secret methods originate with himself, and he has cured illnesses that had not been cured for a few decades. I have seen and heard their divine effects several times. To those people who know his special skills, they are vivid.

Wu then lamented that medical talent truly useful to society often remained unknown and unused.[88] Wu spoke highly of another Daoist monk, Chen Zijing 陳子靖, who also excelled in medicine. Writing a preface to Chen's medical book, Wu praised it by saying, "[the book] compiled all the prescriptions that have been tested and found effective. It is thorough but not complicated. It is succinct but not simplistic."[89] In an inscription dedicated to a Daoist monastery, *Zhaoyin tang* 招隱堂, Wu praised a monk, Liu Tianrui 劉天瑞, who specialized in ophthalmology. According to Wu, it was reputed that Liu was able to help the blind to "see the sun and the moon," and that "he had divine skills and a benevolent heart." Therefore, he said, people went to the monastery to buy his drugs, just as "they would go to a market." Wu continued his adulation by stating that Liu donated the money that he earned to the monastery. Moreover, he had other monks manage the fund so that he would not be suspected of appropriating it.[90]

Wu Cheng had several terms to describe superb doctors. Wu once referred to the *Classic of Difficult Questions*, which said,

> When a doctor sees [a patient] and understands [the illness], he is divine (*shen* 神). If he listens [to a patient's voice] and understands [the illness], he is called sacred (*sheng* 聖). If he asks [a patient what he likes to eat] and understands [the illness], he is sophisticated (*gong* 工). If he feels [a patient's pulse] and understands [the illness], he is a virtuoso (*qiao* 巧).[91]

Wu said, "Now that the three methods—divine, sacred, and sophisticated—have been lost, only virtuoso doctors practice in the world the method of feeling the pulse to understand the *qi*."[92]

As such, Wu saved the term "divine doctor" (*shenyi* 神醫) for a legendary figure, Qin Yueren 秦越人, also called Bianque 扁鵲. According to Sima Qian's *The Records of the Grand Historian*, he had the ability to see inside the human body.[93] Wu said, for example, "An ancient divine doctor, Qin Yueren, authored *Eighty-One Difficult Questions* (*Bashiyi nan* 八十一難, i.e., the *Classic of Difficult Questions*)."[94] Or, as Wu argued in another essay, a good doctor did not always come from a family that had produced generations of doctors: he pointed to the fact that Bianque became a divine doctor by receiving a secret potion from a total stranger, Changsangjun 長桑君, not by receiving family instruction.[95]

When he was past eighty *sui*, Wu Cheng met two doctors who he believed were virtuosi: Dong Qiqian 董起潛 and Zhang Boming 章伯明. Both of them cured Wu's illnesses and the former also cured his great-nephew's. Wu argued that he had traveled all around the empire for seventy years but that he had never seen doctors as good as they were. He said, "I was already happy when I met Dong. I am even happier now that I am acquainted with Zhang. It is very surprising that I met two virtuoso doctors at an old age!" Citing the *Rites of Zhou*, Wu praised Dong Qiqian for being able to accurately predict which illnesses he could cure. Zhang, according to Wu, had studied not just medical classics and prescriptions from the ancient period but also books written by doctors in North China. Dong and Zhang were both learned doctors from eminent families in his prefecture, which had produced generations of *jinshi* degree holders.[96] Wu Cheng apparently thought, however, that the term "virtuoso doctors," physicians skilled in their own art, was a better compliment than the term "Confucian doctors."

The other terms that Wu Cheng used were an "eminent doctor" (*mingyi* 名醫) and a "good doctor" (*liangyi* 良醫). For example, in his preface to the *Great Compendium of Medical Prescriptions* (*Yifang dacheng* 醫方大成), he said the book referred to the achievements of the ancient sage gods (*shanggu shengshen* 上古聖神) and latter-day eminent doctors (*houshi mingyi* 後世名醫).[97] In a preface for the above-mentioned Zhang Boming, Wu said the doctor had read books written by "recent eminent doctors in the Central Plains" (*jindai Zhongyuan zhu mingyi* 近代中原諸名醫).[98] When Wu used the term "good doctor," he emphasized the doctor's moral character. For example, Chen Liangyou 陳良友 was a good doctor in Wu's eyes because Chen treated the rich and the poor equally. Interestingly, Wu thought that morality was linked to the quality of a doctor's service. Wu said that Chen's character allowed him to feel spirits (*shenming* 神明) and he was able to dream about proper prescriptions for patients while sleeping.[99]

Wu Cheng used the term "doctor of the realm" (*guoyi*) only once, when he wrote a preface for Peng Ding 彭鼎, who was a famous pediatrician in his town. Wu said, "Why is he called only a town doctor (*liyi* 里醫), even though he could be called a doctor of the realm?"[100] This example shows that Wu placed some importance on empire-wide fame, but the infrequency of his use of the term *guoyi* tells us that it was not his top concern. In fact, he revealed his localist tendency in his preface to Zhang Boming, in which he said:

> I started socializing with people when I was fifteen or sixteen *sui*. Going through major cities from the sacred capital and neighboring provinces, I have been to all the places under Heaven. I was not able to meet some doctors who I heard were famous because they were deceased. Among a thousand doctors whom I met, only two were competent and they are both in my prefecture![101]

The difference between Yuan Haowen, who actively used the term "doctor of the realm," and Wu Cheng probably reflected the cultural and discursive discrepancies between North and South China in the Jin and the Yuan periods. North Chinese people's attention centered around the literary tradition (*wen*) supported more by the imperial powers than by personal connections. The South Chinese, however, often wrote to valorize the cultural traditions of their own localities since the Southern Song period.[102]

Yu Ji (1272–1348)

Wu Cheng's student and Yuan Jue's friend, Yu Ji 虞集, belonged to the generation of elites in South China that actively participated in the central government under the Mongols from the last decade of the thirteenth century onward. A descendant of a Song minister and numerous scholars and officials, he received an excellent education since childhood and had a successful career in the Yuan central government. Just like Wu and Yuan, he had positive opinions about the Yuan policy of promoting medical institutions and had friends and acquaintances who were doctors, to whom he dedicated prose and poetry. Yu Ji also argued that medical practice could be a way to reach sagehood.

Yu Ji was from a well-educated family. Yu's paternal great-grandfather Yu Gangjian 虞鋼簡 studied the learning of the Cheng brothers and Zhu Xi with scholars, such as Wei Liaoweng 魏了翁 (1178–1237), Fan Zhongfu 范仲黼, and Li

Xinzhuan 李心傳 (1167–1240) in what is now Sichuan province. Yu Gangjie later wrote a book titled *Discussions on the Books of Changes, Poetry, and Documents and Analects* (*Yi shi shu lunyu shuo* 易詩書論語說). Yu Ji's grandfather and father were both known for their excellent writing, and the latter gained a position in the Hanlin Academy under the Mongols toward the end of his life. Yu Ji's mother came from a lineage that had been known for their expertise in *Chronicle of Spring and Autumn* (*Chunqiu* 春秋), and her father Yang Wenzhong 楊文仲 (d. 1279) was the Chancellor of the Directorate of Education (*guozi jijiu* 國子祭酒) in Southern Song. She studied with Yang Wenzhong's younger cousin, Yang Dong 楊棟 (*jinshi* 1229), who had also served as the Chancellor of the Directorate of Education and was a follower of the Learning of the Way. According to a funerary inscription for Yu Ji, she "understood all of his theories and there were no contemporary [words] and ancient references that she did not pierce into." As such, when the family fled during the war between the Southern Song and Yuan armies, and when her sons had no books to read, she was able to teach them *Analects*, *Mencius*, and *Zuo's Annotations to the Chronicle of the Spring and Autumn Period* by reciting them from memory. After the fall of the Southern Song, Yu Ji's family settled down in Chongren county 崇仁縣 of Fuzhou circuit 撫州路, the county in which Wu Cheng's family lived. Yu's father became friends with Wu Cheng, who in turn tutored Yu Ji and his brother.[103]

Yu Ji's political career was somewhat similar to Yuan Jue's. Yu received his first governmental position as the professor of the Confucian school in Daidu in 1297 and eventually served in the National Institute (*Guozi jian*), the Hanlin Academy, and the Jixian Academy. He ended his official career as a writer-academician (*shishu xueshi* 侍書學士, 2b) of the Academy of Scholars in the Kuizhang Pavilion (*Kuizhang ge xueshi yuan* 奎章閣學士院).[104]

Serving in the same offices, Yu Ji and Yuan Jue were close friends. Yuan Jue, for example, wrote over thirty poems and several essays for Yu Ji.[105] Yu also dedicated at least thirteen poems to Yuan and wrote a funerary inscription for Yuan's wife.[106] After Yuan died in 1317, Yu wrote an elegy (*jiwen* 祭文) for him, saying, "At the time, there were a lot of great scholar-officials at the court, but you were my only friend, with whom I discussed the world in the ancient times."[107] Ouyang Xuan's 歐陽玄 (1283–1357) funerary inscription for Yu acknowledged their close friendship.[108]

While Yu Ji's primary philosophical self-identity was clearly that of a *Daoxue* scholar, his large circle of friends and acquaintances included Daoist monks. Yu Ji dedicated a considerable amount of prose and poetry to Daoist temples and monks. He wrote some of this as a member of the Hanlin Academy on behalf of the emperor, and some as an acquaintance of individual monks.[109] An example of the latter would be the poem that he wrote for Master Liu upon his return to Mt. Mao (Maoshan 茅山), home of the Supreme Purity (*Shangqing* 上清) sect in present-day Jiangsu province.[110] He also wrote colophons (*zan* 贊) for all the paintings of the forty-five masters (*zongshi* 宗師) in the history of the sect.[111]

Yu Ji was curious about medicine since his youth, but I have so far found no evidence that Yu learned to practice medicine himself. In the prose that he dedicated to a doctor Wu Yiqian 吳益謙, Yu Ji said, "Since I was young, I liked searching for old books and reading them. When I obtained Zhang Zhongjing's *Treatise on Cold Damage Disorders*, I respected it as if [the instructions in the book] were rules made up of gold and jade 敬之如金科玉條." At the same time, he said, he realized that he needed a good teacher in order to understand the meaning of the complex rules and learn to apply them.[112]

Yu had a lifelong friendship with an elite doctor in Chongren county, Yi Xiaoya 易小雅. According to Yu, the Yi family was an "old Confucian official family (*gu rujia shizu* 故儒家仕族)." More specifically speaking, Yi's ancestor was a Judicial Intendant of Changsha prefecture (*Changsha zhilu* 長沙知録) during the Song period and lived in Chongren in his old age. "While maintaining Confucian practice (*shou ruye* 守儒業) until they aged," Yu said, his descendants "helped people live with medicine (*yi yiyao huoren* 以醫藥活人) and were admired as 'good people (*shanren* 善人)' in the region." After moving to Chongren, the Yu and Yi families became acquainted with one another, and Yu Ji and Yi Xiaoya became good friends because they were about the same age. Yi Xiaoya, and eventually all of his four sons, became doctors themselves. The family must have been reasonably well-off as Yu Ji wrote a poem dedicated to the Yis' storied building, named "Building with Refreshing Views (*Zhishuang lou* 致爽樓)." In the preface to this poem, Yu addressed Yi as an "elegant scholar (*yashi* 雅士)." Yi Xiaoya's youngest son, Yi Jin 易晉 (*zi* Yongzhao 用昭), in particular, liked to read books and excelled in writing prose and poetry. He recorded a large number of poems that his father and Yu exchanged over the years and made them into a "big box of books (*juzhi* 巨帙)," according to Yu.[113]

In his essay on medicine (*yishuo* 醫説) dedicated to Yi Jin, Yu Ji argued that medical practice is a way to achieve sagehood. He said:

> Medicine is the Way because it is a matter of nurturing others with benevolence. Because of the beginning of their pity and commiseration, physicians achieve the mastery of their art, help people complete their lives and remove harms from them. Isn't this learning important! (醫之爲道, 仁人之事 因其惻隱之發, 而究於其藝之成, 使人得遂其生而無害焉, 其學亦重矣哉).[114]

Needless to say, one of the Confucian classics, *Mencius*, regarded "the mind of pity and commiseration" (*ceyin zhi xin* 惻隱之心) as the foundation of one of the four sagely virtues, benevolence (*ren* 仁).[115] *Daoxue* scholars worked under the premise that they would truly become benevolent and achieve sagehood if they went through proper self-cultivation processes. Yu Ji was saying in the above quote that physicians cultivated themselves toward sagehood by excelling in their own art.

According to Yu Ji, the members of the Yi family were good doctors not just because they had compassion for patients but also because their benevolence helped them communicate well with one another. He said:

> The Yi family has already been studying [medicine] for a few generations. Between the father and the sons and between the elder and younger brothers, they are warm, relaxed, sincere, and detailed. In protecting their legacies, they

dare not miss anything. When they examine old theories, they dare not be neglectful. When they prescribe medicine, they are always elaborate and dare not be careless. When they diagnose illnesses, they are always thorough and dare not be thoughtless. If a younger brother has something insufficient, he asks his elder brother. If a son does not know something, he asks his father.[116]

Yu Ji probably saw in the Yi family an ideal combination of Confucian doctors and hereditary doctors, although he never used either of the terms. They came from a long-standing elite lineage and had the literary skills to exchange elegant poems with elite clients. They were virtuous, at least in the eyes of their elite clients, and helped one another's medical practices.

Another doctor of Yu Ji's that we know about is Huang Daming 黄大明 (1254–1336, *zi* Dongzhi 東之). He was invited to treat Yu Ji in 1333–34 when he fell ill in the capital of his home circuit, on his way to the imperial capital upon the emperor's summons. Huang had studied medicine with a local doctor, male members of whose family all practiced medicine, and written a few books. He was initially introduced to Yu as You Dongzhi 游東之, not Huang Dongzhi. While treating Yu, Huang explained to Yu why people knew him by a different surname. According to him, his real surname was Huang, but his great-great-grandfather married into his wife's family whose surname was You. Since then his great-grandfather, grandfather, father, and brothers had all taken up You as their surname. At some point, however, Daming came to think that the fact that he and his brothers became strangers to the Huang ancestors was deceiving their ancestor (*wu qizu* 誣其祖). He thus authored a genealogy and changed their surnames from You to Huang. Huang Daming further mentioned that he had adopted his younger brother Shimeng 師孟, who his father had with a woman that was not his mother, as his son because he and his wife had no biological sons. Huang Daming, however, felt unsettled. Thus he adopted Shimeng's son Lüxin 履信 as his own.[117]

This is an interesting example of a doctor learning to be a proper Neo-Confucian elite. Although patrilocality and patrilineality had long been the norm of Chinese families, especially in the elite stratum, there had been a lot of exceptions, including uxorilocal marriages.[118] In this context, *Daoxue* scholars attempted to strengthen and redesign patrilineal and patrilocal families. Zhu Xi, for example, wrote *Family Rituals* (*Jiali* 家禮) to show how the capping ceremonies, weddings, funerals, and ancestral rites should be held.[119] It was the responsibility of male descendants and their wives to worship ancestral spirits regularly. Zhu repeatedly argued to his disciples that the deceased ancestors could sense their patrilineal descendants' prayers because they shared the same *qi*.[120] Huang was thus worried about deceiving his patrilineal ancestors. He acknowledged his "true" ancestors by authoring a genealogy and changing back to the "right" surname. Moreover, he straightened out the familial order by making sure that his brother Shimeng was not recorded as his son in the genealogy. When Huang requested Yu Ji to comment on his actions so that he could put it in his genealogy, Yu said immediately, "[One] knows what is not allowed in the rites and what is making him feel anxious and does not hesitate to return [to the correct state]. Is it not the Way of gentlemen (*junzi zhi dao* 君子之道)?"[121]

When Yu Ji was in North China, he wrote a funeral inscription for Wang Defu 王得福 (1236–1315, *zi* Yizhi 宜之), a committed *Daoxue* scholar who practiced medicine. Yu probably was not his patient but knew him. After Wang's passing, his grandson Shoucheng 守誠, a *jinshi* degree-holder, looked for someone to write a funerary inscription for him, when Lü Sicheng 吕思誠 (1293–1357) from the same circuit recommended his colleague Yu. Wang's grandfather Zhang 漳 (*zi* Boyuan 伯元) had served the Jin dynasty. The inscription says Wang Zhang wore a golden symbol (*pei jinfu* 佩金符). Also called a golden fish bag (*jinyu dai* 金魚袋), it was a small ornament that the emperor gave to officials of rank four or higher during the Jin period.[122]

Yu cites several examples that showed that Wang had been a committed *Daoxue* scholar. For example, after his parents had passed away, he and his brothers continued living together and shared their limited resources peacefully. When he bought family gravesites in the capital, he bought extra land next to it for relatives who did not have descendants to bury them. In his old age, he was willing to teach anyone, not just his grandson. The most extraordinary episode in the inscription was about his response when he saw his father shed tears looking at other families' gravesites when he was only fourteen *sui*. It was after the family had fled from Yingzhou 應州 to Yangqu 陽曲 (both in the present-day Shanxi 山西 province) at the end of the Jin period, leaving behind their ancestral gravesites, where Defu's grandparents and great-grandparents had been buried. Wang Defu asked his father exactly where the gravesites were, left for Yingzhou immediately on the following day, and later brought back their remains.[123] The inscription also talked about Wang's reaction when he found a precious pearl that a wealthy merchant from the western region (*xiyu dagu* 西域大賈) had left. When the merchant came back and after Wang confirmed that the merchant owned the pearl, Wang nonchalantly returned it to him. Although the merchant offered a large sum of money to thank him, Wang did not take it.[124]

Wang learned to practice medicine after recovering from a serious illness. He read medical classics and studied with a prominent doctor, Mr. He 和氏. He became so good at medicine that a prime minister (*zaixiang* 宰相) asked him to serve in the ministry. Yu Ji never wrote down who the prime minister was and whether or not Wang received an official position. Yu, however, recorded that Wang treated people there and that he was careful not to receive the gifts the patients tried to give as tokens of gratitude. He was eventually offered a position as the Superintendent of Medicine of Several Circuits (*zhulu guanyi tiju* 諸路官醫提舉), but he declined the offer and left the government. His son later became a Commissioner (*dashi* 大使) of the Imperial Pharmaceutical Bureau (*Yuyao yuan* 御藥院), and one of his two daughters was married to a member of the Imperial Academy of Medicine.[125]

The comment that Wang made when he left the government is intriguing: "I, a Confucian, after all become famous because of medicine? 吾儒者, 竟以醫名乎?"[126] Did he somehow think that medical practice was not praiseworthy and thus thought that it was not an appropriate occupation for a Confucian scholar? Did Yu Ji agree with him? I think both of them valued medical practice itself. Having experienced and recovered from a serious illness, Wang knew the value of life and significance of saving people's lives. Yu Ji, as we have seen, repeatedly argued that medical practice could be a path to sagehood. But as a selfless *Daoxue* scholar, Wang probably did not feel comfortable receiving rewards for his service to others, whether from the government or a wealthy merchant. That was why, I think, he did not take the Superintendent position or money for returning the expensive jewelry. Yu Ji found a man like Wang praiseworthy, but he did not expect other doctors to do the same. In the above-mentioned funerary inscription for Huang Daming, for example, Yu mentioned Huang's more practical approach. He did not decline remuneration from the wealthy but did not take anything from the poor.[127]

Yu Ji heard about other excellent doctors from his acquaintances and sent a presentation preface to one of them, even though he had never met the doctor face-to-face. Wu's disciple Yuan Mingshan 袁明善 (*zi* Chengfu 誠夫) and another acquaintance, Xia Mingdao 夏明道, told him about Zhang Boming, whom Wu Cheng thought was one of the two best doctors he had known (see the last section). According to Yuan, Zhang had thoroughly understood books written by Liu Wansu and applied this knowledge to his patients successfully. Xia told Yu about two instances in detail. In the first instance, Xia's son once had an illness that made him unable to speak at all. While other doctors did not know how to cure him, Zhang diagnosed him correctly and cured the illness in less than half a day. In the second instance, Zhang predicted correctly that Xia's servant was to die in half a day or less, while other doctors thought that he could still be saved. Xia then told Yu about another "good doctor" (*shanyi* 善醫), Wu Yiqian 吳益謙, who was serious and "was never lazy in hoping to cure people's illnesses." Yu did not record the details of Wu's medical practice but was so moved by Xia's comments that he wrote the preface. He probably handed it to Xia so that he could give it to Wu.[128]

The title of Yu Ji's preface was, "Preface to Be Sent to Medical Scholar (*yishi* 醫士) Wu Yiqian." Yu probably chose the word *yishi* over words such as *yi* 醫 (medicine, or a medical practitioner) or *yizhe* 醫者 (medical person) in order to show greater respect to Wu Yiqian. Originally referring to the lower-ranking officials, as opposed to *dafu* 大夫 (high-ranking officials), the term *shi* 士 had come to encompass a larger group of people who were educated enough to participate in the civil service examinations by the Song period.[129] Juxtaposed against *min* 民 (ordinary people), *shi* is often translated as "scholar" or "literati." In the Yuan period, when there were multiple ladders into the governmental offices, there were various kinds of *shi*. Wu Yiqian, in Yu Ji's view, was a medical *shi*.

Yu certainly thought that individual Daoist monks could be good medical practitioners, but he might have been skeptical that their belief system could encourage them to advance medical knowledge and skills. In his inscription for a Daoist monk Xiang Zixu's 項子虛 study, "Hall of Enjoying Life" *Yuesheng tang* 悦生堂, Wu praised Xiang's ability to diagnose illnesses and cure them, but he said he was perplexed by the fact that Xiang studied philosophies of Laozi and Zhuangzi because "the former saw the body as a problem and the latter considered life as labor (老子以身爲患, 莊子以生爲勞)."[130] Yu's inscription for a Daoist monk, Huang Yuanji 黃元吉, mentioned that Huang's teacher surnamed Zhu 朱 had excelled in medicine but did not accept patients seeking for cures or Huang's request to teach him medicine. Zhu said that the Way of Medicine (*yidao* 醫道) was so elaborate and subtle that if one practiced without mastering it, he could kill his patients. It was also not good to pursue profit from it. Thus, to continue Zhu's explanation, it was better not to bother with it.[131]

Yu Ji's other writings confirm that medical positions in the Yuan government and medical profession had comfortably been blended into the elite society by the early fourteenth century. His inscription for an ancestral gravesite of a prominent scholar-official Su Tianjue's 蘇天爵 (1294–1352) family, for example, mentioned matter-of-factly that one of its female members was married to an associate professor of a medical school.[132] When Yu wrote a funerary inscription for You Shaoya 游紹雅 (1258–1341, *zi* Ruyi 汝義), a local elite in his home county related to Southern Song *jinshi* holders through his mother and wife, Yu mentioned that one of You's three sons, You Laiweng 游萊翁, was the Superintendent of Physicians in Jianchang circuit 建昌路 (in present-day Jiangxi province). Shaoya himself was not a doctor, but according to Yu, Laiweng "maintained Confucian scholarship and mastered medicine to practice nurturing" (守儒業, 治醫藥以爲養).[133] Yu Ji's funerary inscription for Li Feng 李鳳 (1254–1317), a Preceptor (*zhujiao* 助教) of the National College (*guozi xue* 國子學), said that Li was married to Ms. Wang, a niece of a Director (*yuanshi* 院使) of the Imperial Academy of Medicine. According to Yu, she was versed in "[Confucian] classics and history (*jing shi* 經史)" and was "serious in observing the rites (*du li* 篤禮)."[134]

We know little about Yu Ji's or his family's illnesses, except that he had vision problems toward the end of his life. According to *Yuan History* and the funerary inscription dedicated to him, he was not able to work on a few book projects because of this problem. He wrote two poems titled, "Eye Illness" (*muji* 目疾). He started the first poem by saying, "Letting pomegranate flowers open in the fifth month of the year. They look like smoke and mist. Isn't it spread all the way?" 一任榴花五月開, 看如煙霧亦悠哉. He used the same metaphor, "smoke and mist," in the second poem as well.[135]

Conclusion

Focusing on five literati from the early Yuan to mid-Yuan, this chapter showed that they expressed the emotions of being ill, or having their loved ones become ill, through poems and other forms of writings, just as Yuan Jue did. These emotions, often those of fear and frustrations, as well as practical needs for treatments, motivated the patients and their families to create and maintain good relationships with elite physicians. The interactions between elite doctors and their literati patients often went far beyond the duration of medical treatments.

This chapter has also demonstrated that discourses about doctors were shaped greatly by the political and intellectual history of the time. While North Chinese under the Jurchens were not so interested in depicting a doctor as a Confucian scholar, their descendants and the South Chinese began elaborating on the reasons why a doctor learned in *Daoxue* teachings would make a good doctor. This tendency culminated when a *Daoxue* leader like Wu Cheng, resentful of the arrogant and incapable Southern Song officials who in his view had caused or permitted the demise of the dynasty, argued that a man would be more likely to achieve sagehood by becoming a doctor than by passing the civil service examinations. Also, as a synthesizer of Zhu Xi's and Lu Jiuyuan's philosophies as well as those of Confucian and Daoist teachings, he valued book learning and experience, but at the same time, he believed in the transcendental power that some physicians possessed, such as that of the legendary figure Bianque. In the following chapter, we will see how this political and intellectual history shaped the history of medical books and theories.

Notes

1 *Qinrong*, 21.21b–23b and 48.12b–13a.
2 *Qinrong*, 7.14b.
3 *Qinrong*, 6.14b–15a.
4 Chen Yuan-Peng, *Liang-Song de "shangyi shiren" yu "ruyi"* (Taibei: Guoli Taiwan daxue wenshi congkan, 1997), 240–48.
5 See Chen Wenyi, "Networks, Communities, and Identities: On Discursive Practices of Yuan literati" (Ph.D. diss., Harvard University, 2007) for an excellent discussion on literary networking and its significance on Yuan Chinese elite identity formation.
6 As to the medical case records as a genre, see, for example, Charlotte Furth, "Producing Medical Knowledge Through Cases: History, Evidence, and Action," in *Thinking with Cases: Specialist Knowledge in Chinese Cultural History*, 125–51, ed. Charlotte Furth, Judith T. Zeitlin, and Ping-chen Hsiung (Honolulu: University of Hawai'i Press, 2007); and Christopher Cullen, "Yi'an: The Origins of a Genre of Chinese Medical Literature," in *Innovation in Chinese Medicine*, ed. Elizabeth Hsu (Cambridge: Cambridge University Press, 2001), 297–323.
7 See Chapter 6 for a discussion of the concept "Iron Curtain."
8 Miao Yue, "Yuan Yishan nianpu huizuan," in *Yuan Haowen quanji* by Yuan Haowen (Taiyuan: Shanxi guji chubanshe, 2004, expanded edition), 58.1403 and 1422.
9 Miao, "Yuan Yishan nianpu huizuan," 58.1422–59.1488. On Dongping as a cultural center, see Abe Takeo, "Gensho no chishikijin to kakyo," in his *Gendaishi no kenkyū* (Tokyo: Sōbunsha, 1972), 23–28.
10 Yuan Haowen, *Yuan Haowen quanji*, 49.1171–72.
11 Yuan, *Yuan Haowen quanji*, 37.785–86.
12 See Miao, "Yuan Yishan nianpu huizuan," 59.1454–55, about his trip this year. Yuan's medical case record is in Li Gao, *Dongyuan shixiao fang*, in his *Li Dongyuan yixue quanshu* (Beijing: Zhongguo Zhongyi chubanshe, 2006), 3.230.
13 Li Gao, *Li Dongyuan shixiao fang*, 3.230. The term *xiaomei zhi bian* is more often written 宵寐之變 (change in evening sleep). See, for example, Yang Jizhou, *Zhenjiu daquan* (Beijing: Zhongyi guji chubanshe, 1998), 6.294, and Jiang Guan, *Mingyi lei'an* (Beijing: Zhongguo Zhongyiyao chubanshe, 1996), 8:172
14 Li, *Li Donguan shixiao fang*, 3.230.
15 Yuan, *Yuan Haowen quanji*, 37.787.
16 Yuan, *Yuan Haowen quanji*, 24.534.

17 Yuan, *Yuan Haowen quanji*, 37.782.
18 Yuan, *Yuan Haowen quanji*, 10.249.
19 Yuan, *Yuan Haowen quanji*, 24.523.
20 Yuan, *Yuan Haowen quanji*, 37.783.
21 On the earliest occurrence of the term *"ruyi,"* see Chen, *Liang-Song de "Shanyi shiren" yu "ruyi,"* 186–87.
22 Yuan, *Yuan Haowen quanji*, 37.786.
23 Yuan, *Yuan Haowen quanji*, 37.786.
24 Tuotuo et al., *Jinshi* (Beijing: Zhonghua shuju, 1975), 51.1130–32; Yoshikawa Kōjirō, "Shushigaku hokuden zenshi: Kinchō to Shushi gaku," in *Uno Tetsuto sensei hakuju shukuga kinen Tōyōgaku ronsō*, ed. Uno Tetsuto hakuju shukuga kinenkai (Tokyo: Uno Tetsujin hakuju shukuga kinenkai, 1974), 1254–57.
25 Yuan, *Yuan Haowen quanji*, 34.724.
26 Tao Yuanming, "Yinjiu qi shiyi," in *Tō Enmei shū zenshaku*, trans. and annot. Tabei Fumio and Ueda Takeshi (Tokyo: Meiji Shoin, 2001), 175–77.
27 Fan Ye, *Hou Hanshu* (Beijing: Zhonghua shuju, 1965), 39.1315; Ban Gu, *Hanshu* (Beijing: Zhonghua shudian, 1962), 67.2907.
28 Yuan Haowen, *Yuan Haowen quanji*, 34.724.
29 Yan Jian, "Dongyuan Laoren zhuan," in Li Gao, *Dongyuan shixiao fang* (Shanghai: Shanghai kexue jishu chubanshe, 1984). For a Japanese translation, see Mayanagi Makoto, "*Naigaishō benwaku ron, Hi'i ron, Ranshitu hizō kaidai*," online at http://mayanagi.hum.ibaraki.ac.jp/paper01/toenkaidai.html.
30 Yoshikawa, "Shushigaku hokuden zenshi," 10–13.
31 Peter Bol, "Chao Ping-wen (1159–1232): Foundations for Literati Learning," in *China under Jurchen Rule*, ed. Hoyt Cleveland Tillman and Stephen H. West (Albany: State University of New York Press, 1995), 116 and 124.
32 Yuan, *Yuan Haowen quanji*, 400–04; Bol, "Chao Ping-wen," 120–25.
33 Miura Shūichi, *Chūgoku shingaku no ryōsen* (Tokyo: Kenbun shuppan, 2003), 107–18.
34 Su Tianjue, *Zixi Wengao* (Beijing: Zhonghua shuju, 1997), 7.106–09. For Huang Gan's life and career, see Kondō Kazunari, *Sōdai Chūgoku kakyo shakai no kenkyū* (Tokyo: Kyūko shoin, 2009), 287–323.
35 For his political career, see Song et al., *Yuanshi*, 167.3932–37.
36 Wang Yun, *Qiujian xiansheng daquan wenji*, SBCK chubian, 3.11a.
37 Wang, *Qiujian xiansheng daquan wenji*, 20.13b.
38 Wang, *Qiujian xiansheng daquan wenji*, 17.12b–13a.
39 *Daban niepan jingji* 大般涅槃經記, annot. Guangding 灌頂 (Taibei: Xin wenfeng chuban gonsi, 1978), 34.15a.
40 Linghu Defen 令狐德棻, *Zhou Shu* 周書 (Beijing: Zhonghua shuju, 1971), 46.833.
41 Du Fu, "Qiuri Kuifu yuanhuai fengji Zheng jian Li binke yibai yun 秋日夔府詠懷奉寄鄭監李賓客一百韻," in *To shi*, trans. and annot. Suzuki Torao and Kurokawa Yōichi, vol. 7 (Tokyo: Iwanami shoten, 1966), 143.
42 Sun Simiao, *Essential Subtleties on the Silver Sea: the Yin-hai jing-wei: A Chinese Classic on Ophthalmology*, trans. and annot. Jürgen Kovacs and Paul U. Unschuld (Berkeley: University of California Press, 1998), 81.
43 Wang, *Qiujian xiansheng daquan wenji*, 32.6b.
44 For the series of the treatments Wang received, see Wang, *Qiujian xiansheng daquan wenji*, 45.18b–19b. For his whereabouts when he received the treatments, see Song et al., *Yuanshi*, 167.3932–33.
45 Wang, *Qiujian xiansheng daquan wenji*, 45.18b–19b.
46 Wang, *Qiujian xiansheng daquan wenji*, 19.5b.
47 Song et al., *Yuanshi*, 167.3934.
48 Wang, *Qiujian xiansheng daquan wenji*, 46.6a–7a.
49 Wang, *Qiujian xiansheng daquan wenji*, 49.6b and 61.6b–7b. For a brief explanation of the Taiyi sect, see Yokote Yutaka, *Chūgoku dōkyō no tenkai* (Tokyo: Yamakawa shuppansha, 2008), 69.

50 Wang, *Qiujian xiansheng daquan wenji*, 7b–8b.
51 Miura, *Chūgoku shingaku no ryōsen*, 115.
52 Wang, *Qiujian xiansheng daquan wenji*, 42.11b–12a; Miura, *Chūgoku shingaku no ryōsen*, 205–06.
53 Wang, *Qiujian xiansheng daquan wenji*, 59.10a–10b.
54 Wang, *Qiujian xiansheng daquan wenji*, 19.5b.
55 Wang, *Qiujian xiansheng daquan wenji*, 20.10b.
56 Wang, *Qiujian xiansheng daquan wenji*, 92.6a.
57 Wang, *Qiujian xiansheng daquan wenji*, 73.1b.
58 Wang, *Qiujian xiansheng daquan wenji*, 73.1b.
59 Wang, *Qiujian xiansheng daquan wenji*, 41.20a.
60 Wang, *Qiujian xiansheng daquan wenji*, 41.17a.
61 Yu Ji, *Yu Ji Quanji* (Tianjin: Tianjin guji chubanshe, 2007), *xia*: 865.
62 Chen, *Liang-Song de "Shanyi shiren" yu "ruyi,"* 242.
63 David Gedalecia, *The Philosophy of Wu Cheng* (Bloomington, IN: Research Institute for Inner Asian Studies, Indiana University, 1999), 5.
64 Gedalecia, *The Philosophy of Wu Cheng*, 11.
65 Gedalecia, *The Philosophy of Wu Cheng*, 17.
66 Miura, *Chūgoku shingaku no ryōsen*, 273.
67 David Gedalecia, *A Solitary Crane in a Spring Grove: The Confucian scholar Wu Ch'eng in Mongol China* (Wiesbaden: Harrassowitz, 2000), 41–46.
68 For brief biographies of doctors in Fuzhou in the Yuan period, see Robert Hymes, "Not Quite Gentlemen?: Doctors in Sung and Yuan," *Chinese Science* 8 (1988): 18–23.
69 Wei Su, *Wei Taipu wen xuji*, YRCK, 3a.
70 Wu Cheng, *Wu Wenzheng gong ji*, YRCK, 46.10a.
71 *Quan Yuanwen*, ed. Li Xiusheng, vol. 14 (Nanjing: Jiangsu guji chubanshe, 1999), *juan* 480, p. 197.
72 *Quan Yuanwen*, 14:477.120.
73 *Quan Yuanwen*, 14:482.277.
74 *Quan Yuanwen*, 14:482.272.
75 *Quan Yuanwen*, 14:477.123.
76 Wei Su, "Linchuan Wu Wenzheng Gong Nianpu xu," 5b in Wu Cheng, *Wu Wenzheng gong ji*, YRCK.
77 *Quan Yuanwen*, 14:477.123–24.
78 *Quan Yuanwen*, 14:477.119. Wu Cheng is citing phrases from the "Aigong wen" 哀公問 chapter in the *Book of Rites. Zuantu huzhu Li ji*, SBCK chubian, 15.5a. Also see *Rai ki (Li ji)*, trans. and annot. Takeuchi Teruo (Tokyo: Meiji shoin, 1979), *ge*: 768.
79 Wu, *Wu Wengzheng gong waiji*, 1.3a–5a.
80 *Quan Yuanwen*, 14:484.327–28.
81 *Quan Yuanwen*, 14:495.642–43.
82 Zhu Xi, *Daxue zhangju*, collected in *Sishu zhangju jizhu* (Beijing: Zhonghua shuju chubanshe, 1983), 9.
83 *Quan Yuanwen*, 14:478.158.
84 *Quan Yuanwen*, 14:478.137–38.
85 *Quan Yuanwen*, 14:477.128–29.
86 *Quan Yuanwen*, 14:481.284.
87 *QuanYuanwen*, 14:476.84. Dedicating a presentation preface was a popular practice, particularly in Yuan China. A literatus dedicated a presentation preface to a specific individual with an assumption that the recipient would show it to others, as a way of introduction or recommendation. See Chen Wenyi, "Networks, Communities, and Identities," chap. 4.
88 *Quan Yuanwen*, 14:481.230–31.
89 *Quan Yuanwen*, 14:486.388.
90 *Quan Yuanwen*, 14:503.169.

91 This quote appears in the 61st question in the *Classic of Difficult Questions*. See *Nanjing jizhu* (SBCK chubian), annotated by Lu Guan et al., 4.39b–40a.

92 *Quan Yuanwen*, 14:480.206.

93 Sima Qian, *Shiji* (Beijing: Zhonghua shudian, 1959), 105.2785.

94 *Quan Yuanwen*, 14:479.177.

95 *Quan Yuanwen*, 14:476.84.

96 *Quan Yuanwen*, 14:477.123–24 and 479.177–78. Also see Hymes, "Not Quite Gentlemen?" 19–20, for their family backgrounds.

97 *Quan Yuanwen*, 14:486.388.

98 *Quan Yuanwen*, 14:479.176.

99 *Quan Yuanwen*, 14:478.143.

100 *Quan Yuanwen*, 14:479.184.

101 *Quan Yuanwen*, 14:479.178.

102 Chen Wenyi, "Networks, Communities, and Identities," in particular chaps. 2 and 3.

103 Song et al., *Yuanshi*, 181.4174–82 and Yu Ji, *Yu Ji quanji, xia*: 1290–1301. The quote is from Yu Ji, *Yu Ji quanji, xia:*1291. Also, see biographies of Yu Yunwen 虞允文, Yang Wenzhong, and Yang Dong in Tuotuo et al., *Songshi* (Beijing: Zhonghua shuju, 1977), 383.11791–1800, 425.12684–87, and 421.12585–87.

104 *Yuanshi*, 181.4174–82.

105 Yu Ji, *Yu Ji quanji, xia*: 1223–30.

106 Yu Ji, *Yu Ji quangji, shang*: 31–32, 33, 92, and 275.

107 Yu Ji, *Yu Ji quanji, shang*: 302–03.

108 Yu Ji, *Yu Ji quanji, xia*: 1250.

109 See, for example, Yu Ji, *Yu Ji quanji*, 820–31.

110 Yu Ji, *Yu Ji quanji, shang*: 156.

111 Yu Ji, *Yu Ji quanji, shang*: 330–39.

112 Yu Ji, *Yu Ji quanji, shang*: 582.

113 Yu Ji, *Yu Ji quanji, shang*: 116, 126, and 366–67.

114 Yu Ji, *Yu Ji quanji, shang*: 366.

115 This point is discussed in "Gaozi shang 告子上" section of *Mengzi* 孟子. See Mencius, *Mencius*, trans. Irene Bloom and P.J. Ivanhoo (New York: Columbia University Press, 2011), 124.

116 Yu Ji, *Yu Ji quanji, shang*: 366–67.

117 Yu Ji, *Yu Ji quanji, xia*: 953.

118 See, for example, Kawamura Yasushi, "Sōdai zeisei shōkō," in Yanagida Setsuko sensei koki kinen, ed., *Chūgoku no dentō to kazoku* (Tokyo: Kyūko shoin, 1993), 347–63, and Beverly Bossler, "'A Daughter Is a Daughter All Her Life': Affinal Relations and Women's Networks in Song and Late Imperial China," *Late Imperial China*, 21.1 (2000): 77–106.

119 See Patricia Ebrey, *Chu Hsi's "Family Rituals": A Twelfth-Century Chinese Manual for the Performance of Cappings, Weddings, Funerals, and Ancestral Rites* (Princeton, NJ: Princeton University Press, 1990).

120 See, for example, Li Jingde, *Zhuzi yu lei* (Beijing: Zhonghua shuju, 1986), 1:37; and Kakiuchi Keiko and Onda Hiromasa, eds., *"Shushi gorui" yakuchū, kan 1–3* (Tokyo: Kyūko shoin, 2007), 281.

121 Yu Ji, *Yu Ji quanji, xia*: 953.

122 Yu Ji, *Yu Ji quanji, xia*: 902–03. *Jinshi*, 43.982–83.

123 Yu Ji, *Yu Ji quanji, xia*: 902–03. The distance between the two places is about 200 km.

124 Yu Ji, *Yu Ji quanji, xia*: 903.

125 Yu Ji, *Yu Ji quanji, xia*: 903.

126 Yu Ji, *Yu Ji quanji, xia*: 903.

127 Yu Ji, *Yu Ji quanji, xia*: 953.

128 Yu Ji, *Yu Ji quanji, shang*: 582.

129　Peter Bol, "The Sung Examination System and the *Shih*," *Asia Major* 3.2 (1992), in particular 168–69.

130　Yu Ji, *Yu Ji quanji, xia*: 753. Neither *Daode jing* nor *Zhuangzi* has exact quotes like Yu's comment, but he was probably referring to the thirteenth chapter of *Daode jing* ("The reason I have great trouble is that I have a body. When I no longer have a body, what trouble have I? 吾所以有大患者，爲吾有身，及吾無身，吾有何患") and the chapter on "The Teacher Who Is the Ultimate Ancestor" (Da zongshi 大宗師) in *Zhuangzi* ("The hugest of clumps of soil loads me with a body, has me toiling through a life, eases me with old age, rests me with death 夫大塊載我以形，勞我以生，佚我以老，息我以死"). See D.C. Lau, trans. *Tao Te Ching: A Bilingual Translation* (Hong Kong: the Chinese University Press, 1963), 18; and A.C. Graham, trans. *Chuang-tzŭ: The Seven Inner Chapters and Other Writings From the Book* Chuang-tzŭ (London: George Allen & Unwin, 1981), 86.

131　Yu Ji, *Yu Ji quanji, xia*: 974.

132　Yu Ji, *Yu Ji quanji, xia,* 1142.

133　Yu Ji, *Yu Ji quanji, xia:* 953.

134　Yu Ji, *Yu Ji quanji, xia:* 878.

135　Yu Ji, *Yu Ji quanji, xia*: 130.

6   Medical books and theories

In a letter to a young doctor surnamed Chen 陳 from his home county of Yin, Yuan Jue reminded him how wonderful their local elite medical culture was. According to Yuan, men from the most flourishing families in this county lived close to each other and often gathered to discuss medicine. Together they would read ancient medical texts carefully and exchange opinions regarding why the treatments were effective at the time when the texts were written. Whenever the elite men found that someone was sick, they would first check the patient's conditions and record them. Taking the timing of the illness into consideration, they would choose an appropriate medicine and wait to see a good result.[1]

As he continued his letter, however, Yuan Jue lamented a new situation that had emerged as the South Chinese began serving as officials in Daidu. They would often eat food and take medicine that northerners liked. This was a problem, in Yuan Jue's eyes, because northerners tended to be taller and stronger, and were able to tolerate aggressive "cooling" (*hanliang* 寒凉) drugs better than southerners did. He urged the young doctor, whose grandfather and father had also been excellent physicians, to study well and practice medicine suited to the time and place that they lived in.[2]

This example shows that South Chinese doctors and patients were placed in a new environment after the Mongols conquered much of the Eurasian continent and unified China. They were exposed to new food, drugs, and medical theories. They also thought they were seeing human bodies that were somewhat different from their own. While Yuan Jue's letter was referring to the differences between North and South China, some other Chinese had opportunities to observe food, drugs, treatment methods, and human bodies from Central and West Asia. How did this new environment, along with institutional and social changes that we have already discussed, affect the history of Chinese medical theories and practices? Focusing on the spread of medical books, movement of doctors, and development of medical theories from the Northern Song to the Yuan, this chapter will show that the Mongol conquest of China and the subsequent new configuration of power had a substantial impact on medical theories and practices. I will start with medical innovations during the Northern Song period, then discuss the developments during the time when China was split into the Jin and Southern Song domains, and finally point to the advantages that the Yuan doctors had as subjects of the large empire.

Medical innovations in the Northern Song

Recent scholarship has clarified that the Northern Song physicians had produced innovative medical theories: the system of the five circulatory phases and six seasonal influences (*wuyun liuqi* 五運六気, hereafter the *yunqi* 運気 system) and "Guiding Channels" (*yinjing* 引經, also called "Affinity Channels" *guijing* 歸經). These theories were advanced at the time when printing technology allowed elite physicians easier access to medical classics, such as the *Basic Questions in Huangdi's Inner Classic* (*Huangdi neijing suwen* 黃帝內經素問) and the *Treatise on Cold Damage Disorders* (*Shanghan lun*). In response to the copious information that they now had at hand, physicians conceived of a large encompassing medical theory that would integrate abstract understanding of the relations among the human body, the cosmos, and treatments as presented in the *Basic Questions* with the practical prescriptions of medical formulas (*fang* 方) found in the *Treatise*. Also, one physician began theorizing simples found in the *materia medica* (*bencao* 本草) by using concepts in the *Treatise* and *Divine Pivot in Huangdi's Inner Classic* (*Huangdi neijing lingshu* 黃帝內經靈樞).

The Northern Song government led the publication of medical classics and created an environment in which doctors and the elite became increasingly interested in them. Emperor Taizu 太祖 (r. 960–76) ordered *A New Detailed Materia Medica Compiled in the Kaibao Era* (*Kaibao xin xiangding bencao* 開寶新詳定本草) to be printed in 973 and its revision in the following year. By decree of Emperor Renzong 仁宗 (r. 1022–62), the *Basic Questions*, the *Classic of Difficulties* (*Nanjing* 難經), and Chao Yuanfang's 巢元方 *On the Origins and Symptoms of Diseases* (*Zhubing yuanhou lun* 諸病源候論) were printed in the late 1020s. In the 1060s, during the reigns of Yingzong 英宗 (r. 1063–66) and Shenzong 神宗 (r. 1066–84), the scholar-officials in the Agency of Collating Medical Books (*jiaozheng yishu ju* 校正醫書局)—Lin Yi 林億, Sun Qi 孫奇, and Gao Baoheng 高保衡—collated and printed at least nine books: *Treatise on Cold Damage Disorders* (*Shanghan lun*), *Classic of the Golden Casket and the Jade Box* (*Jingui yuhan jing* 金匱玉函經), *Essentials of the Golden Casket* (*Jingui yaolüe* 金匱要略), *Prescriptions Worth a Thousand* (*Beiji qianjin yao-fang* 備急千金要方), *Additions to the Prescriptions Worth a Thousand* (*Qianjin yifang* 千金翼方), *Classic of the Pulse* (*Mai jing* 脉經), the *Basic Questions*, *The A-B Classic of Acupuncture and Moxibustion* (*Jiayi jing* 甲乙經), and *Secret and Essential Prescriptions of an Outer Censor* (*Waitai miyao fang* 外臺秘要方).[3] The Directorate of Education (*Guozi jian* 國子監) published these books not only in luxurious versions but also in affordable "small-character versions" (*xiaozi ben* 小字本), allowing not-so-wealthy literati easy access to these books.[4]

The publications of the *Basic Questions*, *Classic of Difficulties*, and the *Treatise on Cold Damage Disorders* marked a shift in doctors' interest; those from the Six Dynasties to the Tang valued medical prescriptions based on experiences, but in the Northern Song, physicians became interested in medical principles detailed in the medical classics.[5] In particular, the Northern Song physicians were fascinated by chapters 66–71 and 74 of the *Basic Questions*, which elaborate on the *yunqi* system. Catherine Despeux defines the *yunqi* system as a cosmological system based upon astro-calendary elements of the sexagesimal cycle; upon a calculation of the development of *yin* and *yang* according to the six modalities taken into consideration by Chinese medicine . . . ; and upon a calculation of the evolution of the Five Phases (wood, fire, earth, metal, water), and the six influences (wind, fire, summer heat, dampness, dryness, and coldness).[6]

From the late tenth century to the eleventh century, commentaries to the *Basic Questions* with occasional mention of pharmacotherapy began to appear, and in the early twelfth century questions regarding the *yunqi* system were asked in examinations for students in the government-run medical schools. Four commentaries to the *Basic Questions*, written in the Northern Song period, are extant: *Master Qixuan's Use of the Calendar of the Original Harmony* (*Qixuan zi yuanhe jiyong jing* 啟玄子元和紀用經, late tenth century), *Secret Words of Master Mysterious Pearl on the Six Influences According to the "Basic Questions"* (*Suwen liuqi Xuanzhu miyu* 素問六氣玄珠密語, tenth to eleventh centuries), Liu Wenshu's 劉温舒 *Marvelous Introductory Remarks on the Theory of the Circulatory Phases and the Six Influences According to the "Basic Questions"* (*Suwen rushi yunqi lun'ao* 素問入式運氣論奧, prefaced 1099), and *Recovered Chapters of the "Basic Questions in Huangdi's Inner Classic"* (*Huangdi neijing Suwen yipian* 黃帝內經素問遺篇, late eleventh century). Particularly noteworthy is *Master Qixuan's Use of the Calendar* and Liu Wenshu's *Marvelous Introductory Remarks*, which used the *yunqi* system to explain pharmacotherapy.[7] In the early twelfth century, after the medical school system was reorganized during the Chongning 崇寧 period (1102–06), the examination questions for the medical school students in the capital began to include questions on the *yunqi* system.[8]

The culmination of the Northern Song promotion of the *yunqi* system was the compilation of a *magnus opus*, 200 volumes of the *Comprehensive Record of Sagely Benefaction* (*Shengji zonglu*), under the leadership of Emperor Huizong 徽宗 (r. 1100–25). The first two chapters of this book were titled "The Circulatory Phases and the Seasonal Influences (*Yunqi*)," indicating that the authors had adopted the system as their basic principle. The manuscript of this book was completed during the Zhenghe 政和 era (1111–18), and the government had begun to have it carved on woodblocks when the Jin army captured the Northern Song capital in 1127.[9]

During the time when the above-mentioned commentaries on the *Basic Questions* were written, authors such as Han Zhihe 韓祗和 (fl. 1086), Zhu Gong, and Pang Anshi 龐安時 (1042–99) analyzed the *Treatise on Cold Damage Disorders*. The *Treatise* was originally written by Zhang Ji 張機 (second century CE, *hao* Zhongjing 仲景) to treat Cold Damage Disorders. Zhang's original text describes the illness in six stages and prescribes various formulas for each stage.[10] Between 1065, when the government printed the *Treatise*, and the end of the Northern Song, at least twenty-four studies devoted to the *Treatise* were published.[11]

A few factors apparently shaped the Northern Song's decision to print medical books, which caused the *yunqi* system and the *Treatise on the Cold Damage Disorder* to become popular among elites. First, the government used woodblock printing as a way of codifying knowledge, not just medical knowledge. The government's use of woodblock printing had started during the period of the Five Dynasties and Six Kingdoms (907–60), and the Northern Song government printed a large number of books, including Buddhist Tripitaka, *Imperial Readings of the Taiping Era* (*Taiping yulun* 太平御覽), *Extensive Records of the Taiping Era* (*Taiping guangji* 太平廣記), *Finest Blossoms in the Garden of Literature* (*Wenyuan yinghua* 文苑英華), *Prime Tortoise of the Record Bureau* (*Cefu Yuangui* 册府元龜), and Confucian classics.[12]

Second, commercialization, urbanization, and southward migration of people appear to have increased the reports, if not actual incidents, of epidemics, prompting the government to respond to them. Although it is hard to know whether there was an increase in epidemic cases, because we have far fewer primary sources for pre-Song periods than for the Song period, a list created by Asaf Goldschmidt shows forty-four cases were reported to the central government from 963 to 1137 from various places under the Song rule.[13] While epidemics in South China had been commonly attributed to the ferocity of demons, and treated by Daoist monks, spirit mediums, and other such religious healers, the Song government and elite claimed that authentic medical learning based on medical classics could and should be used to treat epidemics.[14]

Third, epidemics not necessarily linked to southward migration or urbanization also prompted the interest of the Northern Song government and elites in the *yunqi* system and the *Treatise on the Cold Damage Disorders*. For example, Pang Anshi's *Discussions on the Cold Damage Disorders and Miscellaneous Illnesses* discusses a disease called "Sudden Closure of Throats" (*jihou bi* 急喉閉), characterized by swollen throat. According to Pang, this disease killed "8 or 9 out of 10 patients in as little as half a day to one day" in Qi 蘄 prefecture (in present-day Anhui province) and Huang 黃 prefecture (in present-day Hubei 湖北 province).[15] A few modern historians, such as Fan Xingzhun and Ishida Hidemi, see similarities between the symptoms of *jihou bi* and the bubonic plague.[16] Although it is impossible to tell from such fragmented information whether or not *jihou bi* was equivalent of the "Black Death" in fourteenth-century Europe or *Yersina pestis* infections recognized by modern Western-style medicine,[17] the facts that *jihou bi* occurred in the regions not far from the Huai River 淮河, a geographical marker normally considered as separating North and South China, and that it does not appear to have occurred in major cities, remind us that the causes of epidemics were probably more complex than just southward migration or urbanization, and so were the reasons for the government's and the elite's interest in the *yunqi* system and the *Treatise on the Cold Damage Disorders*.

Reflecting the great popularity of the *Treatise on the Cold Damage Disorders*, which explains the stages of the disorder by showing which one of the Twelve Channels 十二經 is ailing and prescribes different medical formulas for each stage, the Northern Song *bencao* literature, or *materia medica*, listing the simples (*yao* 藥, also "drugs") also began showing their relationships to the channels. For example, Kou Zongshi's 寇宗奭 *Extending Meanings for Materia Medica* (*Bencao yanyi* 本草衍義) says:

Water-plantain (*zexie* 澤瀉): its contribution is that it is strong in letting water flow. Zhang Zhongjing said, "When water is pulled toward the inside of the body (*shui chu* 水搐), and [a patient] has thirst and a hard time urinating, whether [a patient should be forced to] throw up or to be drained, Five Fungi Powder (*wuling san* 五苓散) should be used as the primary formula." The formula uses *zexie*, so [we would] know that its function is that it is strong in letting water flow. *Shennong's Materia Medica* also cites Bianque, who said, "If taken in a large quantity, it causes eye diseases." This is certainly because water-plantains remove the water [from eyes]. Zhang Zhongjin's Eight Flavor Pill (*bawei wan* 八味丸) contains it because [it] guides cinnamon, aconite, etc., to reach the liver channel (*yinjie guifu deng, guijiu shenjing* 引接桂附 等, 歸就腎經). There were no other reasons.[18]

Certainly, the idea of associating simples with the channels pre-dated Kou's *Extending Meanings*. For example, *Shengnong's Materia Medica* says, "Dried nutmeg (*dazao* 大棗) nurtures spleen and helps the Twelve Channels."[19] Kou's *Extending Meanings*, however, was different because it specified which channels simples had effects on. Kou's book also mentioned *Treatise on the Cold Damage Disorders*. Doctors who followed him, especially those in North China, further elaborated on the idea of Guiding Channels, the idea that certain drugs have an affinity for a specific one of the Twelve Channels and that they act by entering into channels and directly affecting the associated organs.[20]

The "Iron Curtain" thesis

The fate of the *Comprehensive Record of Sagely Benefaction* might have represented the fate of medical cultures after the Jin conquest of North China: the obstructed circulation of ideas between North and South China due to what some historians called the "Iron Curtain" along the Huai River. The *Comprehensive Record* had never been printed under the Northern Song regime before 1127, when the Jin army took the woodblocks to the north, along with the retired emperor Huizong, his son Qinzong 欽宗 (r. 1125–27), most of their family members, and many treasures in the Song palace. The Jin government used the woodblocks to distribute the copies of this book, but the Jin imprint never circulated in the Southern Song.[21]

The term "Iron Curtain," referring to the blockage of information between the capitalist and communist countries in the twentieth century, was appropriated by a modern historian, Yoshikawa Kōjirō, as a metaphor for the scarcity of interactions between the literati in the Jin and those in the Southern Song for roughly a century, from 1127 to 1234.[22] Trade between the two domains was allowed only through "monopoly markets" (*quechang* 榷場), and merchants were required to pay high taxes on goods traded there. The markets were closed when the two dynasties were at war. When discovered, smugglers were to be sent into exile for five years, if not executed. The *Jin History* lists only agricultural products among the commodities traded in the markets and does not mention any kinds of books.[23]

In some instances, however, one would find evidence for the "porous" nature of the "Iron Curtain." For example, Yoshikawa and his critic Hoyt Tillman both cite the fact that a Jin literatus, Li Chufu 李純甫 (1177–1223), quoted and refuted the words of Zhu Xi (1130–1200).[24]

Yoshikawa's usage of the term "Iron Curtain" is certainly anachronistic. There are many differences between twentieth-century global politics and the twelfth-century relations among empires in East Asia. That is not, however, the point. The point is that the historiography of Song–Jin–Yuan cultural history behooves medical historians to compare and contrast the history of medicine in North China and that in South China and seriously consider the impact of the geography and politics on medical theories. Thus we will first look at the development of medicine in North China under Jurchen rule and the Mongol impact there. Then we will discuss medicine in the Southern Song.

Medicine under the Jurchens

Doctors under Jurchen rule, or the Jin dynasty, actively continued the attempts to integrate the discussions of the human body, illnesses, and pharmacological principles found in *Huangdi's Inner Classic*, the discourse on symptoms and medical formulas found in the *Treatise on Cold Damage Disorders*, and the knowledge of individual drugs found in *bencao*, or works on *materia medica*. Cheng Wuji 成無己 was a key northern figure during the transitional period from Northern Song to Jin rule. He was born, perhaps in the 1050s, into a family that had produced generations of doctors in Liaoshe 聊攝 in present-day Shandong 山東 province.[25] He wrote three studies on the *Treatise on Cold Damage Disorders*, namely *Annotations to the "Treatise on Cold Damage Disorders"*, (*Zhujie Shanghan lun* 註解傷寒論), *Clarifying the Principles of the "Treatise on Cold Damage Disorders"*, (*Shanghan Mingli lun* 傷寒明理論), and *Discussions on Drugs and Prescriptions Attached to "Clarifying the Principles of the Treatise on Cold Damage Disorders"*, (*Shanghan mingli yaofang lun* 傷寒明理藥方論). He was not, however, particularly eager to publish books during his lifetime. Yan Qizhi 嚴器之 prefaced *Clarifying the Principles of the "Treatise on Cold Damage Disorder"*, in 1142, but it was not printed until 1157. Yan also prefaced his *Annotations to the "Treatise on Cold Damage Disorder"*, in 1144, but it was printed only posthumously in 1172 by Wang Ding 王鼎. According to Wang, Cheng believed that his manuscript was not complete even when he was past ninety *sui*.[26]

Cheng's works marked "a milestone in the development of Chinese medicine."[27] The Northern Song authors, such as Han Zhihe, Zhu Gong, and Pang Anshi, used the terms of the *yunqi* system to explain physiology, diagnostic methods, symptoms, and treatments found in the *Treatise*, but no previous works were as thorough and organized as Cheng's *Annotations to the "Treatise on Cold Damage Disorders."* It provided annotations to every line, if not every word, of the *Treatise*. He also reorganized and collated the original text.[28]

Moreover, Cheng was a forerunner of the Jin physicians, as he took steps a lot further to integrate specialized works on *materia medica* with the medical classics.

Northern Song works on *materia medica*, except for Kou Zongshi's *Extending Meanings for Materia Medica*, were mostly annotated catalogs of a large number of drugs, explaining how they looked, where they could be found, and what kind of illnesses they could cure. Cheng now employed teachings from the *Basic Questions* to theorize the relationship between these individual substances and the multi-ingredient formulas (*fang*) found in the *Treatise on Cold Damage Disorders*. Cheng's preface to *A Discussion of Drugs and Formulas* discussed the Seven Principles of Formulas (*qifang* 七方) originally identified by the *Basic Questions*: large (*da* 大), small (*xiao* 小), slow (*huan* 緩), fast (*ji* 急), odd (*qi* 奇), even (*ou* 耦), and duplicate (*fu* 復). A large formula, for example, was composed of one main drug (*jun* 君, "lord"), three support drugs (*chen* 臣, "minister"), and nine assisting drugs (*zuo* 佐, "assistant"). Just as a kingdom should not have a lot of lords and only a few ministers, Cheng explained, a formula should not have a lot of main drugs and only a few support drugs. After explicating all the Seven Principles in this manner, he analyzed in the main body of the text how individual drugs in 112 formulas in the *Treatise on Cold Damage Disorders* collaborated with one another to cure various symptoms. Moreover, he selected the twenty most important out of the 112 formulas in the *Treatise on Cold Damage Disorders* and analyzed in even more detail how individual drugs worked together in his *Discussions on Drugs and Prescriptions Attached to "Clarifying the Principles of the Treatise on Cold Damage Disorders"*.[29]

Note that the level of concreteness in Cheng's explanations of drugs and prescriptions does not compare with the eleventh-century authors who had just begun seeing the value of the *yunqi* system as a way of explaining medicine. For example, just as Cheng did, Liu Wenshu 劉温舒 had used terms such as "main drug" ("lord"), "support drug" ("minister"), and "assisting drug" ("assistant") from the *Basic Questions*, to explain why a doctor should combine drugs with different flavors, in the chapter titled, "Discussions on Healing Methods" (*zhifa lun* 治法論) in his *Marvelous Introductory Remarks on the Theory of the Circulatory Phases and the Seasonal Influences According to the "Basic Questions"*, (prefaced 1099), but Liu never mentioned specific names of drugs or prescriptions.[30] In contrast, Cheng's *Discussions on Drugs and Prescriptions* uses more than 500 characters to explain why Cinnamomum soup (*guizhi tang* 桂枝湯), for example, worked and how it should be used.[31]

When Cheng's *Clarifying the Principles of the "Treatise on Cold Damage Disorders"* was printed in 1157, the physician Liu Wansu (born between 1126 and 1132) was either in his late twenties or early thirties. Liu was the first of a series of influential innovators who would later be celebrated as the Four Great Masters of Jin-Yuan medicine. Liu's family was from Hejian 河間 in present-day Hebei province. According to his friend Cheng Daoji 程道濟, Liu had indulged in reading medical books since he was a child. In his twenties, he spent three to five years just reading and thinking about *Huangdi's Inner Classic*. Cheng says, "[Liu] stopped sleeping and forgot eating" to understand the principles in the book.[32] Cheng Daoji then goes on to tell about a mysterious experience that Liu went through before he suddenly understood (*kaiwu* 開悟) the *Inner Classic*. Two

Daoist monks (*daoshi* 道士) came into his study one day while Liu was studying and beginning to lose consciousness. They handed him a small drinking cup with good wine in it. The cup turned out to be a magical one that kept on refilling itself as Liu continued drinking. Seeing him puzzled, the monks laughed and told him to spit the wine back into the cup if he did not want to drink any more. When Liu came back to his senses, his face was red and his body smelled of wine, although he could not find the monks. It would have been hard for others to believe this story, so Liu did not tell other people, but "because I am his true friend (*zhiyan* 知言), he sincerely told me [about his experience]," said Cheng.[33]

Although some modern historians categorize him as a "Daoist doctor" because of the above-mentioned anecdotes regarding his interactions with the Daoist monks and because drinking to achieve revelation is a common motif in Daoist biographies,[34] Liu himself argued for the integration of medicine, Daoism, and Confucianism by claiming that Fuxi, Shennong, and Huangdi were the starting points for all three sets of learning. His preface to *Profound Principles and Causes of Illnesses as Seen in the "Basic Questions"* (*Suwen xuanji yuanbingshi* 素問玄機原病式) starts by declaring that medical teaching (*yijiao* 醫教) originated with Fuxi, was disseminated by Shennong, and was explicated by Huangdi. He says that these three legendary figures wrote the *Books of the Three Graves* (*Sanfen* 三墳) based on the Grand Way (*dadao* 大道), which Laozi focused. Confucius studied, to continue his argument, the *Five Canons* (*wudian* 五典) written by the five legendary figures (i.e., Shaohao, Zhuanxu, Gaoxin, Tangyao, and Yuxun), learned the Regular Way (*changdao* 常道), and taught it as Confucian teaching (*rujiao*). Liu argued that all started from the *Books of the Three Graves* and that his intention of writing a study on the *Basic Questions* was to understand Huangdi, one of the Grand Sages (*da shengren* 大聖人).[35] Such an attempt to integrate Daoist and Confucian teaching was common in the Jin period,[36] although Liu was probably unique in placing medicine on the same ground. He cited a Daoist text, the *Record of Western Mountain* (*Xishan ji* 西山記), often in his works on medicine, but he would follow the teachings of the *Basic Questions* when he discovered a discrepancy between the *Record* and the *Basic Questions*.[37]

Just like Cheng Wuji's works, some of Liu's books were not printed until at least a few decades after they were written, if not longer. He completed the manuscript of *Profound Principles and Causes of Illnesses as Seen in the "Basic Questions"* around 1154, but it was not printed until 1182. Although he thought his *Preserving Life Based on Pathology and Pharmacology in the "Basic Questions"* (*Suwen bingji qiyi baoming ji* 素問病機氣宜保命集) had essential information for people's well-being, he ordered his descendants to keep it hidden from unworthy readers. This book was printed for the first time in 1251, half a century after his death and close to two decades after the Mongols' conquest of North China. His *Discussions on the Three Kinds of Exhaustion* (*Sanxiao lun* 三消論) was also printed posthumously in 1244.[38]

Although Liu is normally known for arguing that excessive Fire and Summer Heat in the cosmos were the origins of the majority of illnesses and thus that physicians should use cooling drugs,[39] his contribution to the theorization of pharmacology was equally important. Liu discussed the Seven Principles of Formulas in a chapter, "Discussions on *Materia Medica*," in his *Preserving Life*, but in more detail than Cheng did. In the same chapter, he also explicated ten qualities of drugs (*shiji* 十劑), which appeared in Cheng's book merely in passing: diffusing (*xuan* 宣), opening (*tong* 通), replenishing (*bu* 補), draining (*xie* 瀉), light (*qing* 輕), heavy (*zhong* 重), astringent (*se* 澀), smooth (*hua* 滑), dry (*zao* 燥), and damp (*shi* 濕). He argued that a physician should know the qualities of individual drugs in a formula in order to make necessary adjustments based on his observations. In a chapter titled "Summary on Drugs" (*yaolüe* 藥略), in the same book, he created an annotated list of about sixty drugs and associated some of the individual drugs with the Twelve Channels of the human body, through which they were considered to exert their efficacy. Unlike in Kou Zongshi's *Extending Meanings for Materia Medica* compiled at the end of the Northern Song, which referred to the channels by the organ with which each is associated, Liu's "Summary on Drugs" refers to the channels by their *yin-yang* names such as the Great *Yang* (*taiyang* 太陽) and the Great *Yin* (*taiyin* 太陰) Channels. For example, as mentioned above, Kou Zongshi associated the drug *zexie* with the "liver channel," but Liu linked it to the Lesser *Yin* (*shaoyin* 少陰) Channels.[40]

Being somewhat junior to Liu, Zhang Yuansu 張元素 began studying medicine after he was banned from officialdom at 27 *sui* for using a "taboo character" (i.e., a character that was part of an emperor's name in the Jin dynasty) in his answer to a question in the civil service examination. Zhang was from Yizhou 易州 in present-day Hebei province, about 100 kilometers away from Liu Wansu's hometown. Zhang is said to have written several books, but only two of them are extant: *Disclosing the Origins of Medicine* (*Yixue qiyuan* 医学啓源) and the *Pearl Bag* (*Zhenzhu nang* 珍珠囊). We have little evidence to show that he printed any of his books in his lifetime. Zhang used the first book as a textbook when he taught his students, but the earliest record of its publication is 1244. The history of the second book is completely unknown because of missing prefaces. His son completed their co-authored book, *Jiegu Laoren's Annotations to Wang Shuhe's "Secrets of Pulse"* (*Jiegu laoren zhu Wang Shuhe Maijue* 潔古老人注王叔和脈訣) in 1282.[41]

Although Liu Wansu and Zhang Yuansu are commonly considered to have started different "schools" or "currents" of medical traditions, they interacted through writings and face-to-face communication. For example, the beginning of the second chapter of Zhang's *Disclosing the Origins* is almost identical to the beginning of Liu's *Profound Principles and Causes of Illnesses*.[42] Also, according to a preface to Zhang's *Disclosing the Origins*, Zhang paid a visit to Liu when the latter's disciples could not cure their master's Cold Damage Disorder for eight days. Although Liu did not initially welcome Zhang, he let the guest take his pulse. Based on the result, Zhang rightfully guessed the medicine Liu had taken because he was thoroughly familiar with Liu's theory. Then Zhang said to Li, "The medicine you took tastes cold, sinks [in the body], and penetrates through the Great *Yin* Channels. This results in a decrease in the *yang* influences and perspiration cannot escape. Given your pulse now, you should take such-and-such medicine." Li agreed to take the medicine as prescribed by Zhang and recovered.[43] The author of the preface, Zhang Jifu 張吉甫, was certainly trying to exalt Zhang Yuansu's name, but the anecdote also tells us that they both lived in the same discursive sphere.

Zhuang Yuansu explicated his pharmacological framework in *Disclosing the Origins* based on the *Basic Questions* and used the framework to characterize drugs in *Pearl Bag*'s annotated list of 143 drugs. *Disclosing the Origins* says:

> Flavor (*wei* 味) is *yin*. When its flavor is thick (*hou* 厚), [the drug] is pure *yin* (*chunyin* 純陰). When its flavor is thin (*bo* 薄), [the drug] is *yang* in *yin* (*yinzhong zhi yang* 陰中之陽). *Qi* is *yang*. When its *qi* is thick, [the drug] is pure *yang*. When its *qi* is thin, [the drug] is *yin* in *yang* (*yangzhong zhi yin* 陽中之陰).[44]

This passage was a slight adaptation of the passage from the "Great Essay on Yin-Yang Correspondence" (*Yinyang yingxiang dalun* 陰陽應象大論) chapter of the *Basic Questions*: "When its flavor is thick, [the drug] is *yin*. When thin, [the drug] is *yang* in *yin* (*yin zhi yang* 陰之陽). When its *qi* is thick, [the drug] is *yang*. When its *qi* is thin, [the drug] is *yin* in *yang* (*yang zhi yin* 陽之陰)."[45]

Using these concepts in the *Basic Questions* and elaborating on the classification of drugs' qualities based on the principle of Guiding Channels, Zhang's *Pearl Bag*, for example, says, "Fangfeng 防風: sweet (*gan* 甘); pure yang (*chunyang* 純陽); the original drug of the Great *Yang* Channel (*taiyang jing benyao* 太陽經本藥)," "Huanglian 黃連: bitter (*ku* 苦); pure yin (*chunyin* 純陰)," and "Gegeng 葛根: sweet (*gan* 甘); pure yang (*chunyang* 純陽); the original drug of the Supreme *Yang* Channel (*yangming jing benyao* 陽明經本藥)."[46] According to Okanishi's count, Zhang established such associations between fifteen drugs and the Channels.[47] Just like Liu Wansu, he referred to the Twelve Channels by the *yin-yang* names rather than the names of the organs associated with the channels.

Zhang Zihe 張子和 (1156?–1228?), called Zhang Congzheng 張從正 in his youth, was the second of the Four Masters of Jin-Yuan medicine. He lived in present-day Henan province for most, if not all, of his life. From childhood, he received day-to-day medical instruction from his father. He was a renowned physician, having served in the Jin Imperial Academy of Medicine for a short period of time. The *Jin History* praises him for being sophisticated in medicine and for "piercing through" (*guanchuan* 貫穿) the learning of the *Basic Questions* and *Classic of Difficult Questions*.[48] However, he appears to have not been particularly interested in writing a book. The famous medical text, *Confucians Serve Their Parents* (*Rumen shiqin* 儒門事親), now a fifteen-chapter book, is attributed to Zhang, but he wrote only the first three chapters. In fact, some historians believe that an eminent literatus friend, Ma Jiuchou 麻九疇, wrote them as Zhang dictated the content. The earliest extant edition, and perhaps the first printed version, was published in 1244, after the Mongol conquest of North China. Although he did not study with Liu Wansu directly, Zhang Zihe greatly respected Liu and advanced his theory. In the first section of the *Confucians Serving Parents*, Zhang Zihe expanded and revised the Seven Principles of Formulas and Ten Qualities of drugs. He asserted that doctors should focus on eliminating harmful influences by adopting aggressive treatments: emetics, sweating, and purgation.[49]

The Mongol conquest of North China

The Mongol conquest of the Jin dynasty had an immediate impact on the history of Chinese medical theory in three ways. First, their military campaigns created extreme circumstances under which the third of the Four Masters, Li Gao (1180–1251), highlighted another cause of illness, Internal Damage (*neishang*). Second, in the new regime, which favored doctors, Li Gao's disciple, Wang Haogu 王好古 (fl. 1200–64), gained a position as a local administrator and wrote *Medications Administered as Decoctions* (*Tangye bencao* 湯液本草), the zenith of northern doctors' attempts to explain *materia medica* by the *yunqi* system. Finally, the Mongols' active recruitment of physicians into the military and government, as we have seen in previous chapters, gave another disciple of Li Gao's, Luo Tianyi, opportunities to interact with medical practitioners from other areas, test the master's theories on people from various cultural backgrounds, and eventually take advantage of his position as a member of the Imperial Academy of Medicine to publish Li's manuscripts.

Li Gao was born into a wealthy family in Zhending in present-day Hebei province in 1180 and was well educated in Confucian classics. When he was in his late teens, doctors gave conflicting opinions about his ailing mother, and she died. In search of ways not to repeat the same kind of tragedy, he began studying medicine with Zhang Yuansu. As he served in the Jin government as a regular official and eventually lived in Kaifeng, he slowly came to be known for his talent in the art of medicine.[50]

According to Li Gao's *Explicating the Confusions Between Internal and External Damages*, his attention to Inner Damage (*neishang*) stemmed from his observations during the Mongols' first siege of Kaifeng in 1232. The siege started on the twenty-first day of the third month and lasted until the seventeenth day of the following month, when Mongols and Jurchens reached a temporary peace agreement. Soon after the siege was raised, a large number of people fell ill and died. The *Jin History* claims that about 900,000 people died, while Li Gao said about one million. This experience reminded him that a large number of people had also fallen ill after Mongols' sieges were raised in other places. In his view, their illness was not a "damage" caused by external factors (*waigan* 外感) because such factors were not powerful enough to make such a large number of people suffer in just a few months. Rather, he argued, the Original *Qi* (*yuanqi* 元氣) associated with spleen and stomach became deficient and weak because of irregular eating and drinking as well as exhaustion during the siege. The weak Original *Qi*, to continue his explanation, let the Fire from the heart (*xinhuo* 心火) flare up. To heal these Internal Damages, Li Gao thought physicians should prescribe mild formulas that would replenish the Original *Qi*.[51]

After escaping from Kaifeng, he and his friend the poet Yuan Haowen lived in Dongping in present-day Shandong province. Led by local elites Yan Shi and Song Zizhen 宋子貞, this area hosted "tens of thousands" of refugees from Kaifeng. The leaders were particularly protective of elite refugees, creating an important cultural center of this time. Yuan Haowen was close to Yan Shi, helping Li Gao to be known among the gathering elites, many of whom eventually went to Daidu to serve the Yuan central government.[52]

Li then went back to Zhending in 1243. Between then and his death in 1251, he printed his master Zhang Yuansu's *Disclosing the Origins of Medicine*.[53] During the time he was back in Zhending, Li himself wrote eight books. Four out of the eight are extant: *Clarifying the Confusions Between Inner and Outer Damages* (*Neiwaishang bianhuo lun* 內外傷辨惑論), the *Treatise on Spleen and Stomach* (*Piweilun* 脾胃論), *Secret Treasures in the Orchid Room* (*Lanshi micang* 蘭室秘藏), and *Dongyuan's Tested Formulas* (*Dongyuan shixiao fang* 東垣試効方). Building on Zhang Yuansu's general theory regarding the relations among the Twelve Channels, Organs, formulas, and simples, Li's theory focused on illnesses in the spleen and stomach. As he was writing these books, he confided to his friend Zhou Defu 周德父 one day that he hoped to find a disciple who would pass down the Way. Zhou recommended Luo Tianyi, who studied with him for at least five years before his passing in 1251. As we will see below, Luo printed Li's works for the first time in the 1260s and 1270s. In the case of *Dongyuan's Tested Formulas*, Luo also edited it before printing because Li was not able to complete the manuscript.[54]

Li Gao's earlier disciple, Wang Haogu, came from Zhaozhou 趙州 in present-day Hebei province. He won a *jinshi* degree under the Jin regime when he was young. Wang may have also studied medicine with Zhang Yuansu before the latter's death. Wang and Li were both in Kaifeng when the Mongols occupied it in 1232, but they parted afterwards. Wang returned to Zhaozhou and became the "Zhaozhou professor and superintendent of medical schools in the area" (*Zhaozhou jiaoshou jian tiju guannei yixue* 趙州教授兼提舉管內医學).[55] It is unclear from his official title and scanty biographical data whether he taught in a Confucian school (*ruxue* 儒學) or medical school as a "professor." He would have been able to teach in either kind of school. It is clear, however, that part of his obligation was to supervise local doctors as the superintendent of medical schools in the area.

Wang's stable employment in the new government allowed him to focus on writing books. From the late 1230s to late 1248, he wrote five books.[56] One of them was *Materia Medica of Drugs Used for Decoction Medications* (*Tangye bencao* 湯液本草). As detailed by Ulricke Unschuld and Paul Unschuld as well as Okanishi Tameto, this book culminated the northern doctors' shared enterprise to synthesize the *materia medica* tradition, the principle of Guiding Channels, and the *Basic Questions*.[57] In the first chapter (*juan* 卷) of *Decoction Medications*, he elaborated on Zhang Yuansu's and Li Gao's pharmacological theories. In the following two chapters, he described 242 drugs in detail. About seventy-eight of the drugs that he described were associated with the channels.[58] This is a great increase from Zhuang Yuansu's *Pearl Bag*, which associated only fifteen drugs with the channels.

The Mongols' occupation of North China impacted the medical history of China most dramatically through Luo Tianyi. While studying with Li Gao, Luo was asked by an official of nearby Gaocheng 藁城 prefecture, Dong Wenbing 董文炳 (1217–78, *zi* Yanming 彦明), to cure the boils of the poor at the local administration's expense.[59] Luo's success led to a lifelong relationship with Dong, who brought his followers to join Qubilai Khan's army on its way to conquer Yunnan 雲南 in 1253. Luo also joined Qubilai Khan's army in 1253, serving as a military doctor at least until 1259. Dong Wenbing eventually became junior vice councilor of the Central Secretariat and Luo a member of the Imperial Academy of Medicine.[60]

Luo's career as a military doctor and a member of the Imperial Academy gave him precious opportunities to observe patients of diverse cultural backgrounds. By my count, in thirteen out of seventy-three cases recorded in *A Treasury of the Preservation of Life* (*Weisheng baojian* 衛生寶鑑), clients bore non-Chinese names.[61] Chapter 22 of the book linked a disease roughly equivalent to modern beriberi with an alcoholic drink made from mare's milk (*airag, kumis, comos*). As contemporary European travelers attested, Mongols, especially wealthier Mongols, consumed a large amount of the milk in summer. Luo thought that this drink in addition to humidity in South China contributed to the illness.[62] He was exposed to Mongolian religious ideas when he treated a Mongol man who had suddenly removed his clothes and run around in 1254. Mongols thought that he was possessed by a wind demon (*fengmo* 風魔) and had a shaman pray for him in vain. Luo correctly judged that the patient's body became double *yang* because of the Mongols' favorite meat, lamb, and because of their skin not being used to the southern climate. His effective prescription won him a reputation among Mongols as someone who could fix a wind demon.[63]

Luo also met a number of doctors and exchanged medical information. *A Treasury of the Preservation of Life* records prescriptions and theories that he learned from them in military camps and elsewhere. For example, Luo met Dou Mo in 1253 during Qubilai's campaign to Yunnan and learned acupuncture from him. He recorded Dou's poetry (*fu* 賦) to enable practitioners to memorize acupuncture points. Luo also wrote down twenty formula recipes given by another member of the Imperial Academy of Medicine, Yan Feiqing 顏飛卿, and eighteen recipes obtained from a Mr. Zhang 張 in his hometown.[64]

Luo's successful career helped him disseminate his and his master's medical theory. In 1261, Dong Wenbing, fighting a battle in Ji'nan 濟南 in present-day Shandong province, asked Luo to send medicines for his soldiers suffering from diarrhea. After Dong returned, he reported to Luo how effective the medicines were and encouraged Luo to share the knowledge with others.[65] Luo then edited his master's last book, *Dongyuan's Experimental Formulas*, in 1266. In 1276, he printed Li Gao's *Treatise on Spleen and Stomach* and *Secret Treasures in the Orchid Room* for the first time. He then printed Li's *Dongyuan's Tested Formulas* in 1280. Three years later, Luo completed his own book, *A Treasury of the Preservation of Life*.[66]

Medicine in the Southern Song

During the time of the "Iron Curtain" or, better put, the period of North–South division from 1127 to 1234, the interest of physicians and medical book authors in North and South China appeared to have grown apart as time went on. Thanks to more than 200 publishing centers in the Southern Song, more authors in South China printed their medical books than those in North China during this period. Kosoto Hiroshi has identified forty-three extant medical texts written by thirty-two authors, but we do not see records of the circulation of medical books or the pharmacological theorization in South China similar to what occurred in North China.

There is little evidence that medical books written by the Jin authors were printed or collected in the Southern Song before 1234 or that the Southern Song medical books circulated in the Jin domain. None of the twenty-three important Jin medical books, versions of which have been studied by modern historians Mayanagi Makoto and Kosoto Hiroshi, were printed in the Southern Song prior to the Mongol conquest of North China. At least, they have not found any extant versions printed in the Southern Song before 1234.[67] *Records of Readings at the Prefectural Studio* (*Junzhai dushuzhi* 郡齋讀書志), an annotated catalog of the private holdings of a Southern Song scholar-official, Chao Gongwu 晁公武 (?–1171), lists forty-nine medical books, but none of them were written by the Jin authors.[68] Another Southern Song scholar-official, Chen Zhensun 陳振孫 (*c*. 1190–1249+), wrote *Critical Remarks on the Catalog of Straightforward Studio* (Zhizhai shulu jieti 直齋書錄解題) and listed eighty-seven medical books. Again the Jin doctors left no traces in this catalog.[69] The forty-three Southern Song medical books that Kosoto studied were never printed in the Jin domain (see Table 6.1).

Table 6.1 Medical books written during the Southern Song Period

Title	Year
Jifeng puji fang 雞峰普濟方	1133?
Youyou xinshu 幼幼新書	1150
Puji benshi fang 普濟本事方	mid-12th century
Leizheng benshi fang houji 類證本事方後集	mid-12th century
Beiquan zongxiao fang 備全總效方	1154
Hongshi jiyan fang 洪氏集驗方	1170
Shanghan yaozhi 傷寒要旨	1171
Sanyin jiyi bingzheng fanglun 三因極一病證方論	1174
Yangshi jiacang fang 楊氏家藏方	1178
Yijing zheng benshu 醫經正本書	1176
Shanghai buwang lun 傷寒補亡論	1181
Weisheng jiabao chanke beiyao 衛生家寶產科備要	1184
Weisheng jiabao fang 衛生家寶方	1184
Weisheng jiabao tangfang 衛生家寶湯方	1184
Weisheng jiabao xiao'er fang 衛生家寶小兒方	1184

Yeshi luyan fang 葉氏錄驗方	1186
Yishuo 醫說	1189
Shibian liangfang 十便良方	1196
Baiyi xuanfang 百一選方	1197
Fangshi jiyao fang 方氏集要方	1197
Xiao'er weisheng zongwei lunfang 小兒衛生總微論方	1216
Yijian fang 易簡方	12th century (2nd half)
Xu Yijian fanglun 續易簡方論	1243
Xu Yijianfang houji 續易簡方後集	12th century (2nd half)
Xu Yijian fang mailun 續易簡方脈論	1244
Huoren shizheng fang 活人事證方	1216
Huoren shizheng fang houji 活人事證方後集	around 1220
Zhenqiu zisheng jing 鍼灸資生經	1220
Lidai mingyi mengqiu 歷代名醫蒙求	1120
Beiji jiufa 備急灸法	1126
Weishi jiacang fang 魏氏家藏方	1127
Furen daquan liangfang 婦人大全良方	1237
Waike jingyao 外科精要	1263
Chabing zhinan 察病指南	1241
Xiyuan jilu 洗冤集錄	1247
Yanshi jisheng fang 嚴氏濟生方	1253
Yangshi jisheng xufang 嚴氏濟生續方	1267
Jianyi fanglun 簡易方論	1260
Zhizhi fanglun 直指方論	1264
Xiao'er fanglun 小兒方論	1260
Shanghan leishu huoren zongkuo 傷寒類書活人總括	1262
Yimai zhenjing 醫脈真經	1262
Zhushi jiyan fang 朱氏集驗方	1266

Sources: Kosoto Hiroshi,"Nan-Sōdai no iyaku sho, sono 1," *Gendai Tōyō igaku*, 9.1 (1988): 87–93; "Nan-Sōdai no iyaku sho, sono 2," *Gendai Tōyō igaku*, 9.2 (1988): 79–85; "Nan-Sōdai no iyaku sho, sono 3," *Gendai Tōyō igaku*, 9.3 (1988): 96–104; "Nan-Sōdai no iyaku sho, sono 4," *Gendai Tōyō igaku* 9.4 (1988): 96–103; "Nan-Sōdai no iyaku sho, sono 5," *Gendai Tōyō igaku*, 10.1 (1989): 93–99; and "Nan-Sōdai no iyaku sho, sono 6," *Gendai Tōyō igaku*, 10.2 (1989): 94–103.

   To the best of my knowledge, the only book that might have circulated between North and South China prior to the Mongol conquest of North China is a combined edition of the three works on Cold Damage Disorders written by Cheng Wuji. A Zhang Xiaozhang 張孝忠 supposedly wrote a postscript (*bawen* 跋文) to this collection and printed it in the first year of the Kaixi 開禧 period (1205), one of the Southern Song regnal names. According to the comment, he obtained one of Cheng's texts at a physician's house in the "capital" (*du* 都), perhaps meaning Hangzhou 杭州, in the 1190s and later acquired the remaining two books in present-day Hubei province, close to the Jin–Southern Song border.[70] It is hard for us to tell exactly what happened because the original versions of Cheng's books are not extant. Although there is certainly a possibility that the postscript was falsified in a later period, I would say the books probably crossed the Jin–Southern Song border.

Soon after the Mongols conquered the Jin dynasty in 1234, they sent troops to the Southern Song border and had them bring a large number of books and scholars as early as 1235 from South to North China, as discussed in Chapter 2. Thus they began dismantling the "Iron Curtain" right after the fall of the Jin dynasty, long before the fall of the Southern Song in 1276. An example of early medical interactions between North and South China under Mongol rule is what the National Library of China calls the "Jin imprint" (*Jin ke ben* 金刻本) of the *Basic Questions in Huangdi's Inner Classic*. This is the earliest extant copy of the book, so far found only in the Library. Interestingly, Mayanagi showed recently that the "Jin imprint" used another version of the same text printed in the Shaoxing 紹興 era (1131–62) in the Southern Song as the base text and incorporated annotations from other versions compiled in the Northern Song, judging by the ways different versions annotated the pronunciations of unusual Chinese characters. Because the "Jin imprint" lacks prefaces and a table of contents, it is impossible for us to come up with a definitive answer as to when it was printed. If it was printed before 1234, as the Library assumes, then the Shaoxing imprint must have crossed the border prior to that. If the Jin imprint was actually printed after 1234, then the Shaoxing imprint was likely to have crossed the border after the Mongols had dismantled the "Iron Curtain." The key is the list of twenty-odd woodblock carvers' names, as shown in the centerfold of each sheet, of the "Jin imprint." All but one of them were the same as the names of the carvers of another book, *Revised Edition of Classified Materia Medica of the Zhengh Era* (*Chongxiu Zhenghe jingshi zhenglei beiyong bencao* 重修政和経史証類備用本草), printed in 1249 in Pingshui 平水 in present-day Shandong province.[71] I am tempted to think that the "Jin imprint" was carved after 1234, and thus the Shaoxing imprint was *not* an example of the porous nature of the Curtain, because it is unlikely that two books printed at least fifteen years apart would be the products of the same set of carvers.

In addition to obstructing circulation of the vast majority of medical books, the "Iron Curtain" during the Jin period prevented medical theoreticians in the two domains from having face-to-face interactions. This was problematic at a time when printing one's book was an expensive project.[72] Also, at this time, different sectors of Chinese society were still grappling with the idea of publicizing their manuscripts beyond their friends and students. For example, the Complete Reality Sect (*Quanzhen zong*), a popular Daoist group of this time, believed that their esteemed text, Zhang Boduan's 張伯端 (d. 1082) *Awakening to Reality* (*Wuzhen pian* 悟眞篇), could be transmitted only to deserving disciples; otherwise the revealer would receive the Heavenly Punishment (*tianqian* 天譴). This changed only when Bai Yuchan 白玉蟾 (1194–1229?), the leader of the southern branch of this sect, successfully broke this taboo by arguing that the printing should be regarded as a Heavenly Gift (*tianci* 天賜) because it would allow the sect to inform men in remote places that they also had a talent to be an immortal (*xianfen* 仙分).[73] Doctors before the Song also lived in a "world where master-discipline lineage and religious charisma were central to the production of medical knowledge and authority." In this world, private manuscript texts were transmitted by a master to a relatively small number of trusted followers.[74] Not all the doctors and their teachers even in the Jin domain felt comfortable printing their books, making it hard for the new ideas to cross the Jin–Southern Song border.

Some of the Southern Song authors, especially those active in early Southern Song, inherited the Northern Song doctors' interest in the *Treatise on Cold Damage Disorders* and the *yunqi* system. For example, Xu Shuwei 許淑微 (d. 1154) wrote *One Hundred Mnemonic Verses on Cold Damage Manifestations* (*Shanghan bai zheng ge* 傷寒百證歌) to help the readers remember the basics of the *Treatise* and two other books on the *Treatise* (*Shanghan fawei lun* 傷寒發微論 and *Shanghan jiushi lun* 傷寒九十論) that incorporated a large number of case studies.[75] Chen Yan 陳言 (*zi* Wuze 無擇, fl. 1161–74), supposedly from Qingtian 青田 prefecture in the present-day Zhejiang province, used the *yunqi* system to explain etiology in his *Prescriptions Elucidated on the Premise That All Pathological Symptoms Have Only Three Primary Causes* (*Sanyin jiyibin zheng fang lun* 三因極一病證方論). Based on his broad knowledge of medical classics and other writings on medicine, he divided the causes of illnesses into three categories: internal, external, or "neither internal nor external" causes.[76]

The Southern Song doctors, however, were much less interested in the principle of Guiding Channels compared to their Jin counterparts. Xu Shuwei's *Original Formulary for Popular Relief* (*Puji benshi fang* 普濟本事方) mentions the guiding principle a couple of times. For example, Xu said, "'Mother of Pearl' (*zhenzhumu* 眞珠母) enters the liver channel (*ganjing* 肝經) and is the dominant ingredient."[77] Xu also talked about Sichuan pepper (*chuanjiao* 川椒) having a quality to guide kidney *qi* to return to the channel.[78] Note that he referred to the channels that the simples worked on by the name of the organs they were associated with, just like Kou Zongshi's *Extending Meanings for Materia Medica* at the end of the Northern Song. This was different from Liu Wansu and Zhang Yuansu, who linked the simples to the channels called by the *yin-yang* names, such as Great *Yang* Channel, Lesser *Yin* Channel, or even more precisely the Hand's Great *Yang* Channel. Also, Xu associated many fewer drugs with the channels than North Chinese doctors did.

Chen Yan never analyzed individual drugs in the formulas in the ways the Jin doctors did. His followers, such as Wang Shuo 王碩, Sun Zhining 孫志寧, Shi Fa 施發, Lu Zuchang 盧祖常, and Wang Wei 王暐, located in Wenzhou in present-day Zhejiang province, were more interested in writing practical books that conveniently packaged medical treatments than elaborating on theories. According to a modern historian, Liu Shijue, their prescriptions were heavily influenced by those set by the Charitable Pharmacies.[79] Liao Yujun, Fu Fang, and Zheng Jinsheng argue that the "simplification trend" (*jianhua zhi feng* 簡化之風) of medical learning at the time followed the similar trend in Confucian learning.[80]

Needless to say, what appears to be the growing difference between the Jin and the Southern Song domains should not be interpreted as meaning that one was better than the other. It simply means the political and sometimes military confrontations of the regimes during the period forced upon doctors a communication gap, whether or not we choose to dramatize it by calling it the "Iron Curtain." The Mongols helped doctors fill this gap by unifying China.

Central and West Asian medicine

In addition to tearing down the "Iron Curtain" between North and South China, the Mongols' conquest promoted dialogues between Central and West Asian and Chinese medicines. Although it was certainly not the first time in history that this had happened, the importation was more systematic in the Yuan period than in other periods because of the Mongol rulers and *Semu* (Central and West Asian) officials.[81] Most importantly, 'Īsā, a *Semu* official, built medical institutions offering West Asian medical service in the Yuan capitals. Also, traders imported drugs from Central and West Asia through the so-called Silk Road and sea routes. As a result, Chinese people were curious and knowledgeable about the foreign drugs and treatments.

'Īsā built the Office of Medicine of the Western Regions (Xiyu yiyaosi 西域醫藥司) in 1263,[82] and the name of this office changed to the Office of Broad Grace (Guanghui si 廣惠司) in 1270.[83] The role of this office was to prepare "Islamic medicines for the emperor and to treat imperial guards as well as the lonely and poor in the capital."[84] In 1292, two offices specializing in "supervising matters of Islamic pharmaceuticals"—the Islamic Pharmaceutical Bureau in Daidu (*Daidu Huihui yaowuyuan* 大都回回藥物院) and the Islamic Pharmaceutical Bureau in Shangdu (*Shangdu huihui yaowu yuan* 上都回回藥物院) were also built in the two Yuan capitals. They eventually came under the supervision of the Office of Broad Grace in 1322.[85] Certainly, "Islamic medicine" was not accurate nomenclature because 'Īsā was a Nestorian Christian, but the visibility of West Asian medicine in China at this time is indisputable.

It is likely that 'Īsā modeled the Office of Broad Grace after West Asian hospitals. According to Emilie Savage-Smith, hospitals were constructed and flourished "throughout Islamic lands." The first recorded hospital established by an Islamic ruler was built in Baghdad either in the late eighth or early ninth century, and five more were built within 200 years. The network of hospitals continued to thrive at least until the twelfth century, when a traveler described a hospital there as being like an "enormous palace in size." In Cairo, a hospital was built in the ninth century, and then probably three other ones before the Mansūrī hospital, the largest of them all, was established. According to Savage-Smith, these Islamic hospitals served several purposes; they were centers for medical treatment, convalescent homes for the sick and injured, asylums for the insane, and retirement homes "for the aged and infirm who lacked a family to care for them."[86]

One of the major intellectual achievements of the Islamic medical institutions in the Yuan capitals was the fourteenth-century compilation of *Islamic Pharmacology* (*Huihui yaofang* 回回藥方). It lists more than 400 drugs that originated in the West Asian medical tradition, according to a modern historian Song Xian's count. In this text, Chinese characters and West Asian scripts were written side by side, fusing Chinese and Islamic medical traditions.[87] In addition, *The Correct Essence of Drinking and Eating* (*Yinshan zhengyao* 飲膳正要) was compiled by Hu Sihui 忽思慧, a *Semu* palace dietician. It was a book on dietary medicine that combined food preparation traditions in China, Mongolia, and other parts of the Eurasian continent.[88]

The Mongol domination of Eurasia activated various forms of material exchanges between Yuan China and other regions: formal tributes, government trade, private trade, and proceeds for the Mongol royalty from their allotted territories dispersed in China and Inner Asia. The goods were transferred through land and sea routes. The *Yuan History* says Qubilai dispatched envoys with a large amount of gold to purchase drugs in Ceylon (*Shizi guo* 獅子國).[89] Aromatics to be used as drugs, spices, incense, cosmetics, and decorations were particularly important because of their high value. Maritime trade for these aromatics centered around Quanzhou 泉州 (in present-day Fujian 福建 province). In this port city, traders whose ancestors had come from Arabia, Persia, and India took leadership during the Mongol period.[90]

In this intensely multicultural environment, the Chinese were curious about West Asian doctors and gained some knowledge of their practice. For example, Tao Zongyi 陶宗儀 in the late Yuan recorded a case in which an Islamic medical official (*huihui yiguan* 回回醫官) opened up the forehead of a child who had a severe headache. It stopped after the doctor took out what was possibly a tumor, which looked like a small "crab," from the child's brain. In another instance, a doctor took out a tumor from a leg of a horse that could not stand. After the operation, the horse recovered and was able to run again. In Tao's list of Yuan-period drama scripts, one can find titles that suggest that a protagonist might have been a practitioner of West Asian medicine.[91] A rather obvious example would be *Islamic Bureau of Pear Flowers* (*Huihui lihua yuan* 回回梨花院), which probably was a euphemism for the Islamic Pharmaceutical Bureau. Also, *An Aromatic Cart* (*Xiangyao che* 香藥車) and *The Eye Doctor* (*Yanyao gu* 眼藥孤) might have dealt with West Asian medicine because, according to Song Xian, *Semu* peddlers often put aromatics on carts and sold them; West Asian medicine was known for efficacious ophthalmology.[92]

Electuary sherbet, or syrup, was a good example of a category of "drugs" from West Asia popularized in China during the Yuan period. Prepared from fruits or flower petals with sugar, *sharbat* (deriving from an Arabic verb, *sharāb*, "to drink") was eaten as a concentrate or diluted in water as a drink. Unlike modern sherbet in the U.S. and elsewhere, it was never frozen, but West Asians and later Indians sometimes cooled it down before drinking if they had means to do so. Analyzing uses of sherbet in *One Thousand and One Nights*, a collection of stories originating from Arabic, Persian, Indian, Egyptian, and Mesopotamian folklores, Maejima Shinji has shown that West Asians before the sixteenth century enjoyed this drink in the following five kinds of situations: (1) after a banquet or dinner; (2) when ill or tired; (3) after taking a steam bath; (4) at a wedding banquet; (5) after a long trip or a triumphant return from a battle.[93] *The Canon of Medicine*, written by Ibn Sina (b. 980–1037, born in present-day Uzbekistan and known as Avicenna in Europe), lists more than fifty kinds of syrup.[94]

The Mongol royal family created an office devoted to making sherbet, initially appointing a Nestorian Christian doctor, who cured Chinggis Khan's ailing son with this drink. The doctor's grandson, Mar Sergis (Ma Xuelijisi 馬薛里吉 思), settled down in Zhenjiang (in present-day Jiangsu province) as an assistant *darughachi* and a sherbet maker.[95] Hu Sihui, the palace dietician in the Yuan court, listed ten kinds of syrup in his *The Correct Essence of Drinking and Eating* (*Yinshan zhengyao*). To make cherry syrup, Hu says, for example, one would boil cherries (50 *jin*) and white granulated sugar (24 *jin*, refined) together.[96] Quanzhou, the port city with a lot of *Semu* traders, sent sherbet as their tribute to the last emperor of the Yuan dynasty, Toghan Temür (1320–70, r. 1333–68).[97]

This sweet drink was obviously popular outside of the palace and beyond the circle of Central and West Asians in the Yuan capitals. The *Guide to Domestic Operations* (*Jujia biyong shilei* 居家必用事類), published in the late Yuan for a Chinese literati audience, listed seven varieties of *keshui* 渴水, the book's translation of *shelibai* or sherbet.[98] While the *Correct Essence* called for sugar to be mixed with fruit, the *Guide* suggested the use of honey. The difference was probably a reflection of the fact that refined sugar was a precious commodity at this time. As we will see below, Zhu Zhenheng deplored the popularity of this drink as he saw problems, rather than benefits, with sugar intake.

Chinese doctors in the Mongol empire

After the Yuan conquest of South China, doctors in North and South China were placed in an environment different from their predecessors'. Printing continued to flourish and doctors were now free to travel between North and South China. The Yuan government adopted the *Comprehensive Record of Sagely Benefaction* as the primary textbook for medical schools and supported publications of other medical texts. Commercial presses saw medicine as a profit-making genre, publishing books written by of contemporary and earlier times. Doctors now saw and heard about treatments from West Asia. In this context, the Yuan doctors had a larger pool of theories and treatments to choose from.

Recent studies have shown that publishing culture continued to flourish in the Yuan period, especially from the early fourteenth century. Miya Noriko points to a Yuan picture of a street vendor (*huolang tu* 貨郎圖) and Song pictures of vendors as some illuminating examples. While the Song vendor carts did not carry any books, the Yuan cart carried quite a few, suggesting that printed texts became more accessible to readers by the Yuan.[99] She also mentions that mid-Ming literatus Lu Rong 陸容 (1436–94) pointed to the vigor of the Yuan publishing culture and made suggestions as to how publishing systems in his time should be improved to return to the Yuan level.[100] According to Inoue Susumu, *The Catalog of Ancient Rare Books in China* (*Zhongguo guji shanben shumu* 中國古籍善本書目) lists an average of 43.2 extant Southern Song books per decade, 45.2 Yuan books, and 44.1 early Ming books.[101] Although it is hard to determine how many books were printed by using numbers of currently extant books, Inoue's data is intriguing because normally the earlier a time period is, the less likely books from the period remain preserved. More books appear to have been printed in the Yuan than in early Ming, if not than in Southern Song.

Moreover, the percentage of medical books vis-à-vis the total extant books increased from the Song to the Yuan. According to Lucille Chia, 8.6 percent of the Yuan imprints from the Jianyang 建陽 publishers were medical texts as opposed to 4.7 percent of the Song equivalent.[102] Other historians have also noted that medical books were a more visible genre in the Yuan than in the Song.[103] Kosoto Hiroshi has identified twenty-eight extant books written by Yuan doctors.[104] In addition, books written by authors of previous dynasties, including unpublished manuscripts of the Jin doctors as mentioned above, were printed in the Yuan.

The development of medical institutions and increased support for doctors in the Yuan contributed to the publication of medical books. The *Comprehensive Record of Sagely Benefaction*, the book that was commissioned by Emperor Huizong of the Northern Song and taken by the Jurchens, came to be designated as a textbook for the Yuan medical schools and was reprinted in 1300.[105] When an examination system to recruit members of the Yuan Imperial Academy of Medicine was approved in 1307, the examinees had to be familiar with the *Comprehensive Record*, among a few other classics.[106] Some local medical schools and the Temples of the Three Progenitors kept copies of this book.[107] The continued operation of the Charitable Pharmacies produced as many as seven Yuan imprints of the prescription book, *Taiping-Era Formulary for Charitable Bureau of Compounding Medicine* (*Taiping Huimin Heji ju fang* 太平惠民和劑局方).[108]

Wei Yilin's *Effective Pharmaceutical Recipies by a Hereditary Physician* (*Shiyi dexiao fang*) gives us a window onto how the Imperial Academy of Medicine printed Yuan authors' books. Born into a family that had produced a large number of doctors in Nanfeng prefecture, Wei Yilin first served as the associate professor of the prefecture's medical school and then later the associate superintendent of physicians. He collected recipes used by the doctors in his family and organized them according to the thirteen subjects, as adopted in the medical schools. Upon completion of the book, the medical school professor of Nanfeng recommended this book to the regional Superintendency of Physicians, who in turn recommended it to the Academy.[109] This process was similar to the way books on Confucianism such as Cheng Fuxin's 程復心 *Illustrated Chapters of the Four Books* (*Sishu zhang tu* 四書章圖) were printed by the Hanlin Academy.[110]

Thanks to the unification of China, Ge Yinglei 葛應雷 (1264–1323) in Pinjiang circuit 平江路 (present-day Suzhou) had not only access to Jin doctors' books but also opportunities to converse with Mr. Li 李, a doctor and official originally from the north. According to his biographer, Ge was well read in *Huangdi's Inner Classic*, used the *yunqi* system to understand patients' conditions, and adopted treatments different from the ones other doctors used in the south. One day when Mr. Li's father was ill, he asked Ge's opinion. Mr. Li and his father were surprised that they could find a learned doctor like Ge in the south. They shared with Ge all the books of Liu Wansu and Zhang Yuansu that they owned. They could not find any topics on which Ge and the Jin doctors disagreed. So, the story goes, this was how Liu's and Zhang's learning started to be spread in South China. Ge became the professor of Pingjiang medical school in 1306 and later served in the Superintendency of Physicians in the Jiangzhe 江浙 area. His son was a good friend of Zhu Zhenheng.[111] Because Ge's biographer did not record the content of the conversation between him and Li and because Ge's book is no longer extant, we have no way of knowing the true commonalities and differences between Ge's and the Jin doctors' theories. This story suggests, however, that doctors in the north and the south benefited from the fact that they were the inheritors of the Northern Song legacies. They at least had the language of the medical classics to initiate a dialogue. However, the following example of Zhu Zhenheng (1282–1358), the last of the Four Masters of Jin-Yuan medicine, shows that his relationship to Jin medicine was far more complex than what we can learn from Ge Yinling's story.

Zhu Zhenheng

Zhu Zhenheng was exposed to a broad spectrum of medical theories and treatments, thanks to the Mongol empire. He was born into an elite family in Yiwu county 義烏縣 in Wuzhou circuit 婺州路 (in present-day Zhejiang province). While his early education apparently was focused on Confucian texts, he began studying medicine on his own when he was 30 *sui* in 1310. He read *Basic Questions* for five years until he was finally able to cure his mother's illness. In 1316, he began studying with Xu Qian 許謙 (1270–1337), one of the leading Neo-Confucian scholars of the time. Because of Xu's encouragement and his own two unsuccessful attempts to pass the newly reinstated civil service examinations, Zhu decided to focus on medicine when he was 40 *sui* in 1323.[112]

In addition to the *Basic Questions*, Zhu read the *Formulary for the Charitable Pharmacies* as he began studying medicine. Dissatisfied with "theories without formula and formula without theories," he soon became attracted to the works of the doctors from the north. While in his hometown, he gained access to Zhang Zihe's book and adopted the latter's aggressive treatments. Zhu, however, soon discovered the discrepancy between Zhang's book and the *Basic Questions*. He began traveling in search of a good teacher, but he could not find any in the neighboring prefectures. He found Liu Wansu's *Original Forms of Illness in the Obscurity of the "Basic Questions"* and the manuscript of Li Gao's prescriptions in Dingcheng 定城 in present-day Henan province, just south of Wei River.[113]

Upon hearing that Luo Zhiti 羅知悌 was an excellent doctor, Zhu visited him in Hangzhou 杭州 in 1325. Luo had studied with Liu Wansu's disciple, a Buddhist monk called Jingshan futu 荊山浮屠, in Daidu. Having been a eunuch in the Southern Song court, Luo had been taken to the Yuan capital. After initial hesitation, Luo took Zhu as an apprentice and soon became reliant on him. When a patient came in, Zhu would take his pulse and report it to Luo. Lying down, Luo would listen to Zhu, give him instructions on which drugs to use, and explain the reasons why. Zhu discovered that Luo's prescriptions were never the same during the year and a half they worked together. One day Luo compared curing present illnesses with past formulas to tearing down an old house and inserting the pieces into a new house. The materials were not exactly the same, and a good carpenter was absolutely necessary. To become a good carpenter of medicine, Zhu studied Li Gao's manuscripts by copying them by hand.[114] The act of copying a book by one's own hand was considered an important method of learning. After Luo's death in 1327, Zhu went back to his hometown to practice medicine. Twenty years later, when he was in his seventies, he wrote seven books, three of which are extant: *Further Views on Extending Knowledge* (*Gezhi yulun* 格致餘論), *Expounding the Formulary for the Charitable Pharmacies* (*Jufang fahui* 局方發揮), and *Supplement to Extending the Meanings for Materia Medica* (*Bencao yanyi buyi* 本草衍義補遺).[115]

Zhu's main contribution was that he synthesized Liu Wansu's and Li Gao's seemingly competing theories. On the one hand, Liu had considered that Fire was the dominant circulatory phase in the cosmos, directly affecting the human body and causing the body to shake, feel dizzy, have fever, etc., and thus believed that patients should take medicines with cooling effects. On the other hand, Li Gao had not thought cosmological Fire could affect humans so directly; he had thought illnesses occurred when the Original *Qi* was depleted, allowing the Fire in the human body to flare up. Thus, Li had maintained that doctors should give medicines that would replenish the *qi*. To fuse the two theories, Zhu elaborated on the discussion of cosmology to differentiate the cases when Liu's or Li's treatment strategies were applicable. He said that Heaven, which created the *yang qi*, was larger than Earth, producer of *yin qi*, because in the cosmological understanding of the time, the former wrapped up the latter. Thus, Zhu argued that *yang qi* tended to be superabundant and *yin qi* insufficient (*yang youyu yin buzu* 陽有餘陰不足). Cosmological *yang qi* created the *qi* in the human body and cosmological *yin* created Blood. To continue Zhu's explanation, Blood increased and decreased in a human's life, just as the moon waxed and waned. The young and the old had less Blood, while mature adults with the ability to reproduce had more. Also, the seasons, eating habits, sexual behaviors, and many other factors affected how much *yin* the patient had. While Liu's aggressive strategy might work for adults who did not suffer from the depletion of *yin qi*, Li's strategy to replenish the Original *Qi* needed to be adopted in other cases. A doctor should keep a keen eye on the level of the patient's *yin qi* as he tailored prescriptions on an individual basis.[116]

As a disciple of an eminent *Daoxue* (Learning of the Way) scholar, Zhu Zhenheng showed to other *Daoxue* followers that his medical theory would help them achieve their Way. He entitled his book *Gezhi yulun* (*Further Views on Extending Knowledge*). *Gezhi* 格致 (extending knowledge) is a short form of *gewu zhizhi* 格物致知 (investigation of things and extending knowledge), a basic tenet of the Learning of the Way. He started the preface of his book by saying:

> The *Basic Questions* is a book that records the Way. The words [in the book] are simple, but their meanings are profound. However, as [the time] went farther from the ancient times, there seem to have been errors in characters and sentences. That is why only we Confucians can read it.

While Liu Wansu's preface to his *Profound Principle* discussed earlier in this chapter had presented the *Basic Questions* as a book that would integrate Daoism, Confucianism, and medicine, Zhu argued that the *Basic Questions* was a book for Confucian scholars. "The Preface to Warning Poems on Drinking and Eating and on Sexual Desire" (*Yinshi seyu zhen xu* 飲食色欲箴序) in his *Further Views* starts with a citation from one of the Confucian classics, the *Book of Rites* (*Li ji*), "A person's great desire lies in eating, drinking, and sexual desires."[117] The poems made references to the *Book of Changes*, the *Book of Poems*, *Analects*, the *Doctrine of the Mean*, *Mencius*, and the *Basic Questions*. He also cited writings by Neo-Confucian scholars such as Lü Dalin 呂大臨 (eleventh century) and Zhu Xi but no books associated with other religions.[118]

As Charlotte Furth's excellent study has shown, Zhu linked the medical concepts of managing Sovereign Fire (*junhuo* 君火) and Ministerial Fires (*xianghuo* 相火) to the *Daoxue* concept of "mastering the heart" (*xiuxin* 脩心) or "correcting the heart" (*zhengxin* 正心). The primary characteristics of Fire, as Zhu understood, was the fact that it moved. The Sovereign Fire was located in the heart, which in his and his contemporaries' view, oversaw consciousness. The Ministerial Fires were hidden in the kidney and the liver. If one was overly sexually active, the water in the kidney depleted and the Ministerial Fire there took over, following the "cycle of mutual generation of the Five Phases" (*wuxing xiangsheng* 五行相生), a central doctrine in Chinese cosmology and systems of correspondence medicine. If one over-ate, his stomach (categorized as Earth in the *Basic Questions*) weakened, activating its rival liver (categorized Wood), following the "overcoming cycle of the Five Phases" (*wuxing xiangsheng* 五行相克), another doctrine in the systems of correspondence. Then the Wood fed the Ministerial Fire in the liver. Whether in the kidney or liver, the overactive Ministerial Fire provoked the Sovereign Fire in the heart, resulting in emotional instability and mistaken judgments. Thus, Zhu Zhenheng argued, if one were to master the heart, or to stay calm, one should regulate sexual and eating habits.[119]

As Zhu synthesized the medical theories developed in North China and *Daoxue* concepts of the body and cosmology, he was critical of the *Formulary for the Charitable Pharmacies*, which was particularly popular in the south. At the beginning of his *Expounding the Formulary for the Charitable Pharmacies*, Zhu made cynical comments: if people read the *Formulary for the Charitable Pharmacies*, "they would not need doctors and would not need to create formulas." He continued by saying that if one took a medicine recorded in this book, all pain would be gone. Thus, he commented, "we can say that [the government's] benevolence for the people has reached the highest level!" He was critical of the Pharmacy's approach for two reasons. First, he thought curing illnesses was a much more complex process than it assumed. Second, he was opposed to the book's overuse of medicines categorized as hot and humid.[120]

Zhu's criticism toward the Pharmacy's approaches meant that he was critical of the Southern Song medical legacy, which had been heavily influenced by the *Formulary for the Charitable Pharmacies*. Even Chen Yan, an early Southern Song theoretician who had written *Prescriptions Elucidated on the Premise That*

All Pathological Symptoms Have Only Three Primary Causes, did not satisfy Zhu. In his discussion of the Ministerial Fire (*xianghuo*), a concept found in the *Basic Questions*, Zhu said:

> Even though Chen Wuze (Chen Yan) was well versed and intelligent, he discussed Sovereign Fire as burning warmth and the Ministerial Fire as daily consumed fire, not going into depth. It is no wonder later generations have been blind and deaf. How sad![121]

In contrast, he showed clear respect to Li Gao, Zhang Zihe, and Liu Wansu's interpretations of the Ministerial Fire, by analyzing thoroughly and thinking how the strengths of their ideas could be incorporated into his theory. A modern historian, Liu Shijue, says:

> Although Chen Wuze's theory of the three primary causes was an innovative attempt, it was distant from practice. He focused on categorizing illnesses, and these categories cannot be considered accurate. His instructions for clinical methods, prescriptions, and the uses of individual drugs were not coherent, either.[122]

Liu aptly captured the perception that Zhu Zhenheng and his followers had toward the Southern Song legacies. As a result of their condescending attitudes, many of the medical books produced in the Southern Song were lost in China and are extant only because they were preserved in Japanese private libraries.[123]

Zhu Zhenheng incorporated pharmacological achievements in North China into his *Supplement to Extending the Meanings for Materia Medica* (*Bencao yanyi buyi* 本草衍義補遺). Even though the title of the book sounds as if it was a simple supplement to Kou Zongxi's *Extending Meanings for Materia Medica* written in the late Northern Song period, Zhu often made rather drastic revisions to the content. In particular, Wang Haogu's influence is obvious. He sometimes mentioned Wang by his *hao*, Haicang 海藏, and he sometimes just copied Wang's words without mentioning him. For example, while the "Ginseng" (*renshen* 人參) section of the Northern Song original discussed mostly the difference in quality depending on where ginseng came from, Zhu's section on the drug identified the channel that it was supposed to enter (Hand Lesser Yin; *shou taiyin* 手太陰), as Wang did, and the herb that would work against ginseng if taken together (*lilu* 梨蘆).[124] Also, earlier in this chapter, we saw what the "Water-plantain (*zexie*)" section in Kou's *Extending Meanings* says. Before citing a portion of it, Zhu stated that the drug was "subtle *yang* in *yin* (*yinzhong weiyang* 陰中微陽)" and that it entered the Foot Great *Yang* (*zhu taiyang* 足太陽) and Lesser Yin (*shouyin* 少陰) Channels, following Wang Hao's *Materia Medica of Drugs Used for Decoction Medications*.[125]

In addition to medicine in North China, the Mongol empire exposed Zhu to treatments originating outside of China, and he was open to them. In fact, even before he traveled north to master the theories of Jin doctors, he had adopted a treatment called the "Toppling Granary Method" (*Daocang fa* 倒倉法), which originated from "an extraordinary person of the Western regions" (*xiyu zhi yiren* 西域之異人). He used it to cure his teacher in Confucianism, Xu Qian, who had developed heart and leg pains after he took wrongly prescribed medicines for heart problems. To administer the "Toppling Granary Method," a physician would first have bull's meat boiled in river water until it dissolved into the broth. Then he would have the dregs taken out and simmer the broth until it was amber colored. He would have the patient drink this broth in a large quantity until the latter vomited or had diarrhea. The goal was to clean up all the "flotsam and old rotten substances" in the entire body.[126] In classical Chinese, the term "Western regions" (*xiyu* 西域) meant regions west of Yumen Pass, sometimes referring to the area around Xinjiang and sometimes covering Central and West Asia, India, Eastern Europe, and North Africa.

Zhu, however, was selective in adopting foreign treatments or drugs, just as he was about medical theories and treatments developed in the Jin and the Southern Song. He was critical of West Asia's electuary sherbet, despite its popularity. He argued that sherbet tasted sweet and wonderful but its nature was not harmonious (*zhonghe* 中和). For example, he believed that kumquat sherbet decreased urine, while apricot, cherry, and peach sherbets ignited the stomach Fire. He went as far as to say that these drinks would "commit a crime while smiling pleasantly" (*xixiao zuozui* 嬉笑作罪).[127]

Certainly, Zhu did not have the linguistic abilities or educational opportunities to learn the Galenian medical theory behind West Asian and European medical practice. Thus, despite their foreign origin, he explained the efficacy of foreign treatments, such as the "Toppling Granary Method," by Chinese concepts. Explaining why soup made of a meat taken from a yellow bull was good for the human body, he cited the *Book of Changes* (*Yijing* 易經) as follows:

> Cattle are [ascribed to] "Earth" (*kun* 坤) [according to the *Book of Changes*] and yellow is the color of earth. [Cattle] have the virtue of docility (*shun* 順). Following the rules of the activeness (*jian* 健) [which is "Heaven," or *qian* 乾, according to the *Book of Changes*] and showing the effect are the functions of the bulls.[128]

In other words, Zhu reasoned that the bull soup had a soothing effect because cattle had a quality of docility, or calmness, while the maleness, or *yang*, of the bull made it active. Even though Zhu understood the efficacy of drugs and treatments in Chinese terms, the fact that he chose this method to cure the Confucian teacher whom he respected most, instead of other treatments available in medical practice in South China, exemplified the global perspectives that the Mongols' unification of China and much of the Eurasian continent enabled Zhu and other Yuan doctors to have.

Conclusion

This chapter has demonstrated that medical theories went through transformations from the Northern Song to the Yuan period and that the Mongol conquest of China played important roles. First, the unification of China tore down the so-called Iron Curtain between the Jin and Southern Song and let the cultural legacies of the two regions interact with each other. The history of the *Comprehensive Record of Sagely Benefaction* represented the blockage of information during the Jin–Southern Song period and its circulation in the Yuan period. Second, the Mongols' occupations of northern cities and the resulting sufferings of the residents prompted Li Gao (1180–1251) to focus on illnesses caused by abnormal human behaviors rather than the cosmological influences that his Jin predecessors had paid attention to. Third, the Mongols' active recruitment of physicians into the military and government gave Li Gao's disciple, Luo Tianyi, opportunities to interact with medical practitioners from other areas, test Li's theories, and eventually to publish his book. Finally, Mongols' establishment of the Eurasian empire promoted medical exchanges between China and other parts of the world. West Asians built medical institutions that provided services in the Yuan capital. Leading doctors of the time, Ge Yinglei and Zhu Yuanzheng, in South China were eager to learn from medical traditions in North China and non-Chinese regions.

This chapter also traced the process through which the medical innovations that started out in the Northern Song and developed under the Jurchens merged with the increasingly popular intellectual movement in South China, the Learning of the Way, and the resultant trend to associate doctors with Confucian learning. Although the term "Confucian doctor" had been coined by the late Northern Song, the Jin doctors and their biographers were not as interested in connecting the medical profession and Confucianism. Liu Wansu, for example, aimed at combining Confucian, Daoist, and medical learning, and his friend and biographer Cheng Daoji associated him with Daoism rather than Confucianism. As we have seen in Chapter 5, Yuan Haowen, a famous Jin poet, depicted his friend and doctor Li Gao as a sophisticated literatus with abilities to use elegant metaphors, while Yan Jian, a great-grandson of Zhu Xi, presented Li as a devoted Confucian scholar. Although Zhang Zihe supposedly wrote a medical book titled *Confucians Serving Parents*, the title might have been a post-Jin invention. Zhu Zhenheng was different from the three other "Jin-Yuan Masters of Medicine" because Zhu was born and raised in South China. In his case, he had established a clear sense of self-identity as a *Daoxue* scholar before he took up medicine. He was eager to show that medical theories developed in North China as he synthesized them would help Neo-Confucians achieve the Way.

Notes

1 *Qingrong*, 44.18b.
2 *Qingrong*, 44.19a–b.
3 Kosoto Hiroshi, "Hoku-Sōdai no iyaku sho, sono 1," *Gendai Tōyō igaku*, 9.1 (1988): 86.
4 Okanishi Tameto, "Chūgoku honzō no dentō," in *Sō-Gen jidai no kagaku gijutsu shi*, ed. Yabuuchi Kiyoshi (Kyoto: Kyōtō daigaku jinbun kagaku kenkyūjo, 1967), 207–08.
5 Okanishi Tameto, *Chūgoku isho honzō kō*, cited in Kosoto, "Hoku-Sōdai no iyaku sho, sono 1," 86.
6 Catherine Despeux, "The System of the Five Circulatory Phases and the Six Seasonal Influences (*wuyun liuqi*), a Source of Innovation in Medicine Under the Song (960–1279)," in *Innovation in Chinese Medicine*, ed. Elizabeth Hsu, 122.

7   Despeux, "The System," in particular 130–34.
8   Tuotuo, *Songshi*, 157.3689. Despeux, "The System," 122 footnote 2, quotes this part of *Songshi* to argue that the medical school examinations began asking questions regarding the *yunqi* system when the school was built in 1076. But I disagree with her interpretation. In my view, *Songshi*, 157.3689 shows that the medical school went through two stages. When it was first established during Emperor Shengzong's 神宗 reign (1067–84), the instructors taught three different subjects: sphygmology (*fangmai ke* 方脈科), acupuncture (*zhen ke* 鍼科), and ulcers (*yang ke* 瘍科). The examinations in the spring were optional. The textbooks for each subject are mentioned but not the examination questions. Then the medical school was reformed during the Chongning era (1102–06). Now the Three Hall system for medical schools was implemented, and the students had to take examinations to move from one hall to the next hall. This was when, according to *Songshi*, the examiners asked questions regarding the general essence of the *yunqi* system.
9   Kosoto Hiroshi, "Hoku-Sōdai no iyaku sho, sono 2," *Gendai Tōyō igaku* 8.4 (1987): 93–95.
10 Kosoto Hiroshi, *Chūgoku igaku koten to Nihon: shoshi to denshō* (Tokyo: Hanawa shobō, 1996), 267–71.
11 Asaf Goldschmidt, *The Evolution of Chinese Medicine* (London: Routledge, 2009), 73, Table 3.1.
12 See, for example, Inoue Susumu, *Chūgoku shuppan bunka shi: shomotsu sekai to chi no fūkei* (Nagoya: Nagoya daigaku shuppankai, 2002), 106–11; Ming-sun Poon, "Books and Printing in Sung China (960–1279)" (Ph.D. diss., University of Chicago, 1979), 113–27; Lucille Chia and Hilde de Weerdt's introduction to their *Knowledge and Text Production in the Age of Print: China, 900–1400* (Leiden: Brill, 2011), in particular 9–13.
13 Miyashita Saburō, "Sō-Gen no iryō," in *Sō-Gen jidai no kagaku gijutsu shi*, ed. Yabuuchi Kiyoshi (Kyoto: Kyoto daigaku jinbun kagaku kenkyūjo, 1967), 124–34; Despeux, "The System," 143–47; and Goldschmidt, *The Evolution of Chinese Medicine*, Chapter 3, in particular Table 3.3.
14 Despeux, "The System," 146; and T.J. Hinrich, "The Song and Jin Periods," in *Chinese Medicine and Healing: An Illustrated History*, ed. T.J. Hinrichs and Linda L. Barnes (Cambridge, MA: Harvard University Press, 2013), 108–15. Also see, Hinrich, "Governance Through Medical Texts and the Role of Print," in Chia and de Weerdt, *Knowledge and Text Production*, 217–38.
15 Pang Anshi, *Shanghan zongbin lun* (Beijing: Renmin weisheng chubanshe, 1989), 3.94.
16 Ishida Hidemi, *Chūgoku igaku shisō shi: mōhitotsu no igaku* (Tokyo: Tokyo daigaku shuppankai, 1992), 253–55, and Fan Xingzhun, *Zhongguo yixueshi lüe* (Beijing: Zhongyi guji chubanshe, 1986), 241.
17 For an excellent discussion on the difficulty of identifying bubonic plagues in pre-19th-century China, see Carol Benedict, *Bubonic Plague in Nineteenth-Century China* (Stanford, CA: Stanford University Press, 1996), 7–11.
18 Kou Zongshi, *Bencao yanyi* (Beijing: Renmin weisheng chubanshe, 1990), 7:46–47. Wuling san 五苓散 appears in "Bian Taiyang bing maizheng bing zhi 辨太陽病脈證并治" section in Shanghan lun; and Bawei wan 八味丸 in "Zhongfeng lijiebing maizheng bing zhi" 中風歷節病脈證并治 section of Jinkui yaolüe 金匱要略. See Zhang Ji, *Shanghan lun jiaozhu*, ed. Liu Duzhou (Beijing: Renmin weisheng chubanshe, 1990), 3: 89–91; and Zhang Ji, *Jinkui yaolüe jiaozhu*, ed. He Ren (Beijing: Renmin weisheng chubanshe, 1990), *shang*.56.
19 *Bencao jing jizhu*, comp. Tao Hongjing, Kojima Shōshin, Mori Tatsuyuki, and Okanishi Tameto (Ōsaka: Minami Ōsaka insatu sentā, 1972), 7.120.
20 See Endō Jirō, Nakamura Teruko, Mayanagi Makoto, and Kubodera Takako, "Inkei hōshi setsu no shiteki kentō: kikei, inkei, tsūkei, gyōkei no igi," *Yakushigaku zasshi*, 32.2 (1997): 169–77, for the history of "Guiding Channels."

21 Kosoto,"Hoku-Sōdai no iyaku sho, sono 2," 93–95.
22 Yoshikawa Kōjirō, "Shushigaku hokuden zenshi," in *Uno Tetsuto sensei hakuju shukuga kinen Tōyōgaku ronsō*, ed. Uno Tetsuto hakuju shukuga kinenkai (Tokyo: Uno Tetsujin hakuju shukuga kinenkai, 1974), 1237–58.
23 Tuotuo et al., *Jinshi*, 50.1113–15. For a detailed discussion on the monopoly markets, see Sotoyama Gunji, *Kinchōshi Kenkyū* (Kyoto: Tōyōshi kenkyūkai, 1964), 384–87.
24 Yoshikawa, "Shushigaku hokuden zenshi," 1243; Hoyt Cleveland Tillman, "Confucianism under the Chin and the Impact of Sung Confucian Tao-Hsüeh," in *China under the Jurchen Rule: Essays on Chin Intellectual and Cultural History*, ed. Hoyt Cleveland Tillman and Stephen H. West (Albany: State University of New York Press, 1995), 72.
25 Li Yuqing and Goldschmidt argue that Cheng's birth year was between 1044 and 1052, earlier than the conventional understanding which puts it in the 1060s. Li's and Goldschmidt's basis is Wang Ding's 1172 preface to the *Annotations to the Treatise on Cold Damage Disorders*. Wang says that he met Cheng when he was over 90 *sui*, and 17 years later someone else brought Wang a copy of the book. Scholars prior to Li thought the book was published immediately after Wang received the copy and thus calculated that Cheng must have been born in the early 1060s. However, as Li correctly points out, Wang's postscript says that it took him *yuji* 逾紀 to find means to print it. Li understands the word *yuji* literally and argues that it must have been more than 12 years prior to the conventionally assumed birth year. See Li Yuqing, "Cheng Wuji shengping ji *Zhujie Shanghanlu xuanzhu* niandai kao," *Zhonghua yishi zazhi* 27.4 (Oct. 1997), 250; Goldschmidt, *The Evolution of Chinese Medicine*, 168; and Zhang Jinwu, *Airi jinglu cangshu zhi*, in *Qian Zunwang Dushu minqiuji jiaozheng, Airi jinglu canshu zhi* (Beijing: Zhonghua shuju, 1990), 22.4b–5a. I think the word *yuji* might have simply meant "a long time" rather than strictly "more than 12 years" because the Sibu congkan database shows that contemporary sources used expressions like *leinian yuji* 累年逾紀 to refer to a good length of time.
26 See Mayanagi Makoto, "*Shōkan meiri ron, Shōkan meiri yakuhō ron* kaidai," http://mayanagi.hum.ibaraki.ac.jp/paper01/meirironkaidai.html, originally published in *Somon nyushiki unki ron'ō, Shōkan meiri ron, Shōkan meiri yakuhō ron, Shōni yakushō chokketsu, San'in kyokuitsu byōshō hōron*, WKIS, vol. 1 (1988). Mayanagi and Kosoto, "Kindai no iyaku sho, sono 1," *Gendai Tōyō igaku* 10.3 (1989): 101–07. Zhang Jinwu, *Airi jinglu cangshu zhi*, 22.4b–5a.
27 Goldschmidt, *The Evolution of Chinese Medicine*, 171.
28 For the contributions of Han Zhihe, Pang Anshi, and Zhu Gong, see Han Zhihe, *Shanghan weizhi lun*, SKQS; Zhu Gong and Pang Anshi, *Zhu Gong Pang Anshi yixue quanshu* (Beijing: Zhongguo Zhongyiyao chubanshe, 2006); Kosoto, "Hoku-Sōdai no iyaku sho, sono 1," 87–88; Kosoto, "Hoku-Sōdai no iyaku sho, sono 2," 88–90; and Goldschmidt, *The Evolution of Chinese Medicine*, 153–63. For Cheng Wuji, see his *Cheng Wuji yixue quanshu* (Beijing: Zhongguo Zhong yiyao chubanshe, 2004); Okanishi, "Chūgoku honzō no dentō to Kin-Gen no honzō," 204–05. According to Mayanagi, Cheng's *Clarifying the Principles of the "Treatise of Cold Damage Disorders"* cites the *Inner Classic* 138 times; see his "*Chūkai Shōkan ron* kaidai," http://mayanagi.hum.ibaraki.ac.jp/paper01/chukai.html, originally published in *Shōkan ron kōjōben, Chūkai Shōkan ron, Chūkei zensho*,WKIS, vol. 16 (1992).
29 Cheng Wuji's preface to his *Shanghan mingli yaofang*, in his *Cheng Wuji yixue quanshu*, 154. Okanishi, "Chūgoku honzō no dentō to Kin-Gen no honzō," 204–05.
30 Despeux, "The System," 132–33. Okanishi, "Chūgoku honzō no dentō to Kin-Gen no honzō," 204–05. Liu Wenshu, "Zhifa lun 治法論," in *Suwen rushi yunqi lun'ao*, SKQS, *xia*.27b–32a.
31 Cheng Wuji, *Shanghan mingli yaofang*, in his *Cheng Wuji yixue quanshu*, 182.
32 Cheng Daoji's preface to Liu Wansu's *Suwen xuanji yuanbing shi*, in Tanba Mototane, *Chūgoku iseki kō*, 648–49.

33 Cheng, preface to Liu, *Suwen xuanji yuanbing shi*, in Tanba, *Chūgoku iseki kō*, 648–49.

34 I thank Liao Chao-Heng 廖肇亨 and Hsieh Shu-Wei 謝世維 for drawing my attention to the relation between drinking and Daoist revelation (personal communication, summer 2007). Cheng Yajun, *Jin-Yuan sida yijia yu daojia daojiao* (Chengdu: Bashu shushe, 2006), cites this episode as a piece of evidence that Liu Wansu was a pure Daoist doctor (*chunzheng daoyi* 纯正道医), but he does not consider Liu's intention to integrate Daoism, Confucianism, and medicine.

35 Liu Wansu, *Liu Wansu yixue quanshu* (Beijing: Zhongguo Zhong yiyao chubanshe, 2006), 81.

36 Miura Shūichi, *Chūgoku shingaku no ryōsen: Genchō no chishikijin to Ju Dō Butsu sankyō* (Tokyo: Kenbun shuppansha, 2003), esp. 51–57.

37 Okuno Shigeo, "Ryū Kanso to *Seizan gunsen kaishin ki*," *Tōhō shūkyō* 121 (2013): 24–44.

38 Mayanagi, "*Somon genki genbyō shiki, Kōtei Somon senmei ron* kaidai." http://mayanagi.hum.ibaraki.ac.jp/paper01/liuwansu.html, originally published in *Fusai honji hō, Fusai Honji hō zokushū, Jumon jishin, Somon genki genbyō shiki, senmeiron hō*, WKIS, vol. 2 (1988). Mayanagi and Kosoto, "Kindai no iyaku sho, sono 2 *Gendai Tōyō igaku* 10.4 (1989): 105–12.

39 See, for example, Paul Unschuld, *Medicine in China: A History of Ideas* (Berkeley: University of California Press, 1985), 172–73; Ishida Hidemi, *Chūgoku igaku shisō shi: mōhitotsu no igaku* (Tokyo: Tokyo daigaku shuppan kai, 1992), 260–61; Mayanagi, "*Somon genki genbyō shiki, Kōtei Somon senmei ron* kaidai"; and Song Naiguang et al., "Liu Wansu yixue xueshu sixiang yanjiu," in Liu Wansu, *Liu Wansu yixue quanshu*, 315–16. The most thorough discussion of Liu's theory can be found in Ding Guangdi, *Jin-Yuan yixue pingxi* (Beijing: Renmin weisheng chubanshe, 1999), 100–43.

40 Liu Wansu, *Suwen bingji qiyi baoming ji*, shang.127–28 and xia.169 in *Liu Wansu yixue quanshu*. Also see Okanishi, "Chūgoku honzō no dentō to Kin-Gen no honzō," 205–07.

41 Mayanagi and Kosoto, "Kindai no iyaku sho, sono 2."

42 Zhang Yuansu, *Yixue qiyuan*, zhong.29 in *Zhang Yuansu yixue quanshu* (Beijing: Zhongguo Zhong yiyao chubanshe, 2006) and Liu Wansu, *Suwen xuanji yuanbing shi*, 88 in *Liu Wansu yixue quanshu*.

43 Zhang Yuansu, *Yixue qiyuan*, p. 12.

44 Zhang Yuansu, *Yixue qiyuan*, xia.48.

45 Ishida Hidemi, Shimada Ryūji, Shōji Yoshifumi, Suzuki Hiroshi, Fujiyama Kazuko et al. trans., *Gendai go yaku Kōtei daikei somon (jō)* (Chiba: Tōyōgaku shuppansha, 1991), 103.

46 Zhang Yuansu, *Zhenzhu nang*, 67 and 68 in *Zhang Yuansu yixue quanshu*.

47 Okanishi, "Chūgoku honzō no dentō to Kin-Gen no honzō," 194.

48 Tuotuo, *Jinshi*, 131.2812.

49 Mayanagi Makoto, "*Jumon jishin* kaidai," http://mayanagi.hum.ibaraki.ac.jp/paper01/jumonjishin.html, originally published in *Fusai honji hō, Fusai Honji hō zokushū, Jumon jishin, Somon genki genbyō shiki, senmeiron hō*, WKIS, vol. 2 (1988). Also, Mayanagi and Kosoto, "Kindai no iyaku sho, sono 3, *Gendai Tōyō igaku* 11.1 (1990): 108–13.

50 Mayanagi and Kosoto, "Kindai no iyaku sho, sono 4, *Gendai Tōyō igaku* 11.2 (1990): 99–105; and Mayanagi, "*Naigaishō benwaku ron, Hi'i ron, Ranshitu hizō* kaidai," http://mayanagi.hum.ibaraki.ac.jp/paper01/toenkaidai.html, originally published in *Myakketsu, Naigaishō benwaku ron, Hi'i ron, Ranshitu hizō, Tōeki honzō, Shiji nanchi, Kakuchi yoron, Kyokuhō hakki, Geka seigi, Ikei sokai shū*, WKIS, vol. 6 (1989). Also see Ding Guangdi, *Jin-Yuan yixue pingxi*, 192.

51 Li Gao, *Neiwaishang bianhuo lun*, in *Li Dongyuan yixue quanshu* 1–26 (Beijing: Zhongguo Zhongyi chubanshe, 2006), shang.6–7; Tuotuo, *Jinshi*, 17.386–87. Also see Sotoyama, *Kinchōshi kenkyū*, 52–55, for the summary of the process that led to the fall of the Jin dynasty.

Discrediting Li Gao's observation that the large number of Kaifeng residents died due to the use of strong and poisonous drugs like Purging Croton (*badou*), Fan Xingzhun and Robert Hymes have argued that *Yersinia Pestis* might have caused so many deaths in 1232 Kaifeng. Fan pointed out that the symptoms of the illness at the time as described in another book, *Maijue zhizhang bingshi tushuo* 脉訣指掌病式图説, which might have been written by Li Gao, were likely those of pneumonic plague (Fan, *Zhongguo yixueshi lüe*, [Beijing: Zhongyi guji chubanshe, 1986], 163 and 188. See Mayanagi and Kosoto, "Kindai no iyakusho, sono 4," on the issues of the authorship of *Maijue zhizhang bingshi tushuo*). Hymes suggests that the fact that the illness was spread after the siege was raised might mean that the Mongol troops were the carriers of the bacterium (Hymes, "Epilogue: A Hypothesis on the East Asian Beginnings of the *Yersinia Pestis* Polytomy," *The Medieval Globe*, 1 [2014], in particular 289–91). Whereas Fan thought that the plague arrived in China earlier than the Mongol conquest (see the discussion of the possible case of the plague in Northern Song earlier in this chapter), Hymes is attempting to establish the direct causal relationship between the conquest and the plague. Paul Buell, "Qubilai and the Rats," *Sudhoffs Archiv* 96.2 (2012): 127–44 does not consider the 1232 Kaifeng case but analyzes other evidence to question the possibility that the plague existed in China during the Mongol era. Given the state of the field, it is too early for me to list the plague as the impact of Mongol conquest of China in this chapter.

52 On leaders and culture in Dongping, see Abe Takeo, "Gensho no chishiki jin to kakyo," in *Gendaishi no kenkyū* (Tokyo: Sōbunsha, 1972), 15–30.

53 Mayanagi and Kosoto, "Kindai no iyakusho, sono 2."

54 Mayanagi and Kosoto, "Kindai no iyakusho, sono 4." Mayanagi, *"Naigaishō benwaku ron, Hi'i ron, Ranshitu hizō* kaidai." Ding, *Jin-Yuan yixue pingxi*, pp. 200–07.

55 Some historians have argued that Wang studied with Zhang Yuansu because Wang calls him *xianshi* (Former Teacher); see Mayanagi Makoto, *"Tan'eki honzō, Shiji nanchi* kaidai," http://mayanagi.hum.ibaraki.ac.jp/paper01/okoko.html, originally published in *Myakketsu, Naigaishō benwaku ron, Hi'i ron, Ranshitu hizō, Tōeki honzō, Shiji nanchi, Kakuchi yoron, Kyokuhō hakki, Geka seigi, Ikei sokai shū*, WKIS, vol. 6 (1989). I think, however, that Wang was simply showing respect to him because the term *xianshi* could mean "respected sages, or role models", in the past.

56 Mayanagi,*"Tan'eki honzō, Shiji nanchi* kaidai."

57 Ulrike Unschuld, "Traditional Chinese Pharmacology: An Analysis of Its Development in the Thirteenth Century," *Isis* 68.2 (1977): 229–42; Paul Unschuld, *Medicine in China: A History of Pharmacology* (Berkeley: University of California Press, 1986), 108–17; Okanishi, "Chūgoku honzō no dentō to Kin-Gen no honzō," 196–202.

58 Okanishi, "Chūgoku honzō no dentō to Kin-Gen no honzō," 201–02.

59 Luo Tianyi, *Weisheng baojian*, in *Luo Tianyi yixue quanshu* (Beijing: Zhongguo Zhongyi chubanshe, 2006), 13.104.

60 For Dong Wenbing's biography, see Song Lian et al., *Yuanshi* (Beijing: Zhonghua shuju, 1976), 156.3667–76. For Luo's biography, see Kosoto, "Gendai no iyaku sho, sono 2," *Gendai Tōyō igaku* 11.4 (1990): 76–78. Luo often gave the exact place, time, patients' names, and/or the names of the doctors with whom he conversed. His activities recorded in the following pages of his *Weisheng baojian* took place during his career as a military doctor: 4.47 (1253), 13.112 (1253), 15.133 (1253), 6.59 (1254), 22.190 (1256), 22.190–91 (1256), 2.37 (1257), 13.108 (1257), 3.39–40 (1258), 13.109–10 (1258), 16.141–42 (1258), 22.191 (1258), and 12.100–01 (1259). "4.47 (1253)" here means the case is recorded on *juan* 4, page 47, and it took place in 1253.

61 The thirteen cases are recorded in Luo Tianyi, *Weisheng baojian*, 4.47–48, 5.56, 6.59, 12.100–01, 14.128, 15.133, 16.141–42, 16.144, 17.150, 22.190–91, and 24.198–99.

62 Luo Tianyi, *Weisheng baojian*, 22.189. As to the Mongols' diet, see William of Rubruck, *The Mission of Friar William of Rubruck*, trans. Peter Jackson, introduction,

notes, and appendices by Peter Jackson with David Morgan (London: The Hakluyt Society, 1990), 79. Also see Sorunguto Ba Jigmudo, *Mongoru igakushi*, trans. Ju Runga and Takenaka Ryōji (Tokyo: Nōsan Gyoson bunka kyōkai, 1991), 61–64 and 196–98.

63 Luo Tianyi, *Weisheng baojian*, 6.59.

64 Luo Tianyi, *Weisheng baojian*, 13.112–14, 14.120, and 20.177–78.

65 Luo Tianyi, *Weisheng baojian*, 4.42.

66 For the publication years of Li Gao's books, see Mayanagi and Kosoto, "Kindai no iyaku sho, sono 4" and Mayanagi, "*Naigaishō benwaku ron, Hi'i ron, Ranshitu hizō* kaidai." For the publication year of *Weisheng baojian*, see Kosoto, "Gendai no iyaku sho, sono 2," 76–78.

67 Mayanagi and Kosoto, "Kindai no iyaku sho, sono 1," "Kindai no iyaku sho, sono 2," "Kindai no iyaku sho, sono 3," and "Kindai no iyaku sho, sono 4."

68 Chao Gongwu, *Junzhai dushuzhi jiaozheng* (Shanghai: Shanghai guji chubanshe, 1990), 15:701–36.

69 Chen Zhensun, *Zhizhai shulu jieti* (Shanghai: Shanghai guji chubanshe, 1987). 13:382–98.

70 Tanba Mototane, *Chūgoku iseki kō*, 319–20. Also, see note no. 1 in Hasebe Eiichi, Shinno Reiko, Uemura Asami, Matsushita Michinobu, and Onda Hiromasa, Kakuchi yoron *chūshaku* (Tokyo: Iseisha, 2014), 145–46.

71 Mayanagi Makoto, "*Somon* hanpon kenkyū (sono 2)," *Kikan daikei*, 189 (2012): 31–42.

72 According to Inoue Susumu's calculation, it cost 75,000 *wen* to print a 100-page book in the early Ming. This amounts to the wage that a farm laborer would earn in ten years. See his *Chūgoku shuppan bunka shi*, 198–201.

73 Matsushita Michinobu, "Haku Gyokusen to sono shuppan katsudō: Zenshin kyō nanshū ni okeru shiju ishiki no kokufuku," *Tōhō shūkyō* 104 (2004): 23–42.

74 Charlotte Furth, "Producing Medical Knowledge through Cases: History, Evidence, and Action," in *Thinking with Cases: Specialist Knowledge in Chinese Cultural History*, ed. Charlotte Furth, Judith T. Zeitlin, and Ping-chen Hsiung (Honolulu: University of Hawai'i Press, 2007), 129.

75 See Goldschmidt, *Evolution of Chinese Medicine*, chapters 5 and 6, for more discussions on Xu's contributions.

76 Paul U. Unschuld, *Medicine in China: A History of Ideas*, 175–77; Lucille Chia, *Printing for Profit: The Commercial Publishers of Jianyang, Fujian (11th–17th centuries)* (Cambridge, MA: Harvard University Asia Center, 2002), 286; and Kosoto Hiroshi, "Nan-Sō dai no iyaku sho, sono 1–sono 6, *Gendai Tōyō igaku*, 9.1 (1988): 87–93, 9.2 (1988): 79–85, 9.3 (1988): 96–104, 9.4 (1988): 96–103, 10.1 (1989): 93–99, and 10.2 (1989): 94–103.

77 Xu Shuwei, *Puji benshifang*, 1.91 in his *Xu Shuwei Yixue Quanshu* (Beijing: Zhongguo Zhongyiyao chubanshe, 2006). Cited in Goldschmidt, *Evolution of Chinese Medicine*, 190.

78 Xu Shuwei, *Puji benshifang*, 2.103.

79 Liu Shijue, *Yongjia yipai yanjiu* (Beijing: Zhongguo guji chubanshe, 2000), 61–72. Also see Kosoto, "Nan-Sōdai no iyaku sho, sono 4."

80 Liao Yujun, Fu Fang, and Zheng Jinsheng, *Zhongguo kexue jishu shi: yixue juan* (Beijing: Kexue chubanshe, 1998), 345.

81 See, for example, Shiu Ying Hu, "History of the Introduction of Exotic Elements into Traditional Chinese Medicine," *Journal of the Arnold Arboretum* 71 (Oct. 1990): 487–526, which analyzes a large number of drugs that traveled between regions over history. Not being able to know which exotic drugs in *materia medica*s were used and which were simply recorded, Hu seems to unfairly exalt the encyclopedic *materia medica*s in the Song and downplays their compact and theoretical equivalent in the Yuan. His study shows, however, that it was a norm rather than an exception for medicinal plants to travel between regions.

82 Song et al., *Yuanshi*, 134.3249. The same book, however, simply calls the institution which later became the Office of Broad Grace *yiyaoyuan* (*Yuanshi*, 8.147). I am assuming that *yiyaoyuan* was a short form of *Xiyu yiyaosi*.
83 Song et al., *Yuanshi*, 88.2221.
84 Song et al., *Yuanshi*, 88.2221.
85 Song et al., *Yuanshi*, 88.2221.
86 Emilie Savage-Smith, "Medicine," in *Encylopedia of the History of Arabic Science*, ed. Roshdi Rashed (New York: Routledge, 1996), vol. 3, 903–62.
87 See Song Xian, *Huihui yaofang kaoshi*, 2 vols (Beijing: Zhonghua shuju, 2000); and Paul D. Buell, "How did Persian and Other Western Medical Knowledge Move East, and Chinese West? A Look at the Role of Rashīd al-Dīn and Others," *Asian Medicine: Tradition and Modernity*, 3 (2007): 279–95. A good overview of the content of *Huihuai yaofang* and *Yinshan zhengyao* can be found in Qiu Shusen et al., eds., *Zhongguo Huizu shi* (Yinchuan: Ningxia chubanshe, 1996), 1:290–300.
88 Paul D. Buell and Eugene N. Anderson, *A Soup for the Qan: Chinese Dietary Medicine of the Mongol Era as Seen in Hu Szu-hi's Yin-shan cheng-yao* (New York: Kegan Paul International, 2000).
89 Song et al., *Yuanshi*, 8.148; and Thomas T. Allsen, *Culture and Conquest in Mongol Eurasia* (Cambridge: Cambridge University Press, 2001), 154.
90 Billy K.L. So, *Prosperity, Region, and Institutions in Maritime China: The South Fukien Pattern, 946–1368* (Cambridge, MA: Harvard University Asia Center, 2001), 63 and 114–17.
91 Tao Zongyi, *Nancun chuogeng lu* (Beijing: Zhonghua shuju, 1959), 22.274.
92 Tao Zongyi, *Nancun chuogeng lu*, 25.309; Song Xian, *Gudai Bosi yixue yu Zhongguo*, 43.
93 Maejima Shinji, "Shiroppu kō," *Gekkan kaikyōken*, 2.6 (1939): 12–13.
94 Ibn Sina, *The Canon of Medicine* (Saab Medical Library, American University of Beirut, http://ddc.aub.edu.lb/projects/saab/avicenna/index.html), Book V ("Compound drugs, Formulary"), Treatise 6 ("On potions and thickened juices").
95 Thomas T. Allsen, *Culture and Conquest*, 155–56; Yu Xilu, *Zhishun Zhenjiang zhi* (Taibei: Huawen Shuju, 1968), 9.365–66; Maejima Shinji, *Tōzai bunka koryū no shosō* (Tokyo: Tōzai bunka koryū no shosō kankōkai, 1971), 695–98.
96 Buell and Anderson, *A Soup for the Qan*, 327–28 and 386–89.
97 Wang Qi, *Xu wenxian tongkao* (Beijing: Xiandai chubanshe, 1986), 32.479. *Xu wenxian tongkao*, commissioned by Qianlong Emperor, 28.3057.
98 *Jujia biyong shilei* (Kyoto: Chūbun shuppansha, 1984), 240–41.
99 Miya Noriko, *Mongoru jidai no shuppan bunka* (Nagoya: Nagoya daigaku shuppankai, 2006), 1–4.
100 Miya, *Mongoru jidai no shuppan bunka*, 372.
101 Inoue, *Chūgoku shuppan bunka shi*, 181.
102 Chia, *Printing for Profit*, 111 and 312.
103 For Inoue's negative views on Yuan printing culture, see his *Chūgoku shuppan bunka shi*, chaps. 12–14. Miya Noriko vehemently disagrees with such views in her 732-page book, *Mongoru jidai no shuppan bunka*. Both of them, however, agree that a larger number of medical books were printed in the Yuan than in the Song. See Inoue, *Chūgoku shuppan bunka shi*, 176, and Miya, *Mongoru jidai no shuppan bunka*, 15.
104 Kosoto, "Gendai no iyaku sho, sono 1–sono 5," *Gendai Tōyō igaku*, 11.3 (1990): 92–96, 11.4 (1990): 76–82, 12.1 (1991): 78–85, 12.2 (1991): 93–99, and 12.3 (1991): 94–101.
105 Kosoto, "Hoku-Sōdai no iyaku sho, sono 2," 93–94.
106 YDZ, 32.4a–5a.
107 Yu Xilu, *Zhishun Zhenjiang zhi*, 11.656. Yuan Jue, *Yanyou Siming zhi*, 14.17a.
108 Kosoto Hiroshi, "*Taihei keimin wazai kyoku hō* kaidai," in WKIS, vol., 5.
109 Wei Yilin, *Wei Yilin yixue quanshu* (Beijing: Zhongguo Zhong yiyao chubanshe, 2006), 9.
110 As to the process through which Cheng Fuxi's book was printed, see Miya, *Mongoru jidai no shuppan bunka*, chap. 7.

111   Huang Jin, *Jinhua Huang xiansheng wenji* (reprint, SBCK chubian), 38.7a–9a. Also see Liao Yujun, et al., *Zhongguo kexue jishu shi*, 354.

112   "Fu; Zhu Danxi nianpu," in Zhu Zhenheng, *Danxi yiji*, ed. Zhejiang sheng Zhong yiyao yanjiuyuan wenxian yanjiushi (Beijing: Renmin weisheng chubanshe, 1993), 1019–25.

113   "Fu; Zhu Danxi nianpu," 1025–28.

114   Zhu Zhenheng, "Zhang Zihe gongji zhu lun," 張子和攻擊注論 in his *Gezhi Yulun*, in his *Danxi yiji*, compiled by Zhejiang sheng Zhongyiyao yanjiuyuan wenxian yanjiushi (Beijing: Renmin weisheng chubanshe, 1993), 44; Hasebe et al., Kakuchi yoron *chūshaku*, 238–39; Yang Shou-zhong and Duan Wu-jin, *Extra Treatises Based on Investigation and Inquiry: A Translation of Zhu Dan-xi's* Ge Zhi Yu Lun (Boulder, CO: Blue Poppy Press, 1994), 128–31.

115   Mayanagi, "*Kakuchi yoron, Kyokuhō hakki* kaidai." http://mayanagi.hum.ibaraki. ac.jp/paper01/kakuchikaidai.html. Originally published in *Myakketsu, Naigaishō benwaku ron, Hi'i ron, Ranshitu hizō, Tōeki honzō, Shiji nanchi, Kakuchi yoron, Kyokuhō hakki, Geka seigi, Ikei sokai shū*, WKIS, vol. 6 (1989).

116   Zhu Zhenheng, "Yang youyu yin buzu lun," 陽有餘陰不足論 in his *Gezhi Yulun*, 10–11; Hasebe et al., Kakuchi yoron *chūshaku*, 15–21; Yang and Duan, *Extra Treatises Based on Investigation and Inquiry*, 4–8. See Christopher Cullen, *Astronomy and Mathematics in Ancient China: The Zhou bi Suan Jing* (Cambridge: Cambridge University Press, 1996), 65, for an illustration of the *huntian* 渾天 universe that Zhu apparently lived in.

117   The quote is from the "Li Yun" 禮運 chapter of the *Book of Rites*. *Zuantu huzhu Li ji*, SBCK chubian, 7a.

118   For the references in the poems, see Hasebe et al., Kakuchi yoron *chūshaku*, 9–14.

119   For detailed discussions on Zhu's understanding of sexual desires, see Charlotte Furth, "The Physician as Philosopher of the Way: Zhu Zhenheng (1282–1358)," *Harvard Journal of Asiatic Studies* 66.2 (2006): 441–51. For his understanding of over-eating, see, for example, Zhu Zhenheng, "Rudan lun 茹淡論" and "Eni lun 呃逆論," in *Gezhi yulun*, 40–42. Also, see Hasebe et al., Kakuchi yoron *chūshaku*, 211–27.

120   Zhu Zhenheng, *Jufang fahui*, in his *Danxi yiji*, compiled by Zhejiang sheng Zhongyiyao yanjiuyuan wenxian yanjiushi (Beijing: Renmin weisheng chubanshe, 1993), 47.

121   Zhu Zhenheng, "Xianghuo lun," 相火論 in his *Gezhi Yulun*, 39–40. The English translation is adopted from Yang and Duan, *Extra Treatises Based on Investigation and Inquiry*, 115, but I changed part of it based on the Japanese translation by Hasebe et al., Kakuchi yoron *chūshaku*, 204–05.

122   Liu Shijue, *Yongjia yipai yanjiu*, 63.

123   Liu Shijue, *Yongjia yipai yanjiu*, 2–3.

124   Kou Zongshi, *Bencao yanyi*, 7:48. Zhu Zhenheng, *Bencao yanyi buyi*, in his *Danxi yiji*, comp. Zhejiang sheng Zhong yiyao yanjiuyuan wenxian yanjiushi (Beijing: Renmin weisheng chubanshe, 1993), 76–77.

125   Zhu Zhenheng, *Bencao yanyi buyi*, 98. Wang Haogu, *Tangye Bencao*, in his *Wang Haogu yixue quanshu* (Beijing: Zhongguo yiyao chubanshe, 2004), 38. Kou Zongshi, *Bencao yanyi*, 7:46–47.

126   Zhu Zhenheng, "Daocang lun," 倒倉論 in his *Gezhi Yulun*, 37–38; Hasebe et al., Kakuchi yoron *chūshaku*, 191–98; Yang and Duan, *Extra Treatises Based on Investigation and Inquiry*, 4–8.

127   Zhu Zhenheng, *Jufang fahui*, 65.

128   Zhu Zhenheng, "Daocang lun," in his *Gezhi Yulun*, 38; The English translation is adopted from Yang and Duan, *Extra Treatises Based on Investigation and Inquiry*, 107, but I changed part of it based on the Japanese translation by Hasebe et al., Kakuchi yoron *chūshaku*, 196.

Epilogue

Toward the end of the Hongwu 洪武 period (1368–98), under the rulership of the first emperor of the Ming dynasty, Zhu Yuanzhang 朱元璋 (Hongwu emperor, 1328–98, r. 1368–98), a scholar-official named Wang Jin 王璡 came to the former Qingyuan circuit, now Ningbo prefecture 寧波府, as the governor. According to the *Ming History*, he woke up early every morning to read books and made sure that the students in the governmental school did the same. He destroyed inappropriate temples (*yinci* 淫祠), among which were the temples for the Three Progenitors. When someone questioned his judgment, he said, "Only the Son of Heaven can worship the Three Progenitors. The Progenitors have nothing to do with elites and commoners. Why do you question [my] destroying them?"[1]

A Brief Record of Ningbo Prefecture (*Ningbofu jianyaozhi* 寧波府簡要志), compiled in the Chenghua 成化 era (1465–87), agrees with this story that the Temples of the Three Progenitors in the Ningbo prefecture was abolished after the fall of the Yuan period, except that it says that the abolition occurred early in the Hongwu period. A new building for the school was built in 1411. The building was later taken over by a branch office of the Provincial Administration Commission (*buzheng fensi* 布政分司), so the directorates of the medical schools moved to the Charitable Pharmacy. Medical temple-schools of Cixi, Fenghua, Dinghai, and Xiangshan counties of the Ningbo prefecture had all been abandoned by the time the *Brief Record* was compiled and, instead, private homes were used as medical schools.[2]

This book has discussed the political, institutional, and cultural history of medicine through the Yuan period. The Mongol rulers recruited and promoted a vast number of doctors in the central government because of their needs as world conquerors, and the medical administrators in turn created and expanded the networks of medical institutions. The Mongols' unification of China also had implications. Now that the "Iron Curtain" that divided the two domains had been lifted, two major cultural trends—the system of the five circulatory phases and six seasonal influences integrated with the principle of Guiding Channels by the Jin doctors and the *Daoxue* philosophy that had flourished in the Southern Song—met with each other. Philosophers used *Daoxue* vocabulary to embellish doctors and medical institutions, while doctors cited Confucian books to justify their medical theories.

The remaining question is what happened afterward. Wang Jin's episode above shows that something certainly changed in the second half of the fourteenth century when China transitioned from the Yuan to the Ming period. To say the least, the Three Progenitors had been monopolized by the Ming emperor and local elites and commoners were not allowed to worship them any longer in the Ming. What happened and how did the changes occur?

Previous studies have shown the complexity of the Yuan-Ming transition. On the one hand, the Ming founder tried to purify the realm by rejecting the legacies of the Mongol rule. For instance, he no longer allowed his subjects to "speak Mongolian, wear Mongolian hats or gowns, follow Mongol marriage or burial practices, or play Mongolian tunes." On the other hand, he in reality adopted many of the Yuan governmental institutions as detailed in David M. Robinson's "The Ming Court and the Legacy of the Yuan Mongols."[3] By the same token, parts of the Yuan medical institutions were abolished while other parts became prototypes for the Ming-Qing institutions.

Zhu Yuanzhang created the Superintendency of Medical Schools and ranked the head of the office, the Superintendent, 5b in 1364, after occupying Jiqing 集慶 circuit (present-day Nanjing) in 1356. The office was renamed the Directorate of Imperial Medicine (*taiyi jian* 太醫監) in 1366 and then the Imperial Academy of Medicine in 1367. The head of the Academy was no longer called *tidian* 提點 but instead *yuanshi* 院使, which used to be the name of the second position in this office in the Yuan period. The rank for the *yuanshi* in the Ming was initially as high as 3a, but was lowered to 5a in 1381.[4] Under the supervision of the Academy, the medical service examinations continued. A doctor's son would be taught and tested so that he might be recruited into the Academy. The tests were given once every three to five years and a candidate was allowed to take a test at most three times.[5] A year after the Yongle emperor (1360–24, r. 1402–24) moved the capital to Beijing in 1420, he established the Imperial Academy of Medicine there while keeping the one in Nanjing as well. The latter was placed under the Court of the Imperial Clan in Nanjing (*Nanjing zongren fu* 南京宗人府) and focused on caring for the members of the imperial clan.[6] The Qing dynasty established an Imperial Academy of Medicine similar to its predecessor in Beijing during the Ming period and abolished the one in Nanjing. Instead the Qing Imperial Academy in Beijing was divided into two branches, one that served the imperial family and another that administered medical matters outside of the court. The head of the Academy was again called *yuanshi*, initially ranked 5a and later 4a (in 1909).[7]

When Zhu Yuanzhang created a house registration system for his empire in 1381, he might have maintained the "medical household" category. The *Ming History* says:

> There were three ranks for households: ordinary households (*minhu* 民戶), military households (*junhu* 軍戶), and artisan households (*jianghu* 匠戶). Ordinary households included [households of] Confucians, doctors, and diviners . . . Everyone should have his occupation recorded in the register.[8]

Just like the Yuan government, the Ming government in its early times needed to know what kind of service labor the adult male members of the households were capable of offering. Therefore, they recorded the occupation of the head of each family. The need for occupational categories apparently disappeared as the Ming government began to collect silver tax instead of having its population engage in service labor in the sixteenth century,[9] but the concept of "medical registration" (*yiji* 醫籍) remained throughout the Ming period. The Ming lists of the *jinshi* degree holders consistently include a few whose households were registered as such.[10] In contrast, the "Household and Population" (*hukou* 戶口) section of the *Draft History of Qing* makes no mention of medical households or medical registration.[11]

Medical temple-schools went through major changes. The greatest change, as we have already seen through the case of Ningbo prefecture above, was that the Temples of the Three Progenitors were no longer part of local medical schools. In 1368, when the Ming dynasty was established, the Hongwu emperor decreed that the Three Progenitors should be worshiped in the capital and in the following year he said they should be accompanied by their legendary assistants, Goumang, Zhurong, Fenghou, and Limu. Then, in 1371, the Ministry of Rites reported that it was highly improper to worship the Three Progenitors in prefectures and counties because the Tang dynasty had established a temple for the Three Progenitors and the Five Emperors only in the capital. The ministry's intention was to construct the lineage of the emperors of China starting with the Three Progenitors and to place the Hongwu emperor in the lineage, to justify his enthronement.[12] Despite the ministry's claim, the Ming institution was not a simple revival of the Tang institution because the latter was much more selective as to which emperors were to be worshiped there than was the former.[13] Doctors were allowed to worship the Three Progenitors again in 1542, but only members of the Imperial Academy of Medicine.[14] The local buildings for the Temples of the Three Progenitors appear to have followed diverse paths. Some of them, like the one in Ningbo as seen above, were destroyed. Some were eventually turned into Temples of the Medical King (*yaowang miao* 藥王廟) by the Qing period.[15] I have also found that Fuzhou 撫州 in present-day Jiangxi province kept part of the building as a Temple of the Three Progenitors at least until 1503, despite the central government's effort to ban them.[16]

As the Ming government took the Temples of the Three Progenitors away from local medical schools, it also deprived the medical schools of the prestige attaching to *xuexiao* 學校 (schools). Unlike the *Yuan History* and *Yuan Dianzhang*, neither the *Ming History* nor the *Draft History of Qing* lists medical schools in their sections on schools. Medical instructors, moreover, no longer received any salary, while their Yuan counterparts had received as much as Confucian school instructors did. The medical school instructors in the Ming-Qing period also lost the titles of *jiaoshou* 教授 (professor), *xuelu* 學錄 (associate professor), and *xuezheng* 學正 (assistant professor) and instead gained titles like *zhengke* 正科 (subject correctors), *dianke* 典科 (subject standardizers), and *xunke* 訓科

(subject trainers).[17] The new titles give an impression that the instructors were still supposedly making efforts to standardize medical knowledge, but that their presence no longer carried the scholarly weight that their counterparts in the Yuan had.

Despite the diminished prestige of the medical schools and the lack of salaries for instructors, the positions were still attractive enough in the early Ming to motivate some families to continue medical practice and dominate it with a few other families in the same localities.[18] The prestige of the positions, however, was further undermined as they were placed on sale, or to be precise, became available to those who made contributions to the government from the 1450s onward.[19] Late Ming to Qing authors often lamented the low level of medical knowledge that the instructors possessed.[20]

Although the Yuan local medical institutions were largely altered or abolished by the mid-Ming, the *yunqi* system and the principle of Guiding Channels, the medical theories that the Yuan culture had helped grow, now established themselves as the foundation of medical knowledge and practice in the Ming-Qing period. The "Biographies of Craftsmen" (*fangji zhuan* 方伎傳) section in the *Yuan History* compiled by Song Lian 宋濂 (1310–81), who had authored a funerary inscription for Zhu Zhenheng and later joined the entourage of the first Ming emperor, included only one doctor: Li Gao.[21] Zhu's disciple Dai Sigong 戴思恭 (1324–1405) served the Hongwu emperor and became his favorite doctor.[22] When the Shizong emperor ordered the Imperial Academy of Medicine to worship the Three Progenitors in 1536, Li Gao, Liu Wansu, Zhang Yuansu, and Zhu Zhenheng were among the twenty-eight doctors in history to be worshiped. The list included two Northern Song doctors (Qian Yi 錢乙 and Zhu Gong), but no Southern Song doctors.[23] The "Biographies of Craftsmen" in the *Ming History* compiled by the Qing court started out with four doctors who studied books written by Liu Wansu and Li Gao in the late Yuan to the early Ming: Hua Shou 滑壽, Ge Gansun 葛乾孫, Lü Fu 呂復, and Ni Weide 倪維德 (1303–77). Zhu Zhenheng's disciple, Wang Lü 王履, also had his biographies included in the *Ming History*.[24] It is true that the scholarly descendants of the Jin-Yuan doctors debated over and over whose theories were better than the others and challenged some parts of them quite passionately.[25] The knowledge of their theories and books, however, was an important way for elite doctors to claim the legitimacy of their medical knowledge and skills, especially when they did not come from a family that had practiced medicine for generations.[26]

Yuan Jue, our protagonist, wrote the gazetteer for the Qingyuan circuit at 55 *sui* in 1320. Three years later in 1323, he was called back to Daidu to serve in the Hanlin Academy again and received the position of *shijiang xueshi* 侍講學士 (expositor, 2b). Receiving posthumous titles for his ancestors might have motivated him to renovate his family graveyard; at least his funerary inscription for his grandfather is dated the year of his return to his hometown, 1324. When he passed away in 1327 at 62 *sui* because of an unknown illness, he was survived by one son, a few daughters, and several grandchildren, one of whom eventually achieved a high status in the Yuan court.[27] The local medical temple-schools that he and his Chinese, Mongol, and Central and West Asian contemporaries created and maintained changed in form after the descendants of Chinggis Khan left China. However, the medical culture that they built together nurtured a long-lasting legacy in the history of medicine in China: a medical theory that is the foundation of East Asian medicine to this day.

Notes

1 Zhang Tingyu et al., *Mingshi* (Beijing: Zhonghua shuju, 1975), 143.4061.
2 Huang Runyu, *Ningbofu jianyaozhi* (Siming congshu edition), 2.4a.
3 In *Culture, Courtiers, and Competition: The Ming Court (1368–1644)*, ed. David M. Robinson (Cambridge, MA: Harvard University Press, 2008). The quote is on p. 367.
4 Liang Jun, *Zhongguo gudai yizhen shilue* (Hohht: Nei Mengu renmin chubanshe, 1995), 145; Zhang et al., *Mingshi*, 74.1813.
5 Zhang et al., *Mingshi*, 74.1812.
6 Liang, *Zhongguo gudai yizhen shilue*, 145; Zhang et al., *Mingshi*, 75.1836.
7 Liang, *Zhongguo gudai yizhen shilue*, 172. Zhao Erxun et al., *Qingshi gao* (Beijing: Zhonghua shuju, 1976), 115.3326.
8 Zhang et al., *Mingshi*, 77.1878.
9 A large number of studies on service labor during the Ming period have been published in Japan. For the list of these works, see Tonami Mamoru et al., eds., *Chūgoku Rekishi kenkyū nyūmon* (Nagoya: Nagoya daigaku shuppankai, 2006), 195.
10 Tsuchiya Yūko, "Mindai no tai'i in seki ni tsuite," *Ajia shi kenkyū* 34 (2010), esp. 191–92.
11 Zhao et al., *Qingshi gao*, 120.3480–82.
12 Yüan-ling Chao, *Medicine and Society in Late Imperial China: A Study of Physicians in Suzhou, 1600-1850* (New York: Peter Lang, 2009), 65–70.
13 See my Chapter 3 for the discussion of the Temple of the Three Progenitors and the Five Emperors in the Tang period.
14 Chao, *Medicine and Society*, 65–70.
15 Chao, *Medicine and Society*, 70–74.
16 Li Zhe et al., *Hongzhi Fuzhoufu zhi* (TYG Xubian), 25.705.
17 Zhang et al., *Mingshi*, 75.1853; Zhao et al., *Qingshi Gao*, 135.3360. See my Chapters 2 and 3 for the Yuan titles.
18 Qiu Zhonglin, "Mianmian guadie: guanyu Mingdai Jiansu shiyi de chubu kaocha," *Chugoku shigaku* 13 (2003): 62.
19 Qiu, "Mianmian guadie," 64–66.
20 Angela Ki Che Leung, "Organized Medicine in Ming-Qing China: State and Private Medical Institutions in Lower Yangzi Region," *Late Imperial China* 8.1 (1987): 140.
21 Song et al., *Yuanshi* (Beijing: Zhonghua shuju, 1976), 203.4540. See Zhang et al., *Mingshi*, 128.3784–88, for Song Lian's career. His funerary inscription for Zhu Zhenheng is in Song Lian, *Song Lian Quanji* (Hangzhou: Zhejiang guji chubanshe, 1999), 4.2131–38. Also, for an excellent analysis of Song Lian's inscription, see Charlotte Furth, "The Physician as the Philosopher of the Way: Zhu Zhenheng (1282–1385)," *HJAS* 66.2 (2006): 434–41.
22 Zhang et al., *Mingshi*, 299.7645.
23 Li Dongyang et al., *Da Ming huidian* (Guofeng chubanshe, 1963), 92.12b (p. 1456).
24 Zhang et al., *Mingshi*, 299.7634–38.
25 For example, while Zhu Zhenheng did not talk about physical differences between the North and South Chinese, his followers found ways to incorporate their perceptions of the differences into Zhu's theory. See Dai Liang's biography of Zhu in *Quan Yuanwen*, in particular 53:1638.438; Marta Hansen, *Speaking of Epidemics: the Disease and Geographic Imagination in Late Imperial China* (London: Routledge, 2011); and Zhang Xueqian, "Yuan-Ming ruyi sixiang yu shijian de shehuishi: yi Zhu Zhenheng ji

'Danxi xuepai' wei zhongxin" (Ph.D. diss., Xianggang Zhongwen Daxue, 2012), in particular Chapter 1.

26 Numerous books and articles have been written on Ming-Qing medicine. Examples of the books in English are Paul U. Unschuld, *Medicine in China: A History of Ideas* (Berkeley: University of California Press, 1985); Volker Scheid, *Currents of Tradition in Chinese Medicine, 1626–2006* (Seattle, WA: East Land Press, 2007); and Yi-Li Wu, *Reproducing Women: Medicine, Metaphor, and Childbirth in Late Imperial China* (Berkeley: University of California Press, 2010).

27 Su Tianjue, *Zixi wengao* (Beijing: Zhonghua shuju, 1997), 9.134 and 136; *Qingrong*, 33.4b.

Appendix I

Locations of medical temple-schools and times of the construction and renovations

The following table shows when and where buildings for medical temple-school complexes were constructed or renovated. If an inscription says that a small and shabby temple existed prior to the construction of the major building, the former is counted as the original building and the latter is counted as its "renovation." A renovation might have taken place either at the same location or somewhere in the same city. However, when an inscription says, for example, that local physicians had met at a temporary place for spring and autumn rituals prior to the construction of a building, the temporary meeting place is not counted. A question mark means that the date of construction or renovation is unknown.

Location	Year built	Dates of renovations	Sources
METROPOLITAN AREA (ZHONGSHUSHENG 中書省)			
Daidulu 大都路	1295		Xu Youren 許有壬, *Zhizheng ji* 至正集, SKQS, 44.5b–9a.
Daidulu Qianweitunying 前衛屯營	1336		Su Tianjue 蘇天爵, *Zixi wengao* 滋溪文稿, SKQS, 2.16a–18b.
Quanninglu 全寧路	1317		Liu Guan 柳貫, *Daizhi ji* 待制集, SKQS, 14.4b–5b.
Baodinglu Yizhou Dingxingxian 保定路易州定興縣	1210	1302	Yan Fu 閻復, *Jingxuan ji* 靜軒集, YRCK, 4.23b–25a.
Zhangdelu 彰德路	1288		Hu Zhiyu 胡祗遹, *Chaishan daquanji* 柴山大全集, SKQS, 10.2b–4a.
Weihuilu 衞輝路	Early Yuan	1300–01	Wang Yun 王惲, *Qiujian ji* 秋澗集, SKQS, 59.1a–4a.
Hejianlu Xianzhou Jiaohexian 河閒路獻州交河縣	?	1312–13	*Qingrong*, 25.2b–4b.
Yidulu Yizhou 益都路沂州	?	1324	Zhang Yanghao 張養浩, *Guitian leigao* 歸田類稿, SKQS, 4.3b–6a.
Jinanlu 濟南路	?	1322	Zhang, *Guitian leigao*, 4.1a–3b.

(continued)

Location	Year built	Dates of renovations	Sources
Tai'anzhou Laiwuxian 泰安州萊蕪縣	?	1327	Zhang, *Guitian leigao*, 4.6a–8a.

HENAN-JIANGBEI BRANCH CENTRAL SECRETARIAT 河南江北行省

Bianlianglu 汴梁路	?		Li Lian 李濂, *Bianjing yiji zhi* 汴京遺蹟志, SKQS, 15.19b–22a.
Runingfu Xinyangzhou Luoshanxian 汝寧府信陽州羅山縣	?	1342?	Su Tianjue, *Zixi wengao*, 4.3b–5b.
Huai'anlu Hainingzhou 淮安路海寧州	1319	1342	Huang Jin, *Jinhua Huang xiansheng wenji* 金華黃先生文集, SBCK chubian, 10.5a–6a.

SHANXI BRANCH CENTRAL SECRETARIAT 陝西行省

Fengyuanlu 奉元路	1297		Luo Tianxiang 駱天驤, *Leibian Chang'an zhi* 類編長安志, SYD Xubian, 5.81–82 and 6.141. Li Haowen 李好文, *Chang'an zhitu* 長安志圖, SKQS, *shang*.11b–12a.
Xingyuanlu 興元路	1292	1330	Pu Daoyuan 蒲道源, *Xianju conggao* 閑居叢稿, SKQS, 14.16a–18a.
Xingyuanlu Fengzhou 鳳州	?		Pu Daoyuan, *Xianju conggao*, 14.18a–19b.
Xingyuanlu Yangzhou 洋州	?	?	Pu Daoyuan, *Xianju conggao*, 14.19b–21a.

JIANGZHE BRANCH CENTRAL SECRETARIAT 江浙行省

Hangzhoulu 杭州路	?	1349	Liu Ji 劉基, *Chengyibo wenji* 誠意伯文集, SKQS, 9.15b–17a.
Pingjianglu 平江路	?	1302, 1331 1347, 1358	Qian Gu 錢穀, ed. *Wudu wencui xuji* 吳都文粹續集, SKQS, 17.1a–5b. Chen Ji 陳基, *Yibaizhai gao* 夷白齋稿, SKQS, 30.1a–3b.
Pingjianglu Changshuzhou 常熟州	1317	1337, 1362	Qian Gu, ed. *Wudu wencui xuji*, 17.5a–6b.
Pingjianglu Jiadingzhou 嘉定州	1326	1340–41	Qian Gu, ed. *Wudu wencui xuji*, 17.6b–8b.
Pingjianglu Kunshanzhou 崑山州	?	?, 1359	Qian Gu, ed. *Wudu wencui xuji*, 17.8b–10b. Yang Hui 楊譓, *Zhizheng Kunshan zhi* 至正崑山志, Sanshiqi, 1.4a
Changzhoulu Wuxizhou 常州路無錫州	?		*Wuxi zhi* 無錫志, SYD xubian, 1.15a.

Zhenjianglu 鎮江路	?		Yu Xilu 俞希魯, *Zhishun Zhenjiang zhi* 至順鎮江志 (Taibei: Huawen Shuju, 1968), 8.483–84, 11.656, and 17.914–16.
Zhenjianglu Danyangxian 丹陽縣	?		Yu Xilu, *Zhishun Zhenjiang zhi*, 8.501.
Zhenjianglu Jintanxian 金壇縣	?		Yu Xilu, *Zhishun Zhenjiang zhi*, 8.514.
Qingyuanlu 慶元路	1291	1315, 1353	*Qingrong*, 18.10b–11b. Wu Sidao 烏斯道, *Chuncaozhai ji* 春草齋集, SKQS, 1.15a–17a. Yuan Jue 袁桷, *Yanyou Siming zhi* 延祐四明志, ZGFZCS (vol. 578), 14.12b–17a. Wang Yuangong 王元恭, *Zhizheng Siming xuzhi* 至正四明續志, ZGFZCS, 8.1a–2a.
Qingyuanlu Fenghuazhou 奉化州	1314	1319 (twice)	*Qingrong*, 25.4b–6a. Yuan Jue, *Yanyou Siming zhi*, 14.17a–19b. Wang Yuangong, *Zhizheng Siming xuzhi*, 8.2a–3a.
Qingyuanlu Changguozhou 昌國州	1292	1324	*Qingrong*, 18.15b–17a. Yuan Jue, *Yanyou Siming zhi*, 14.19b–21a. Wang Yuangong, *Zhizheng Siming xuzhi*, 3.20a and 8.3b. Feng Fujing 馮福京 et al., *Dade Changguozhou tuzhi* 大德昌國州圖志, ZGFZCS, 2.13b–14a.
Qingyuanlu Cixixian 慈溪縣	1288	1314	Yuan Jue, *Yanyou Siming zhi*, 14.21a–21b. Wang Yuangong, *Zhizheng Siming xuzhi*, 8.5a.
Qingyuanlu Dinghaixian 定海縣	?		Wang Yuangong, *Zhizheng Siming xuzhi*, 9.14b–16a.
Quzhoulu 衢州路	1324		*Qingrong*, 25.6a–8a.
Wuzhoulu Pujiangxian 婺州路浦江縣	1321?	1328–29, 1332	Huang Jin, *Jinhua Huang xiansheng wenji*, SBCK chubian, 10.4a–5a.
Huizhoulu Jixixian 徽州路績溪縣	1335		Zheng Yu 鄭玉, *Shishan ji* 師山集, SKQS, 5.1a–2a. Wu Cheng 吳澄, *Wu Wenzheng gong ji* 吳文正公集, YRCK, 21.1a–3a.
Jiankanglu 建康路 (= Jiqinglu 集慶路)	?	1318–19	Zhang Xuan 張鉉, *Zhizheng Jinling xinzhi* 至正金陵新志, Song-Yuan fangzhi congkan 宋元方志叢刊 (Beijing: Zhonghua shuju, 1990), 1.19a.
Jiankanglu Lishuizhou 溧水州	?	?	Zhang Xuan, *Zhizheng Jinling xinzhi*, Song-yuan fangzhi congkan, 1.32a.

(continued)

(continued)

Location	Year built	Dates of renovations	Sources
Xinzhoulu Yongfengxian 信州路永豐縣	1300	1302	Liu Yueshen 劉岳申, *Shenzhai ji* 申齋集, SKQS, 7.1a–3b.
Jiangyinlu 江陰路	1286		Lu Wengui 陸文圭, *Qiangdong leigao* 牆東類稿, SKQS, 8.14b–15b.
Jiandelu 建德路	1298		He Menggui 何夢桂, *Qianzhai wenji* 潛齋文集, SKQS, 9.16b–18b.
Shaowulu Tainingxin 邵武路泰寧縣	?	1342, 1348	Zheng Yu, *Shishan ji*, SKQS, 4.19a–20b.
Fuzhoulu 福州路	?	?	Gong Shitai 貢師泰, *Wanzhai ji* 玩齋集, SKQS, 7.15b–17a.

JIANGXI BRANCH CENTRAL SECRETARIAT 江西行省

Location	Year built	Dates of renovations	Sources
Ji'anlu 吉安路	?	1320, 1336	Liu Shen 劉詵, *Guiyin wenji* 桂隱文集, YRCK, 1.20b–21b. Yu Ji 虞集, *Daoyuan leigao* 道園類藁, YRCK, 25.42a–44a.
Ji'anlu Yongxinzhou 永新州	1313		Cheng Jufu 程鉅夫, *Cheng Xuelou wenji* 程雪樓文集, Huikan, 13.8b–9a.
Yuanzhoulu Fenyixian 袁州路分宜縣	?	1339	Yu Ji, *Daoyuan leigao*, 23.35a–37a.
Fuzhoulu 撫州路	1300?	1331	Wu Cheng, *Wu Wenzheng gong ji*, 21.3a–6a.
Fuzhoulu Yihuangxian 宜黃縣	1313–15		Wu Cheng, *Wu Wenzheng gong ji*, 21.6a–7b.
Fuzhoulu Le'anxian 樂安縣	?	1333	Yu Ji, *Daoyuan leigao*, 23.33a–35a.
Fuzhoulu Chongrenxian 崇仁縣	1304	1336	Yu Ji, *Daoyuan leigao*, 23.29b–33a.
Nanfengzhou 南豐州	1300–1301		Liu Xun 劉壎, *Shuiyuncun gao* 水雲村藁, SKQS, 2.3b–6b.
Guangzhoulu Zengchengxian 廣州路增城縣	1331		Jie Xisi 揭傒斯, *Wen'an ji* 文安集, SKQS, 10.8b–10a.
Chaozhoulu 潮州路	?	?	Wu Hai 吳海, *Wenguozhai ji* 聞過齋集, SKQS, 3.9a–10b.

HUGUANG BRANCH CENTRAL SECRETARIAT 湖廣行省

Location	Year built	Dates of renovations	Sources
Lizhoulu Cilizhou 澧州路慈利州	?		Yu Ji, *Daoyuan leigao*, 27b–29b.
Yuezhoulu 岳州路	?		Cheng Jufu, *Cheng Xuelou wenji*, Huikan, 12.1b–2a.

Appendix II

Medical administrators in *Index to Biographical Materials of Yuan Figures*

The following table lists the Yuan men who served as medical administrators, according to Wang Deyi 王德毅 et al.'s *Index to Biographical Materials of Yuan Figures* (*Yuanren zhuanji ziliao suoyin* 元人傳記資料索引 Taibei: Xinwenfeng chuban gongsi, 1979–82). As discussed in Chapter 4, this list is only a small portion of a large number of Yuan medical administrators; many more men took such positions in reality.

Name	Medical school instructor?	Positions held	Volume: page number
Ding Tingyu 丁廷玉	✓	武義縣醫學教諭	1: 5
Fang Tingjin 方廷瑾		江浙醫學提舉	1: 66
Wang Zong 王宗	✓	保正路醫學正, 衢州路教授, 河間路教授	1: 89
Wang Shan 王善	✓	鎮江路醫學教授	1: 111
Wang Yi 王儀		太醫院判兼教授	1: 131
Wang Renzheng 王仁整	✓	揚州醫學教授	1: 154
Wang Hongyi 王弘毅		太醫院管勾	1: 163
Wang Haogu 王好古	✓	趙州醫學教授	1: 167
Wang Weiyi 王惟一	✓	鎮江路醫學教授	1: 197
Wang Deyu 王德玉	✓	鎮江路醫學教授	1: 210
Shen Jing 申敬		太醫, 御藥院使, 秘書監丞, 秘書少監, 太常卿	1: 258
Wei Yilin 危亦林	✓	南豐州醫學教授	1: 290
Zhu Fu 朱紱	✓	鎮江路醫學教授, 太醫, 諸路醫學副提舉	1: 308
He Feng 何鳳	✓	婺州醫學教授, 江西醫學提舉	1: 344
He Xian 何暹	✓	鎮江路醫學錄	1: 344
He Zirong 何子榮	✓	鎮江路醫學錄	1: 345
Wu Cheng 吳成	✓	新昌州醫學正, 餘干州醫學教授	1: 365

(continued)

(continued)

Name	Medical school instructor?	Positions held	Volume: page number
Song Chao 宋超	✓	大都醫學教授, 翰林侍讀學士	1: 434
Song Yuan 宋淵	✓	義烏醫學教諭	1: 439
Li Gang 李綱	✓	南京路醫學教授, 襄陽路醫學教授	1: 491
Li Kerang 李克讓	✓	滄州醫學正, 河間路醫學教授, 他.	1: 524
Wang Reng 汪礽		太醫院左丞	1: 574
Gu Gao 谷杲		太醫院同簽, 廣平路 總管, 他.	1: 603
Zhou Jizhou 周繼周	✓	平江醫學正	2: 646
Meng Shouhe 孟守和	✓	清河縣醫學教諭	2: 654
Shang Congshan 尚從善		上都惠民局提點, 江浙醫學提舉	2: 661–62
Yu Zhongwen 俞仲溫	✓	平江路醫學錄	2: 723
Yu Shizhong 俞時中		太醫令史, 都水監, 廬江縣尹	2: 727
Shi Dacai 施大才	✓	鎮江路醫學正	2: 747
Hu Shike 胡仕可	✓	瑞州路醫學教授	2: 802
Hu Jiuju 胡就矩	✓	鎮江路醫學正	2: 812
Ni Jujing 倪居敬	✓	杭州路醫學正, 教授, 江浙官醫副提舉, 提舉	2: 842
Gao Wenzhong 郜文忠	✓	大都路醫學教授, 諸路醫學提舉	2: 964
Ma Su 馬肅	✓	福州路醫學教授, 江西醫學提舉	2: 978
Chang Zhong 常中		御醫	2: 1039
Chang Qian 常謙		安西王府醫藥提舉, 開成路 判官, 陝西興元長官吏	2: 1040
Zhang Yu 張煜	✓	鎮江路醫學正	2: 1082
Zhang Qing 張慶	✓	鎮江路醫學教授	2: 1091
Zhang Yi 張翼	✓	鎮江路醫學正	2: 1100
Zhang Yuangui 張元珪	✓	太醫院使	2: 1112
Zhang Yuanshan 張元善		江浙官醫提舉	2: 1112
Zhang Feiqing 張飛卿		監察御使, 太醫院使	2: 1146
Zhang Yinglei 張應雷	✓	太醫, 鎮江路醫學教授	2: 1170
Qi Qinghong 戚慶洪	✓	鎮江路醫學錄	2: 1176
Qi Qingzu 戚慶祖	✓	鎮江路醫學錄, 學正	2: 1176
Xu Yi 許宸		禮部尚書, 太醫院提點, 尚醫大監	2: 1222
Xu Zixun 許子遜		集賢學士兼太醫院使	2: 1228
Xu Guozhen 許國禎		太醫院提點, 禮部尚書	2: 1234
Chen Geng 陳庚		江西官醫提舉司都目	2: 1274

Appendix III

The administrators listed in Wei Yilin's *Effective Pharmaceutical Recipes by a Hereditary Physician*

The following table shows the members of the Imperial Academy of Medicine who endorsed the printing of Wei Yilin's 危亦林 *Effective Pharmaceutical Recipes by a Hereditary Physician* (*Shiyi dexiao fang* 世醫得效方) in 1339. Although biographical materials for the members are not extant, their names allow us to speculate on their ethnic backgrounds.

Name	Honorary titles (sanguan 散官)	Position held in the Imperial Academy of Medicine	Ethnicity? (NC: not Chinese)
Guo Yi 郭毅	奉直大夫 (civil 5B)	General secretary 太醫院都事	
'Alā' al-Dīn 阿老了（丁？）	承直郎 (civil 6A)	General secretary 太醫院都事	NC
Tian Shouxin 田守信	奉直大夫 (civil 5B)	Registrar 太醫院經歷	
Buyan-Temür 卜顔帖木儿	奉直大夫 (civil 5B)	Registrar 太醫院經歷	NC
Lang Shiyan 郎師顔	成和郎 (medical 6B)	Supervisor 太醫院判官	
Qi Xian 齊顯	承直郎 (civil 6A)	Supervisor 太醫院判官	
Hu Deqin 胡得勤	成和郎 (medical 6B)	Deputy junior assistant director 同僉太醫院事	
Gong Shuzheng 弓叔正	成安郎 (medical 6A)	Deputy junior assistant director 同僉太醫院事	
Jia Wenbing 賈文炳	承直郎 (civil 6A)	Assistant director 太醫院事	
Ma Wenjin 馬文瑾	承務郎 (civil 6B)	Junior assistant director 僉太醫院事	
Xu Wenmei 許文美	奉訓大夫 (civil 5B)	Associate director 同知太醫院事	
Zhao Liang 趙良	奉議大夫 (civil 3A)	Associate director 同知太醫院使	
Zhao Weiyin 趙惟寅	嘉議大夫 (civil 3A)	Director 太醫院使	
Zhao Quan 趙權	嘉議大夫 (civil 3A)	Director 太醫院使	

Feng Shi 馮適	嘉議大夫 (civil 3A)	Director 太醫院使	
Jiang Gaiji 蔣溉濟	———	Director 太醫院使	
Zhang Yuangui 張元珪	中奉大夫 (civil 2B)	Director 太醫院使	
Zhang Yuanze 張元澤	資善大夫 (civil 2A)	Director 太醫院使	
Zhang Yi 張翼	資善大夫 (civil 2A)	Director 太醫院使	
Ban'ge 伴哥	資善大夫 (civil 2A)	Director 太醫院使	NC
Wushisi 五十四	資善大夫 (civil 2A)	Director 太醫院使	NC
Shixia'ni 石下尼	資善大夫 (civil 2A)	Director 太醫院使	NC
Qaradai 哈剌歹	資善大夫 (civil 2A)	Director 太醫院使	NC

Source: Wei Yilin, *Wei Yilin yixue quanshu* (Beijing: Zhongguo Zhong yiyao chubanshe, 2006), 3–4.
David M. Farquhar, *The Government of China Under Mongolian Rule: A Reference Guide* (Stuttgart: Steiner, 1990), 24–29.

Bibliography

Abe Takeo 安部健夫. "Gensho chishikijin to kakyo" 元初知識人と科挙. In *Gendaishi no kenkyū* 元代史の研究, 3–53. Tokyo: Sōbunsha, 1972.

Allsen, Thomas T. *Culture and Conquest in Mongol Eurasia*. Cambridge: Cambridge University Press, 2001.

Atwood, Christopher. *Encyclopedia of Mongolia and the Mongol Empire*. New York: Facts on File, 2004.

Balazs, Etienne. *Chinese Civilization and Bureaucracy: Variations on a Theme*. Translated by H.M. Wright. Edited byArthur F. Wright. New Haven, CT: Yale University Press, 1964.

Ban Gu 班固 et al. *Hanshu* 漢書. Beijing: Zhonghua shudian, 1962.

Bei Qiong 貝瓊. *Qingjiang Bei xiansheng ji* 清江貝先生集. SBCK chubian.

Bencao jing jizhu 本草經集注. Comp. Tao Hongjing 陶弘景, Kojima Shōshin 小嶋尚真, Mori Tatsuyuki 森立之, and Okanishi Tameto 岡西為人. Ōsaka: Minami Ōsaka insatu sentā, 1972.

Benedict, Benedict. *Bubonic Plague in Nineteenth-Century China*. Stanford, CA: Stanford University Press.

Bian Shi 邊實. *Yufeng xuzhi* 玉峰續志. 1 *juan*. 1272. Sanshiqi.

Birge, Bettine. "Chu Hsi and Women's Education." In *Neo-Confucian Education: The Formative Stage*, ed. Wm. Theodore de Bary and John W. Chaffee, 325–67. Berkeley: University of California Press, 1989.

——. *Women, Property, and Confucian Reaction in Sung and Yuan China, 960–1368*. Cambridge: Cambridge University Press, 2002.

Bol, Peter K. "Chao Ping-wen (1159–1232): Foundations for Literati Learning," in *China under Jurchen Rule*, ed. Hoyt Cleveland Tillman and Stephen H. West, 115–44. Albany: State University of New York Press, 1995.

——. "The Sung Examination System and the *Shih*," *Asia Major* 3.2 (1992): 149–71.

——. *"This Culture of Ours": Intellectual Transition from T'ang and Sung China*. Stanford, CA: Stanford University Press, 1992.

——. *Neo-Confucianism in History*. Cambridge, MA: Harvard University Asia Center, 2008.

Bossler, Beverly J. "A Daughter is a Daughter All Her Life: Affinal Relations and Women's Networks in Song and Late Imperial China." *Late Imperial China* 21.1 (2000): 77–106.

Buell, Paul D. "How did Persian and Other Western Medical Knowledge Move East, and Chinese West? A Look at the Role of Rashīd al-Dīn and Others." *Asian Medicine: Tradition and Modernity* 3 (2007): 279–95.

——. "Qubilai and the Rats." *Sudhoffs Archiv* 96.2 (2012): 127–44.

Buell, Paul D., and Eugene N. Anderson. *A Soup for the Qan: Chinese Dietary Medicine of the Mongol Era as Seen in Hu Szu-hi's* Yin-shan cheng-yao. New York: Kegan Paul International, 2000.

Chang Bide 昌彼得 et al. *Songren zhuanji ziliao suoyin* 宋人傳記索引. Taibei: Dingwen shuju, 1974–84.

Chang Tang 常棠. *Ganshui zhi* 橄水志. 8 *juan*. 1230. Sanshiqi.

Chao Gongwu 晁公武. *Junzhai dushuzhi jiaozheng* 郡齋讀書志校證. Shanghai: Shanghai guji chubanshe, 1990.

Chao, Yüan-ling 趙元玲. *Medicine and Society in Late Imperial China: A Study of Physicians in Suzhou, 1600–1850*. New York: Peter Lang International Academic Publishers, 2009.

Chen Bangxian 陳邦賢. *Zhongguo yixue shi* 中國醫學史. 1937. Taibei: Taiwan Shangwu yishuguan, 1981.

Chen Dazhen 陳大震. *Dade Nanhai zhi* 大德南海志. 1304. SYD Xubian.

Chen Gaohua 陳高華. "Yuandai de difang guanxue" 元代的地方官學. *Yuanshi luncong* 元史論叢 5 (1993): 160–89.

Chen Gongliang 陳公亮. *Yanzhou tujing* 嚴州圖經. 3 *juan*. 1186. Sanshiqi.

Chen Ji 陳基. *Yibaizhai gao* 夷白齋稿. SKQS.

Chen Junkai 陳君愷. "Songdai yizheng zhi yanjiu" 宋代醫政之研究. Ph.D. diss., Guoli Taiwan Shifan Daxue 國立臺灣師範大學, 1996.

Chen Qiqing 陳耆卿. *Jiading Chicheng zhi* 嘉定赤城志. 40 *juan*. Sanshiqi.

Chen Tianfu 陳天夫. *Nanyue zongsheng ji* 南岳總勝記. 3 *juan*. SYD Xubian.

Chen Wenyi 陳雯怡. "Networks, Communities, and Identities: On Discursive Practices of Yuan Literati." Ph.D. diss., Harvard University, 2007.

Chen Yuan-Peng 陳元朋. "Songdai de ruyi: jianping Robert P. Hymes youguan Song-Yuan yizhe diwede lundian" 宋代的儒醫: 兼評 Robert P. Hymes 有關宋元醫者地位的論點. *Xin shixue* 新史學 6.1 (March 1995): 179–203.

——. *Liang-Song de "shangyi shiren" yu "ruyi": jianlun qizai Jin-Yuan de liubian* 兩宋的「尚醫士人」與「儒醫」: 兼論其在金元的流變. Taibei: Guoli Taiwan daxue wen-shi congkan, 1997.

Chen Zhensun 陳振孫. *Zhizhai shulu jieti* 直齋書錄解題. Shanghai: Shanghai guji chu-banshe, 1987.

Cheng Dachang 程大昌. *Yonglu* 雍録. 10 *juan*. Sanshiqi.

Cheng Hao 程顥 and Cheng Yi 程頤. *Henan Er-Cheng quanji* 河南二程全集. Sibu beiyao.

——. *Henan Chengshi yishu* 河南二程遺書. In their *Er-Cheng ji* 二程全集, Beijing: Zhonghua shuju, 1981, vol. 1.

Cheng Hsiao-wen. "Traveling Stories and Untold Desires: Female Sexuality in Song China, 10th–13th Centuries." Ph.D. diss., University of Washington, 2012.

Cheng Jufu 程鉅夫. *Cheng Xuelou wenji* 程雪樓文集, Huikan, 1970.

——. *Xuelouji* 雪樓集. SKQS.

Cheng Wuji 成無己. *Cheng Wuji yixue quanshu* 成無己醫學全集. Beijing: Zhongguo Zhong yiyao chubanshe, 2004.

Cheng Yajun 程雅君. *Jin-Yuan sida yijia yu daojia daojiao* 金元四大医家与道家道教. Chengdu: Bashu shushe, 2006.

Chia, Lucille. *Printing for Profit: The Commercial Publishers of Jianyang, Fujian (11th–17th Centuries)*. Cambridge, MA: Harvard University Asia Center, 2002.

Chia, Lucille, and Hilde de Weerdt, eds., *Knowledge and Text Production in the Age of Print: China, 900–1400*. Leiden: Brill, 2011.

Chow, Kai-wing. Review of *Manufacturing Confucianism: Chinese Traditions and Universal Civilization*, by Lionel M. Jensen. *American Historical Review* 104.5 (1999): 1645–46.

Chu Ci 楚辞. SBCK chubian.

Classic of Changes, The: A New Translation of the I-Ching as Interpreted by Wang Bi. Translated by Richard John Lynn. New York: Columbia University Press, 1994.

Confucius. *The Analects* (*Lunyu* 論語). Trans. D.C. Lau. Harmondsworth: Penguin Books, 1979.

Cullen, Christopher. *Astronomy and Mathematics in Ancient China: The Zhou bi Suan Jing.* Cambridge: Cambridge University Press, 1996.

——. "Yi'an: The Origins of a Genre of Chinese Medical Literature." In *Innovation in Chinese Medicine*, ed. Elizabeth Hsu, 297–323. Cambridge: Cambridge University Press, 2001.

Czikszentmihalyi, Mark. Review of *Manufacturing Confucianism: Chinese Traditions and Universal Civilization*, by Lionel M. Jensen. *Journal of the American Academy of Religion* 67.3 (1999): 678–81.

——. *Material Virtue: Ethics and the Body in Early China.* Leiden: Brill, 2004.

Da Yuan shengzheng guochao dianzhang 大元聖政國朝典章. 60 *juan*. Yuan dynasty. Taibei: Guoli Gugong bowu yuan, 1976. Also, Taibei: Wenhai chubanshe, 1974 (the version originally published by Shen Jiaben 沈家本, 1840–1913). [Unless mentioned otherwise, I cite from the Gugong bowu yuan version.]

Daban niepan jingji 大般涅槃經記. Annotated by Guanding 灌頂. Taibei: Xin wenfeng chuban gonsi, 1978.

Dai Biaoyuan 戴表元. *Shanyuan wenji* 剡源文集. CSJC.

——. *Shanyuan wenji.* SKQS.

Dardess, John W. *Confucianism and Autocracy: Professional Elites in the Founding of the Ming Dynasty.* Berkeley: University of California Press, 1983.

Davis, Richard L. *Court and Family in Sung China, 960–1279: Bureaucratic Success and Kinship Fortunes for the Shih of Ming-chou.* Durham, NC: Duke University Press, 1986.

——. "Political Success and the Growth of Descent Groups: The Shih of Ming-chou during the Sung." In *Kinship Organization in Late Imperial China 1000–1940*, ed. Patricia B. Ebrey and James L. Watson, 62–94. Berkeley: University of California Press, 1986.

De Bary, Wm. Theodore. "The Rise of Neo-Confucian Orthodoxy in Yüan China." In *Neo-Confucian Orthodoxy in Yüan China*, 1–66. New York: Columbia University Press, 1981.

De Rachewiltz, Igor, et al., eds. *In the Service of the Khan: Eminent Personalities of the Early Mongol-Yüan Period.* Wiesbaden: Harrassowitz, 1993.

——. "Some Reflections on Čingis Qan's Jasay." *East Asian History* 6 (Dec. 1993): 91–104.

De Weerdt, Hilde. "Aspects of Song Intellectual Life: A Preliminary Inquiry into Some Southern Song Encyclopedias." *Papers on Chinese History* 3 (1994): 1–27.

——. *Competition over Content: Negotiating Standards for the Civil Service Examinations in Imperial China (1127–1276).* Cambridge, MA: Harvard University Asia Center, 2007.

Deng Wenyuan 鄧文原. *Baxi ji* 巴西集. SKQS.

Dennis, Joseph. "Early Printing in China Viewed from the Perspectives of Local Gazetteer." In *Knowledge and Text Production in an Age of Print: China, 900–1400*, ed. Lucille Chia and Hilde de Weerdt, 105–34. Leiden: Brill, 2011.

Despeux, Catherine. "The System of the Five Circulatory Phases and the Six Seasonal Influences (*wuyun liuqi*), a Source of Innovation in Medicine Under the Song (960–1279)." In *Innovation in Chinese Medicine*, ed. Elizabeth Shu. Cambridge: Cambridge University Press, 2001.

Ding Guangdi 丁光迪. *Jin-Yuan yixue pingxi* 金元医学評析. Beijing: Renmin weisheng chubanshe, 1999.

Du Fu (To Ho) 杜甫. *To shi* 杜詩. Translated and annotated by Suzuki Torao 鈴木虎雄 and Kurokawa Yōichi 黒川洋一. Tokyo: Iwanami shoten, 1966.

Du You 杜佑. *Tong dian* 通典. Taibei: Xinxing shuju, 1963.

Duara, Prasenjit. "Superscribing Symbols: The Myth of Guandi, Chinese God of War." *Journal of Asian Studies* 47.4 (1988): 778–95.

Ebrey, Patricia. *Chu Hsi's "Family Rituals": A Twelfth-Century Chinese Manual for the Performance of Cappings, Weddings, Funerals, and Ancestral Rites*. Princeton, NJ: Princeton University Press, 1990.

——. *Inner Quarters: Marriage and the Lives of Chinese Women in the Sung Period*. Berkeley: University of California Press, 1992.

——. *China: A Cultural, Social, and Political History*. Wadworth Publishing, 2006.

Elman, Benjamin A. *From Philosophy to Philology: Intellectual and Social Aspects of Change in Late Imperial China*. Cambridge, MA: Council on East Asian Studies, Harvard University, 1984.

——. *Classism, Politics, and Kinship: The Ch'ang-chou School of New Text Confucianism in Late Imperial China*. Berkeley: University of California Press, 1990.

——. "Political, Social, and Cultural Reproduction via Civil Service Examinations in Late Imperial China." *Journal of Asian Studies* 50.1 (1991): 7–28.

Endicott-West, Elizabeth. *Mongolian Rule in China: Local Administration in the Yuan Dynasty*. Cambridge, MA: Council on East Asian Studies, Harvard University, and the Harvard-Yenching Institute, 1989.

Endō Jirō 遠藤次郎, Nakamura Teruko 中村輝子, Mayanagi Makoto 真柳誠, and Kubodera Takako 久保寺峰子. "Inkei hōshi setsu no shiteki kentō: kikei, inkei, tsūkei, gyōkei no igi" 引経報使説の史的検討: 帰経、引経、通経、行経の意義. *Yakushigaku zasshi* 薬史学雑誌 32.2 (1997): 169–77.

Fan Chengda 范成大. *Wujun zhi* 呉郡志. 50 *juan*. 1192. Sanshiqi.

Fan Xingzhun 范行準. *Zhongguo yixueshi lüe* 中國醫學史略. Beijing: Zhongyi guji chubanshe, 1986.

Fan Ye 范曄. *Hou Hanshu* 後漢書. Beijing: Zhonghua shuju, 1965.

Farquhar, David M. *The Government of China Under Mongolian Rule: A Reference Guide*. Stuttgart: Steiner, 1990.

Fei, Si-yen 費絲言. *You dianfan dao guifan: cong Mingdai zhenjielienü de bianshi yu liuchuan kan chenjie guannian de yangehua* 由典範到規範: 從明代貞節烈女的辨識與流傳看貞節觀念的嚴格化. Taibei: Guoli Taiwan daxue wenshi congkan, 1996.

Feng Fujing 馮福京 et al. *Dade Changguozhou tuzhi* 大德昌國州圖志. 7 *juan*. 1298. ZGFZCS.

Franke, Herbert. "Chia Ssu-tao (1213–1275): A 'Bad Last Minister'?" In *Confucian Personalities*, ed. Arthur F. Wright and Denis Twitchett, 146–61. Stanford, CA: Stanford University Press, 1962.

Franke, Herbert, and Denis Twitchett, eds. *Cambridge History of China, vol. 6: Alien Regimes and Border States, 907–1368*. Cambridge: Cambridge University Press, 1994.

Funada Yoshiyuki 舩田善之. "*Gen tenshō* dokkai no tameni: kōgusho, kenkyū bunken ichiran o kanete" 『元典章』読解のために: 工具書・研究文献一覧を兼ねて. *Kai Pian* 開篇 (Waseda University) 18 (1999): 113–28.

——. "Genchō chika no shikimoku jin ni tsuite" 元朝治下の色目人について. *Shigaku zasshi* 史学雑誌 108.9 (Sept. 1999): 43–68.

——. "Review of *Mongoru teikoku to Daigen urusu* by Sugiyama Masaaki" 書評・杉山正明著『モンゴル帝国と大元ウルス』. *Shigaku zasshi* 史学雑誌 113.11: 100–10.

Furth, Charlotte. *Flourishing Yin: Gender in China's Medical History, 960–1665.* Berkeley: University of California Press, 1999.

——. "The Physician as Philosopher of the Way: Zhu Zhenheng (1282–1358)." *Harvard Journal of Asiatic Studies* 66.2 (2006): 423–59.

——. "Producing Medical Knowledge through Cases: History, Evidence, and Action." In *Thinking with Cases: Specialist Knowledge in Chinese Cultural History*, ed. Charlotte Furth, Judith T. Zeitlin, and Ping-chen Hsiung, 125–51. Honolulu: University of Hawai'i Press, 2007.

Gao Sisun 高似孫. *Yanlu* 剡録. 10 *juan*. Sanshiqi.

Gedalecia, David. "Wu Cheng and the Perpetuation of the Classical Heritage in the Yüan." In *China under Mongol Rule*, ed. John D. Langlois, Jr., 186–211. Princeton,, NJ: Princeton University Press, 1981.

——. *The Philosophy of Wu Cheng.* Bloomington: Research Institute for Inner Asian Studies, Indiana University, 1999.

——. *A Solitary Crane in a Spring Grove: The Confucian Scholar Wu Ch'eng in Mongol China.* Wiesbaden: Harrassowitz, 2000.

Goldschmidt, Asaf. "Epidemics and Medicine During the Northern Song Dynasty: The Revival of Cold Damage Disorders (*Shanghan*)." *T'oung Pao* 93.1–3 (2007).

——. *The Evolution of Chinese Medicine: Song Dynasty, 960–1200.* London: Routledge, 2009.

——. "Huizong's Impact on Medicine and on Public History." In *Emperor Huizong and Late Northern Song China: The Politics of Culture and the Culture of Politics*, ed. Patricia Ebrey and Maggie Bickford, 290–91 and 304–08. Cambridge, MA: Harvard University Asia Center, 2006.

Gong Shitai 貢師泰. *Wanzhai ji* 玩齋集. SKQS.

Graham, A.C. trans. *Chuang-tzǔ: The Seven Inner Chapters and Other Writings From the Book* Chuang-tzǔ. London: George Allen & Unwin, 1981.

Gu Jiegang 顧頡剛 and Yang Xiangkui 楊向奎. "Sanhuang kao" 三皇考. In *Gushi bian* 古史辨 7.*zhong* 中, ed. Lü Simian 呂思勉 and Tong Shuye 童書業, 20–282. Shanghai: Kaiming shudian, 1941.

Gujin tushu jicheng 古今圖書集成. Taibei: Dingwen shuju.

Han Yu 韓愈. *Hanyu quanji jiaozhu* 韓愈全集校注. Chengdu: Sichuan daxue chubanshe, 1996.

Han Zhihe 韓祗和. *Shanghan weizhi lun* 傷寒微旨論. SKQS.

Hansen, Marta. *Speaking of Epidemics: The Disease and Geographic Imagination in Late Imperial China.* London: Routledge, 2011.

Hasebe Eiichi 長谷部英一, Shinno Reiko 秦玲子, Uemura Asami 上村元顧, Matsushita Michinobu 松下道信, and Onda Hiromasa 恩田裕正. *Kakuchi yoron chūshaku* 格致餘論注釈. Tokyo: Iseisha, 2014.

He Menggui 何夢桂. *Qianzhai wenji* 潛齋文集. SKQS.

Hinrichs, T.J. "The Medical Transforming of Governance and Southern Customs in Song dynasty China (960–1279 C.E.)." Ph.D. diss., Harvard University, 2003.

——. "Governance Through Medical Texts and the Role of Print." In *Knowledge and Text Production in an Age of Print: China, 900–1400*, ed. Lucia Chia and Hilde de Weerdt, 217–38. Leiden: Brill, 2011.

——. "The Song and Jin Periods." In *Chinese Medicine and Healing: An Illustrated History*, ed. T.J. Hinrichs and Linda L. Barnes, 97–127. Cambridge, MA: Harvard University Press, 2013.

Ho, Ping-ti. *The Ladder of Success in Imperial China: Aspects of Social Mobility, 1368–1911.* New York: Columbia University, 1962.

Honda Seiichi 本田精一. "*Toen saku* kō: sonsho no kenkyū" 「兎園策」攷: 村書の研究. *Tōyōshi ronshū* (*Kyūshū daigaku*) 東洋史論集 (九州大学) 21 (1993): 65–101.

Hori Toshikazu 堀敏一. *Kindensei no kenkyū*: *Chūgoku kodai kokka no tochi seisaku to tochi shoyūsei* 均田制の研究: 中国古代国家の土地政策と土地所有制. Tokyo: Iwanami Shoten, 1975.

Hsia, R. Po-chia. Review of *Manufacturing Confucianism: Chinese Traditions and Universal Civilization*, by Lionel M. Jensen. *History of Religions* 41.1 (2001): 71–73.

Hsiao Ch'i-ch'ing 蕭啓慶. *The Military Establishment of the Yuan Dynasty*. Cambridge, MA: Council on East Asian Studies, Harvard University, 1978.

——. "Yuandai de ruhu: rushi diwei yanbian shi shang de yizhang" 元代的儒戶: 儒士地位演變史上的一章. In *Yuandai shi xintan* 元代史新探, 1–58. Taibei: Xinwenfeng chuban gongsi, 1982.

Hu, Shiu Ying. "History of the Introduction of Exotic Elements into Traditional Chinese Medicine." *Journal of the Arnold Arboretum* 71 (Oct. 1990): 487–526.

Hu Zhiyu 胡祇遹. *Chaishan daquanji* 柴山大全集. SKQS.

Huang Jin 黃溍. *Huang Wenxian gong ji* 黃文獻公集. CSJC chuban.

——. *Jinhua Huang xiansheng wenji* 金華黃先生文集. 43 *juan*. SBCK chuban.

——. *Wenxian ji* 文獻集. SKQS.

Huang Junda 黃俊達. "Yuandai yishi zhidu yanjiu" 元代醫事制度研究. MA thesis, Guoli Qinghua Daxue 国立清華大學, 2011.

Huang Kuanzhong 黃寬重. "Songdai Siming Yuanshi jiazu yanjiu 宋代四明袁氏家族研究." In *Zhongguo jinshi shehui wenhuashi lunwenji* 中国近世社會文化史論文集, ed. Zhongyang yanjiuyuan lishi yuyan yanjiusuo chubanpin bianji weiyuanhui 中央研究院歷史語言研究所出版品編輯委員會, 105–31. Taibei: Zhongyang yanjiuyuan lish yanjiusuo, 1992.

Huang Qinglian 黃清連. *Yuandai huji zhidu yanjiu* 元代戶計制度研究. Taibei: Guoli Taiwan daxue wenxueyuan, 1977.

Huang Runyu 黃潤玉. *Ningbofu jianyaozhi* 寧波府簡要志. Siming congshu 四明叢書.

Huang Yansun 黃巖孫. *Xianxizhi* 仙溪志. 4 *juan*. SYD Xubian.

Huangfu Mi 皇甫謐. *Diwang shiji* 帝王世紀. CSJC chuban.

Huangshan tujing 黃山圖經. 2 *juan*. SYD Xubian.

Hucker, Charles O. *A Dictionary of Official Titles in Imperial China*. Stanford, CA: Stanford University Press, 1985.

Hymes, Robert P. "Not Quite Gentlemen? Doctors in Sung and Yuan." *Chinese Science* 8 (1988): 9–76.

——. "Epilogue: A Hypothesis on the East Asian Beginnings of the *Yersinia Pestis* Polytomy," *The Medieval Globe* 1 (2014): 285–308.

Ibn Sina (Avicenna). *The Canon of Medicine*. Digitized and published by Saab Medical Library, American University of Beirut. http://ddc.aub.edu.lb/projects/saab/avicenna/index.html.

Ichiki Tsuyuhiko 市来津由彦. *Shu Ki monjin shūdan keisei no kenkyū* 朱熹門人集団形成の研究. Tokyo: Sōbunsha, 2002.

Ihara Hiroshi 伊原弘. "Sōdai Meishū ni okeru kanko no kon'in kankei" 宋代明州における官戶の婚姻関係. *Chūō daigaku daigakuin kenkyū nenpō* 中央大学大学院研究年報 1 (March, 1972): 157–58. Reprinted in *Chūgoku kankei ronsetsu shiryō* 中国関係論説資料 14, part 3–2.

Iiyama Tomoyasu 飯山知保. *Kin-Gendai no Kahoku shakai to kakyo seido: Mōhitotsu no "shijin sō"* 金元代の華北社会と科挙制度: もう一つの「士人層」. Tokyo: Waseda daigaku shuppanbu, 2011.

Ikeuchi Isao 池内功. "Genchō no gunken saishi ni tsuite" 元朝の郡県祭祀について. In *Chūgoku ni okeru oshie to kokka* 中国における教と国家, ed. Noguchi Tetsurō 野口鐵郎, 155–79. Tokyo: Yūzankaku shuppan, 1994.

Inoue Susumu 井上進. *Chūgoku shuppan bunka shi: shomotsu sekai to chi no fūkei* 中国出版文化史: 書物世界と知の風景. Nagoya: Nagoya daigaku shuppankai, 2002.

Ishida Hidemi 石田秀実. *Chūgoku igaku shisō shi: mōhitotsu no igaku* 中国医学思想史: もう一つの医学. Tokyo: Tokyo daigaku shuppankai, 1992.

Ishida Hidemi, Shimada Ryūji 島田隆司, Shōji Yoshifumi 庄司良文, Suzuki Hiroshi 鈴木洋, and Fujiyama Kazuko 藤山和子, trans. *Gendai go yaku Kōtei daikei somon (jō)* 現代語訳黄帝内経素問（上）. Chiba: Tōyō gakujutsu shuppansha, 1991.

Ishida Hidemi, Katsuta Masayasu 勝田正泰, Suzuki Hiroshi 鈴木洋, and Hyōdō Akira 兵頭明, trans. *Gendai go yaku Kōtei daikei somon (chū)* 現代語訳黄帝内経素問（中）. Chiba: Tōyō gakujutsu shuppansha, 1992.

Isomae Jun'ichi 磯前順一. *Kindai Nihon no shūkyō gensetsu to sono keifu* 近代日本の宗教言説とその系譜. Tokyo: Iwanami shoten, 2003.

Iwamura Shinobu 岩村忍. "Gen tenshō keibu no kenkyū: keibatsu tetsuzuki" 元典章刑部の研究: 刑罰手続. In *Tōhō gakuhō (Kyoto)* 東方学報 (京都) 24 (1954): 1–114.

Iwamura Shinobu 岩村忍 and Tanaka Kenji 田中謙二. *Gen tenshō keibu* 元典章・刑部, vol. 1. Kyoto: Kyōtō daigaku jinbun kagaku kenkyūjo *Gentenshō* kenkyūhan, 1964.

Jay, Jennifer W. *A Change in Dynasties: Loyalism in Thirteenth-Century China.* Bellingham: Western Washington University, 1991.

Jensen, Lionel M. *Manufacturing Confucianism: Chinese Traditions and Universal Civilization.* Durham, NC: Duke University Press, 1998.

Jian Shuoyou 僭説友. *Xianchun Lin'an zhi* 咸淳臨安志. 100 *juan.* 1268. Sanshiqi.

Jiang Guan 江瓘. *Mingyi lei'an* 名醫類案. Beijing: Zhongguo Zhongyiyao chubanshe, 1996.

Jie Xisi 揭偯斯. *Wen'an ji* 文安集. SKQS.

Jujia biyong shilei: fu Lixue zhinan 居家必用事類: 附吏學指南. Kyoto: Chūbun shuppansha, 1984.

Juvaini, Ata-Malik. *Genghis Khan: The History of the World Conqueror.* Translated by J.A. Boyle with an introduction by David O. Morgan. University of Washington Press, 1997.

Kakiuchi Keiko 垣内景子 and Onda Hiromasa 恩田裕正, eds. *"Shushi gorui" yakuchū, kan 1–3* 『朱子語類』訳注 巻1–3. Tokyo: Kyūko shoin, 2007.

Kawajiri Fumihiko 川尻文彦. "'Zhexue' zai jindai Zhongguo: yi Cai Yuanpei de 'zhexue' wei zhongxin" 「哲学」在近代中国: 以蔡元培的「哲学」为中心. In *Yazhou gai'nian shi yanjiu di 1 ji* 亚洲概念史研究 第1辑. ed. Sun Jiang 孙江and Liu Jianhui 刘建辉, 66–83. Beijing: Shenghuo, Dushu, Xinzhi Sanliang shudian, 2013.

Kawamura Yasushi 川村康. "Sōdai zeisei shōkō 宋代贅壻小考." In *Chūgoku no dentō shakai to kazoku* 中国の伝統社会と家族, ed. Yanagida Setsuko sensei koki kinen ronshū henshū iinkai 柳田節子先生古稀記念論集編集委員会, 347–63. Tokyo: Kyūko shoin, 1993.

Kobayashi Kōshirō 小林高四郎 and Okamoto Keiji 岡本敬二, eds. *Tsūsei jōkaku no kenkyū yakuchū* 通制條格の研究譯注, vol. 1. Tokyo: Kokusho kankōkai, 1964.

Kobayashi Masayoshi 小林正美. *Rikuchō dōkyō shi kenkyū* 六朝道教史研究. Tokyo: Sōbunsha, 1990.

Kondō Kazunari 近藤一成. *Sōdai Chūgoku kakyo shakai no kenkyū* 宋代中国科挙社会の研究. Tokyo: Kyūko shoin, 2009.

Kosoto Hiroshi 小曽戸洋. "Hoku–Sōdai no iyaku sho, sono 1." 北宋代の医薬書, その 1. *Gendai Tōyō igaku* 8.3 現代東洋医学 (1987): 83–91.

——. "Hoku–Sōdai no iyaku sho, sono 2." *Gendai Tōyō igaku* 8.4 (1987): 86–95.

——. "*Taihei keimin wazai kyoku hō* kaidai"『太平恵民和剤局方』解題. In *Zōkō Taihei keimin wazai kyoku hō, Genshi saiseihō, Genshi seisei zokuhō.* 増広太平恵民和剤局方、厳氏済生法、厳氏済生續方, WKIS vol. 4 (1988), *kaisetsu* 1–9.

——. "Nan–Sōdai no iyaku sho, sono 1" 南宋代の医薬書, その 1. *Gendai Tōyō igaku* 9.1 (1988): 87–93.

——. "Nan–Sōdai no iyaku sho, sono 2." *Gendai Tōyō igaku* 9.2 (1988): 79–85.

——. "Nan–Sōdai no iyaku sho, sono 3." *Gendai Tōyō igaku* 9.3 (1988): 96–104.

——. "Nan–Sōdai no iyaku sho, sono 4." *Gendai Tōyō igaku* 9.4 (1988): 96–103.

——. "Nan–Sōdai no iyaku sho, sono 5." *Gendai Tōyō igaku* 10.1 (1989): 93–99.

——. "Nan–Sōdai no iyaku sho, sono 6." *Gendai Tōyō igaku* 10.2 (1989): 94–103.

——. "Gendai no iyakusho, sono 1" 元代の医薬書, その1" *Gendai Tōyō igaku* 11.3 (1990): 92–96.

——. "Gendai no iyakusho, sono 2." *Gendai Tōyō igaku* 11.4 (1990): 76–82.

——. "Gendai no iyakusho, sono 3." *Gendai Tōyō igaku* 12.1 (1991): 78–85.

——. "Gendai no iyakusho, sono 4." *Gendai Tōyō igaku* 12.2 (1991): 93–99.

——. "Gendai no iyakusho, sono 5." *Gendai Tōyō igaku* 12.3 (1991): 94–101.

——. *Chūgoku igaku koten to Nihon: shoshi to denshō* 中国医学古典と日本：書誌と伝承. Tokyo: Hanawa shobō, 1996.

Kou Zongshi 寇宗奭. *Bencao yanyi* 本草衍義. Beijing: Renmin weisheng chubanshe, 1990.

Kyōdai jinbun kagaku kenkyū jo *Gentenshō* kenkyūhan 京大人文科学研究所元典章研究班, ed. *Gen tenshō sakuinkō* 元典章索引稿. 1954. Handwritten manuscript.

Lam, Yuan-chu. "The First Chapter of the 'Treatise on Selection and Recommendation' for the Civil Service in the *Yüan shih.*" Ph.D. diss., Harvard University, 1978.

Langley, C. Bradford. "Wang Ying-lin (1223–1296): A Study in the Political and Intellectual History of the Demise of the Sung." Ph.D. diss., Indiana University, 1980.

Laozi 老子 (attrib.). *Daode jing* 道德經. Translated as *Rōshi* 老子 and annotated by Hachiya Kunio 蜂屋邦夫. Tokyo: Iwanami shoten, 2011.

—— (attrib.). *Daode jing* 道德經. Translated as *The Wisdom of Laotse* and annotated by Lin Yutang. New York: Modern Library, 1976.

Lau, D.C., trans. *Tao Te Ching: A Bilingual Translation.* Hong Kong: The Chinese University Press, 1963.

Lau Nap-yin 柳立言. "Qiantan Songdai funü de shoujie yu zaijia 淺談宋代婦女守節與再嫁." *Xin shixue* 新史學 2.4 (1991): 37–76.

Lee, Sherman E., and Wai-kam Ho. *Chinese Art Under the Mongols: The Yüan Dynasty (1279–1368).* Cleveland, OH: Cleveland Museum of Art, 1968.

Leung, Angela Ki Che 梁其姿 "Organized Medicine in Ming-Qing China: State and Private Medical Institutions in the Lower Yangzi Region." *Late Imperial China* 8.1 (June 1987): 134–66.

——. *Shishan yu jiaohua: Ming-Qing de cishan zuzhi* 施善與教化: 明清的慈善組織. Taibei: Lianjing, 1997.

——. "Medical Learning from the Song to the Ming." In *The Song-Yuan-Ming Transition*, ed. Richard Von Glahn and Paul Smith, 374–98. Cambridge, MA: Harvard University Asia Center, 2003.

Li Dongyang 李東陽 et al. *Da Ming Huidian* 大明會典. Guofeng chubanshe, 1963.

Li Gao 李杲. *Dongyuan shixiao fang* 東垣試效方. Shanghai: Shanghai kexue jishu chubanshe, 1984.

——. *Dongyuan shixiao fang.* In *Li Dongyuan yixue quanshu* 李東垣醫學全書, 195–275. Beijing: Zhongguo Zhongyi chubanshe, 2006.

——. *Neiwaishang bianhuo lun* 內外傷辨惑論. In *Li Dongyuan yixue quanshu*, 1–26. Beijing: Zhongguo Zhongyi chubanshe, 2006.

Li Haowen 李好文. *Chang'an zhitu* 長安志圖. 3 *juan*. 1344–46. ZGFZCS (attached to Song Minqiu, *Chang'an zhi*).

——. *Chang'an zhitu* 長安志圖. 1784 edition in Jingxuntang congshu 經訓堂叢書.

Li Jingde 黎靖德. *Zhuzi yu lei* 朱子語類, vol. 1. Beijing; Zhonghua shuju, 1986.

Li Jingwei 李經緯 et al., eds. *Zhongyi dacidian* 中醫大辭典. Beijing: Renmin weisheng chubanshe. 1995.

Li Lian 李濂. *Bianjing yiji zhi*. 汴京遺蹟志. SKQS.

Li Yuqing 李玉清. "Cheng Wuji shengping ji *Zhujie Shanghanlu xuanzhu* niandai kao 成无己生平及《注解伤寒论》撰注年代考." *Zhonghua yishi zazhi* 中华医史杂志 27.4 (Oct. 1997): 249–51.

Li Zhe 黎喆 et al. *Hongzhi Fuzhoufu zhi* 弘治撫州府志. TYG Xubian.

Liang Jun 梁峻. *Zhongguo gudai yizheng shilüe* 中国古代医政史略. Hohhot: Nei Menggu renmin chubanshe, 1995.

Liang Kejia 梁克家. *Chunxi Sanshan zhi* 淳熙三山志. 42 *juan*. SYD xubian.

Liao Yujun 廖育郡, Fu Fang 傅芳, and Zheng Jinsheng 鄭金生. *Zhongguo kexue jishu shi: yixue juan* 中國科學技術史: 醫学卷. Beijing: Kexue chubanshe, 1998.

Lin Sufen 林素芬. "Boshi yi zhiyong: Wang Yinglin xueshu de zai pingjia" 博識以致用: 王應麟學術的再評價. Master's thesis, Guoli Taiwan daxue, 1994.

Ling Wanqing 陵萬頃. *Yufeng zhi* 玉峰志. 3 *juan*. 1252. Sanshiqi.

Linghu Defen 令狐德棻. *Zhou Shu* 周書. Beijing: Zhonghua shuju, 1971.

Liu Boji 劉伯驥. *Zhongguo yixue shi* 中國醫學史. Yangmingshan: Huagang chubanshe, 1974.

Liu Guan 柳貫. *Daizhi ji* 待制集. SKQS.

Liu, James T.C. *China Turning Inward: Intellectual-Political Changes in the Early Twelfth Century.* Cambridge, MA: Council on East Asian Studies, Harvard University, 1988.

Liu Ji 劉基. *Chengyibo wenji* 誠意伯文集. SKQS.

Liu Minzhong 劉敏中. *Zhong'an xiansheng Liu Wenjian gong wenji* 中庵先生劉文簡公文集. 25 *juan*. Beitu.

Liu Qi 劉祁. *Guiqian zhi* 歸潛志. *Yuan-Ming shiliao biji congkan* 元明史料筆記叢刊 series. Beijing: Zhonghua shuju, 1983.

Liu Shen 劉詵. *Guiyin wenji* 桂隱文集. SKQS.

——. *Guiyin wenji* 桂隱文集, 8 *juan* and *fulu* 1 *juan*. YRCK.

Liu Shijue 刘时觉. *Yongjia yipai yanjiu* 永嘉医派研究. Beijing: Zhongguo guji chubanshe, 2000.

Liu Wansu 劉完素. *Liu Wansu yixue quanshu* 劉完素醫學全書. Beijing: Zhongguo Zhong yiyao chubanshe, 2006.

Liu Wenshu 劉温舒. *Suwen rushi yunqi lun'ao* 素問入式運氣論奧. SKQS.

Liu Xu 劉煦 et al., comp. *Jiu Tangshu* 舊唐書. Beijing: Zhonghua shuju, 1975.

Liu Xun 劉壎. *Shuiyuncun gao* 水雲村槀. SKQS.

Liu Yueshen 劉岳申. *Shenzhai ji* 申齋集. SKQS.

Lü Pu 呂溥. *Zhuqi gao* 竹谿稿. Xu Jinhua congshu 續金華叢書.

Lu Wengui 陸文圭, *Qiangdong leigao* 牆東類稿, SKQS.

Lu Xian 盧憲. *Jiading Zhenjiang zhi* 嘉定鎮江志. 22 *juan*. 1213. Sanshiqi.

Luo Jun 羅濬 et al. *Baoqing Siming zhi* 寶慶四明志. 21 *juan*. 1227. Sanshiqi.

Luo Tianxiang 駱天驤. *Leibian Chang'an zhi* 類編長安志. 10 *juan*. SYD Xubian.

Luo Tianyi 羅天益. *Weisheng baojian* 衛生宝鑑. CSJC chubian.

——. *Weisheng baojian*. In *Luo Tianyi yixue quanshu* 羅天益醫學全書. Beijing: Zhongguo Zhongyi chubanshe, 2006.

Luo Yuan 羅願. *Xin'an zhi* 新安志. 10 *juan*. 1175. Sanshiqi.

Ma Duanlin 馬端臨. *Wenxian tongkao* 文獻通考. Guoxue jiben congshu. Taibei: Xinxing shuju, 1962.

Mabuchi Masaya 馬淵昌也. "Gen-Minsho seirigaku no ichi sokumenn: Shushigaku no biman to Son Saku no shisō" 元・明初性理学の一側面—朱子学の瀰漫と孫作の思想. *Chūgoku tetsugaku* 中国哲学 4 (1992): 60–131.

Maejima Shinji 前嶋信次. "Shiroppu kō 舎利別考." *Gekkan kaikyōken* 月刊回教圏 2.6 (1939): 12–35.

———. *Tōzai bunka koryū no shosō* 東西文化交流の諸相. Tokyo: *Tōzai bunka koryū no shosō* kankōkai, 1971.

Maeno Naoaki 前野直彬, ed. *Chūgoku bungakushi* 中国文学史. Tokyo: Tokyo University Press, 1975.

Matsushita Michinobu. "Haku Gyokusen to sono shuppan katsudō: Zenshin kyō nanshū ni okeru shiju ishiki no kokufuku" 白玉蟾とその出版活動: 全眞教南宗における師授意識の克服 *Tōhō shūkyō* 東方宗教 104 (2004): 23–42.

Mayanagi Makoto 真柳誠. *"Jumon jishin* kaidai" 『儒門事親』解題. http://mayanagi. hum.ibaraki.ac.jp/paper01/jumonjishin.html. Originally published in *Fusai honji hō, Fusai Honji hō zokushū, Jumon jishin, Somon genki genbyō shiki, senmeiron hō* 普済本事方、普済本事方続集、儒門事親、素問玄機原病式、宣明論方, WKIS, vol. 2 (1988).

———. *"Shōkan meiri ron, Shōkan meiri yakuhō ron* kaidai" 『傷寒明理論』『傷寒明理薬方論』解題. http://mayanagi.hum.ibaraki.ac.jp/paper01/meirironkaidai.html. Originally published in *Somon nyushiki unki ron'ō, Shōkan meiri ron, Shōkan meiri yakuhō ron, Shōni yakushō chokketsu, San'in kyokuitsu byōshō hōron* 素問入式運気論奥、傷寒明理論、傷寒明理薬方論、小児薬証直訣、三因極一病証方論, WKIS, vol. 1 (1988).

———. *"Somon genki genbyō shiki, Kōtei Somon senmei ron* kaidai" 『素問玄機原病式』『黄帝素問宣明論』解題. http://mayanagi.hum.ibaraki.ac.jp/paper01/liuwansu.html. Originally published in *Fusai honji hō, Fusai Honji hō zokushū, Jumon jishin, Somon genki genbyō shiki, senmeiron hō*, WKIS, vol. 2 (1988).

———. *"Kakuchi yoron, Kyokuhō hakki* kaidai" 『格致余論』『局方発揮』解題. http:// mayanagi.hum.ibaraki.ac.jp/paper01/kakuchikaidai.html. Originally published in *Myakketsu, Naigaishō benwaku ron, Hi'i ron, Ranshitu hizō, Tōeki honzō, Shiji nanchi, Kakuchi yoron, Kyokuhō hakki, Geka seigi, Ikei sokai shū* 脈訣、内外傷弁惑論、脾胃論、蘭室秘蔵、湯液本草、此事難知、格致余論、局方発揮、外科精義、医経溯洄集, WKIS, vol. 6 (1989).

———. *"Naigaishō benwaku ron, Hi'i ron, Ranshitu hizō* kaidai" 『内外傷弁惑論』『脾胃論』『蘭室秘蔵』解題. http://mayanagi.hum.ibaraki.ac.jp/paper01/toenkaidai.html. Originally published in *Myakketsu, Naigaishō benwaku ron, Hi'i ron, Ranshitu hizō, Tōeki honzō, Shiji nanchi, Kakuchi yoron, Kyokuhō hakki, Geka seigi, Ikei sokai shū*, WKIS, vol. 6 (1989).

———. *"Tan'eki honzō, Shiji nanchi* kaidai" 『湯液本草』『此事難知』解題. http:// mayanagi.hum.ibaraki.ac.jp/paper01/okoko.html. Originally published in *Myakketsu, Naigaishō benwaku ron, Hi'i ron, Ranshitu hizō, Tōeki honzō, Shiji nanchi, Kakuchi yoron, Kyokuhō hakki, Geka seigi, Ikei sokai shū*, WKIS, vol. 6 (1989).

———. *"Chūkai Shōkan ron* kaidai" 『注解傷寒論』解題. http://mayanagi.hum.ibaraki. ac.jp/paper01/chukai.html. Originally published in *Shōkan ron kōjōben, Chūkai Shōkan ron, Chūkei zensho* 傷寒論後条弁、注解傷寒論、仲景全書, WKIS, vol. 16 (1992).

———. "Yakusei ron no kentō (dai 4 hō): Hoku-Sō no keishi kaibō to inkei, kikeisetu no keisei." 薬性論の検討（第4報） 北宋の刑屍解剖と引経・帰経説の形成. http:// mayanagi.hum.ibaraki.ac.jp/paper02/touyou93.html. Originally published in *Nihon Tōyō igaku zasshi* 日本東洋医学雑誌 43.5 (1993): 153.

——."*Somon* hanpon kenkyū (sono 2)" 『素問』版本研究　（その二）. *Kikan daikei* 季刊内經 189 (2012): 4–42.

Mayanagi Makoto 真柳誠 and Kosoto Hiroshi 小曽戸洋. "Kindai no iyaku sho, sono 1" 金代の医薬書, その1. http://mayanagi.hum.ibaraki.ac.jp/paper01/kindai1.html. Originally published in *Gendai Tōyō igaku* 現代東洋医学 10.3 (1989): 101–07.

——. "Kindai no iyaku sho, sono 2." http://mayanagi.hum.ibaraki.ac.jp/paper01/kindai2.html. Originally published in *Gendai Tōyō igaku* 10.4 (1989): 105–12.

———. "Kindai no iyaku sho, sono 3." http://mayanagi.hum.ibaraki.ac.jp/paper01/kindai3.html. Originally published in *Gendai Tōyō igaku* 11.1 (1990): 108–13.

———. "Kindai no iyaku sho, sono 4." http://mayanagi.hum.ibaraki.ac.jp/paper01/kindai4.html. *Gendai Tōyō igaku* 11.2 (1990): 99–105.

——. "Gendai no iyaku sho, sono 6" 元代の医薬書, その6. *Gendai Tōyō igaku* 現代東洋医学 12.4 (October 1991), 103–09.

McKnight, Brian E. *Village and Bureaucracy in Southern Song China*. Chicago, IL: University of Chicago Press, 1971.

Mei Yingfa 梅應發 et al. *Kaiqing Siming xuzhi* 開慶四明續志. 12 *juan*. 1259. Sanshiqi.

Mencius. *Mencius*. Translated by Irene Bloom and P.J. Ivanhoo. New York: Columbia University Press, 2011.

Miao Yue 繆鉞. "Yuan Yishan nianpu huizuan" 元遺山年譜彙纂. In *Yuan Haowen quanji* 元好問全集, by Yuan Haowen 元好問, 57.1339–59. 1448. Expanded edition. Taiyuan: Shanxi guji chubanshe, 2004.

Miura Shūichi 三浦秀一. "Gakusei Go Chō, aruiwa Sōmatu no shoin no kōryō ni tsuite" 学生呉澄，あるいは宋末の書院の興隆について. *Bunka* 文化 60.3–4 (1997): 37–56.

——. *Chūgoku shingaku no ryōsen: Genchō no chishikijin to Ju Dō Butsu sankyō* 中国心学の稜線: 元朝の知識人と儒道仏三教. Tokyo: Kenbun shuppan, 2003.

Miya Noriko 宮紀子. *Mongoru jidai no shuppan bunka* ンゴル時代の出版文化. Nagoya: Nagoya daigaku shuppankai, 2006.

——. "Mongoru ōzoku to kitai no gijutsu shugi shūdan モンゴル王族と漢児の技術主義集団." In *Gakumon no katachi: mōhitotsu no Chūgoku shisōshi* 学問のかたち: もう一つの中国思想史, ed. Kominami Ichirō, 177–222. Tokyo: Kyūko shoin, 2014.

Miyashita Saburō 宮下三郎. "Sō-Gen no iryō" 宋元の医療. In *Sō-Gen jidai no kagaku gijutsu shi* 宋元時代の科学技術史, ed. Yabuuchi Kiyoshi 薮内清, 123–70. Kyoto: Kyoto daigaku jinbun kagaku kenkyūjo, 1967.

Miyazaki Ichisada 宮崎市定. "Sōgen jidai no hōsei to saiban kikō" 宋元時代の法制と裁判機構. *Tōhō gakuhō* 東方学報 24 (Feb. 1954): 115–226.

——."Gakushū no eki zengo" 鄂州之役前後. In *Ajiashi kenkyū* アジア史研究, vol. 1. Kyoto: Tōyōshi kenkyū kai, 1957, 402–14.

——. "Nan-Sō matsu no saishō Ka Jidō" 南宋末の宰相賈似道. In *Ajiashi kenkyū* アジア史研究, vol. 2. Kyoto: Tōyōshi kenkyū kai, 1959, 193–231.

Mizoguchi Yūzō et al., eds. *Chūgoku shisō bunka jiten* 中国思想文化事典. Tokyo: Tokyo daigaku shuppankai, 2001.

Morgan, David. *The Mongols*. Oxford: Basil Blackwell, 1986.

Morita Kenji 森田憲司. *Gendai chishikijin to chiiki shakai* 元代知識人と地域社会. Kyūko shoin, 2004.

Mote, Frederick W. *Imperial China 900–1800*. Cambridge, MA: Harvard University Press, 1999.

Murthy, Viren."On the Emergence of New Concepts in Late Qing China and Meiji Japan: the Case of Religion." In *Sino-Japanese Transculturation: From the Late Nineteenth*

Century to the End of the Pacific War, ed. Richard King, Cody Paulton, and Katsuhiko Endo, 71–97. Lanham, MD: Lexington Books, 2012.

Nanjing jizhu 難經集註, annotated by Lü Guan 呂廣, et al. SBCK chubian.

Neskar, Ellen G. "The Cult of Worthies: A Study of Shrines Honoring Local Confucian Worthies in the Sung Dynasty (960–1279)." Ph.D. diss., Columbia University, 1993.

——. *The Politics of Prayer: Shrines to Local Former Worthies in Sung China* (forthcoming).

Ni, Maoshing, trans. *The Yellow Emperor's Classic of Medicine: A New Translation of the Neijing Suwen with Commentary*. Boston, MA: Shambhala, 1995.

Ni Shouyue 倪守約. *Jinhua Chichengshan zhi* 金華赤城山志. 1 *juan*. SYD Xubian.

Niida Noboru 仁井田陞. "*Gen tenshō no seiritsu to Daitoku tenshō*" 元典章の成立と大德典章. Originally published 1940. Reprinted in *Chūgoku hōseishi kenkyū: hō to kanshū, hō to dōtoku* 中国法制史研究: 法と慣習・法と道徳, 182–99, Tokyo: Tokyo daigaku Tōyō bunka kenkyū jo, 1964.

Niwa Tomosaburō 丹羽友三郎. "Genchō niokeru in, ji, kan nado no seiritsu katei nitsuite" 元朝における院・寺・監等の設立過程について. *Mie Hōkei* 三重法経 24 (Sept. 1970): 13–28.

Oguri Eiichi. "Gen Kōmon to igaku" 元好問と医学. *Gen Kōmon: Chūgaku shijin senshū 2 shū dai 9 kan furoku* 元好問: 中国詩人選集二集第9巻付録. Tokyo: Iwanami shoten, 1963.

Okamoto Keiji 岡本敬二, ed. *Tsūsei jōkaku no kenkyū yakuchū* 通制條格の研究譯注, vol. 2. Tokyo: Kokusho kankōkai, 1975.

——, ed. *Tsūsei jōkaku no kenkyū yakuchū* 通制條格の研究譯注, vol. 3. Tokyo: Kokusho kankōkai, 1976.

Okanishi Tameto 岡西為人. "Chūgoku honzō no dentō to Kin-Gen no honzō" 中国本草の伝統と金元の本草. In *Sō-Gen jidai no kagaku gijutsu shi*, ed. Yabuuchi Kiyoshi, 123–70. Kyoto: Kyoto daigaku jinbun kagaku kenkyūjo, 1967.

Okuno Shigeo 奥野繁生. "Ryū Kanso to *Seizan gunsen kaishin ki*" 劉完素と『西山群仙會眞記』. *Tōhō shūkyō* 東方宗教 121 (2013): 24–44.

Ōshima Ritsuko 大島立子. "Gendai kokei to yōeki" 元代戸計と徭役. *Rekishigaku kenkyū* 歴史学研究 484 (Sept. 1980): 23–32, 60.

——. "Gendai no juko ni tsuite" 元代の儒戸について. In *Nakajima Satoshi sensei koki kinen ronshū* 中嶋敏先生古稀記念論集, ed. Nakajima Satoshi sensei koki kinen jigyōkai 中嶋敏先生古稀記念事業会, vol. 2, 319–39. Tokyo: Kyūko shoin, 1981.

——. *Mongoru no seifuku ōchō* モンゴルの征服王朝. Tokyo: Daitō shuppansha, 1992.

Otagi Matsuo 愛宕松男. "Mōkojin seiken chika no kannchi ni okeru hanseki no mondai" 蒙古人政権治下の漢地に於ける版籍の問題. In *Haneda Hakase shōju kinen Tōyōshi ronsō* 羽田博士頌壽記念東洋史論叢, ed. Haneda hakase kanreki kinenkai 羽田博士還暦記念会 et al. Kyoto: Tōyōshi kenkyûkai, 1950.

Ouyang Xiu 歐陽脩 et al. *Xin Tangshu* 新唐書. Beijing: Zhonghua shuju, 1975.

Pang Anshi 龐安時. *Shanghan zongbin lun* 傷寒總病論. Beijing: Renmin weisheng chubanshe, 1989.

Poon, Ming-sun. "Books and Printing in Sung China (960–1279)." Ph.D. diss., University of Chicago, 1979.

Pu Daoyuan 蒲道源. *Xianju conggao* 閑居叢稿. SKQS.

Qian Gu 錢穀 ed. *Wudu wencui xuji* 呉都文粹續集. SKQS.

Qinding xu wenxian tongkao 欽定續文獻通考. Commissioned by the Qianlong emperor (Qing dynasty). Guoxue jiben congshu.

Qiu Shusen 邱樹森, Wu Yiye 伍貽業, et al., eds. *Zhongguo Huizu shi* 中国回族史. 2 vols. Yinchuan: Ningxia chubanshe, 1996.

Qiu Zhonglin 邱仲麟. "Mianmian guadie: guanyu Mingdai Jiangsu shiyi de chubu kaocha" 綿綿瓜瓞—關於明代江蘇世醫的初步考察. *Chugoku shigaku* 中国史学 13 (2003): 45–67.

Quan Yuanwen 全元文. Ed. Li Xiusheng 李修生 et al. 61 vols. Nanjing: Jiangsu guji chubanshe (vols. 1–25) and Fenghuang chubanshe (vols. 26-61), 1997–2005.

Rai ki (*Li ji*) 禮記. Translated and annotated by Takeuchi Teruo 竹内照夫. Volume *ge* (下). Tokyo: Meiji shoin, 1979.

Rall, Jutta. *Die Vier Grossen Medizinschulen der Mongolzeit: Stand und Entwicklung der Chinesischen Medizin in der Chin-und Yüan-zeit*. Wiesbaden: Franz Steiner Verlag, 1970.

Ratchnevsky, Paul. *Un code des Yuan*. Paris: Libraire Ernest Leroux, 1937.

——. *Historisch-Terminologisches Wörterbuch der Yüan-zeit: Medizinwesen*. Unter Miterbeit von Johann Dill und Doris Heyde. Berlin: Akademie-Verlag, 1967.

——. *Un code des Yuan*, vol. 2. Paris: Presses Universitaire de France, 1972.

——. *Un code des Yuan*, vol. 3. Paris: Presses Universitaire de France, 1977.

——. *Un code des Yuan*, vol. 4. Paris: Presses Universitaire de France, 1985.

Riasanovsky, Valentin A. *Fundamental Principles of Mongol Law*. Bloomington: Indiana University, 1965.

Robinson, David M., ed. *Culture, Courtiers, and Competition: The Ming Court (1368–1644)*. Cambridge, MA: Harvard University Press, 2008.

Rossabi, Morris. *Khubilai Khan: His Life and Times*. Berkeley: University of California Press, 1988.

Rubruck, William of. *The Mission of Friar William of Rubruck: His Journey to the Court of the Great Khan Möngke 1253–1255*. Translated by Peter Jackson. Introduction, notes, and appendices by Peter Jackson with David Morgan. London: The Hakluyt Society, 1990.

Sang Bing 桑兵. "Kindai 'Chūgoku tetsugaku' no kigen" 近代「中国哲学」の起源. Trans. Murata Ei 村田衛. In *Kindai Higashi Ajia niokeru honyaku gainen no tenkai* 近代東アジアにおける翻訳概念の展開, ed. Ishikawa Yoshihiro 石川禎浩 and Hazama Naoki 狭間直樹. Kyoto: Kyoto daigaku jinbun kangaku kenkyūjo fuzoku Chūgoku kenkyū sentā 2013, 143–66.

Savage-Smith, Emilie. "Medicine." In *Encylopedia of the History of Arabic Science*, ed. Roshdi Rashed, vol. 3, 903–62. New York: Routledge, 1996.

Scheid, Volker. *Currents of Tradition in Chinese Medicine, 1626–2006*. Seattle, WA: East Land Press, 2007.

Schurmann, Herbert Franz. *Economic Structure of the Yüan Dynasty: Translation of Chapters 93–94 of the* Yuan shih. Cambridge, MA: Harvard University Press. 1956.

Shi E. 施鍔. *Chunyou Lin'an jiyi* 淳祐臨安輯逸. 8 *juan*. SYD Xubian.

——. *Chunyou Lin'an zhi* 淳祐臨安志. 6 *juan* (incomplete). 1152. Sanshiqi.

Shi Nengzhi 史能之. *Xianchun Piling zhi* 咸淳毘陵志. 30 *juan*. 1268. Sanshiqi.

Shi Su 施宿. *Jiatai Kuaiji zhi* 嘉泰會稽志. 20 *juan*. Sanshiqi.

Shiba Yoshinobu 斯波義信. *Sōdai Kōnan keizaishi no kenkyū* 宋代江南経済史の研究. Tokyo: Kyūko shoin, 1988.

Shimonaka Kunihiko 下中邦彦, ed. *Ajia rekishi jiten* アジア歴史事典 (Encyclopedia of Asian history). 10 vols. Tokyo: Heibonsha, 1959–62.

Shinno, Reiko 秦玲子. "Sōdai no kō to teishi ketteiken" 宋代の后と帝嗣決定権. In *Chūgoku no dentō shakai to kazoku* 中国の伝統社会と家族, ed. Yanagida setsuko sensei kokikinen ronshū henshū iinkai 柳田節子先生古稀記念論集編集委員会, 51–70. Tokyo: Kyūko shoin, 1993.

——. "Sōdai kōgōsei kara mita Chūgoku kafuchōsei" 宋代皇后制から見た中国家父長制. In *Ajia joseishi: hikakushi no kokoromi* アジア女性史: 比較史の試み, ed. Ajia joseishi kokusai shimpojūmu jikkō iinkai アジア女性史国際シンポジウム実行委員会, 297–311. Tokyo: Akashi shoten, 1997.

——. "Promoting Medicine in the Yuan Dynasty (1206–1368): An Aspect of Mongol Rule in China." Ph.D. diss., Stanford University, 2002.

——. "Medical Schools and the Temples for the Three Progenitors in Yuan China: A Case of Cross-Cultural Interactions." *Harvard Journal of Asiatic Studies* 67.1 (2007): 89–133.

Shouchang sheng 壽昌乗. 1 *juan*. SYD Xubian.

Shu Jingde 黍靖德, comp. *Zhuzi Yulei* 朱子語類. Reprinted in 1872, Yingyuan shuyuan 應元書院.

Sima Qian 司馬遷. *Shiji* 史記. Beijing: Zhonghua shudian, 1959.

Simonis, Fabien. "Mad Acts, Mad Speech, and Mad People in Late Imperial Chinese Law and Medicine." Ph.D. diss., Princeton University, 2010.

Sivin, Nathan. "On the Word 'Taoist' as a Source of Perplexity, with Special Reference to the Relations of Science and Religion in Traditional China." *History of Religions* 17.3/4 (1978): 303–30.

——. *Granting the Seasons: The Chinese Astronomical Reform of 1280, With a Study of Its Many Dimensions and an Annotated Translation of Its Records*. New York: Springer, 2010.

So, Billy K.L. *Prosperity, Region, and Institutions in Maritime China: The South Fukien Pattern, 946–1368*. Cambridge, MA: Harvard University Asia Center, 2001.

Song Lian 宋濂. *Song Lian quanji* 宋濂全集. Hangzhou: Zhejiang guji chubanshe, 1999.

Song Lian 宋濂 et al., eds. *Yuanshi* 元史. Beijing: Zhonghua shuju, 1976.

Song Minqiu 宋敏求. *Chang'an zhi* 長安志. 20 *juan*. ZGFZCS.

——, ed. *Tang da zhaoling ji* 唐大詔令集. Beijing: Shangwu yinshuguan, 1959.

Song Naiguang 宋乃光 et al. "Liu Wansu yixue xueshu sixiang yanjiu" 刘完素医学学术思想研究, in Liu Wansu, *Liu Wansu yixue quanshu*, 311–27.

Song Xian 宋峴. *Huihui yaofang kaoshi* 回回藥方考釋, 2 vols. Beijing: Zhonghua shuju, 2000.

——. *Gudai Bosi yixue yu Zhongguo* 古代波斯医学与中国. Beijing: Jingji ribao chubanshe, 2001.

Soronguto Ba Jigumudo 索倫古特・巴・吉格木特. *Mongoru igakushi*モンゴル医学史. Originally titled *Mongyol anyaxu uxayan-u tobei teüke*. Translated from Mongolian to Japanese by Ju Runga 珠荣嘎 and Takenaka Ryōji 竹中良二. Tokyo: Nōsan Gyoson bunka kyōkai, 1991.

Sotoyama Gunji 外山軍治. *Kinchōshi Kenkyū* 金朝史研究. Kyoto: Tōyōshi kenkyūkai, 1964.

Su Tianjue 蘇天爵, ed. *Yuan wenlei* 元文類, 70 *juan*. Guoxue jiben congshu 國學基本叢書 series. Shanghai: Shangwu yinshuguan, 1936. Originally titled *Guochao wenlei* 國朝文類.

——, ed. *Yuanchao mingchen shilüe* 元朝名臣事略. 15 *juan*. Beijing: Zhonghua shuju, 1996. Originally titled *Guochao mingchen shilüe* 國朝名臣事略.

——. *Zixi wengao* 滋溪文稿. SKQS.

——. *Zixi wengao* 滋溪文稿. Beijing: Zhonghua shuju, 1997.

Sugiyama Masaaki 杉山正明. *Yaritsu Sozai to sono jidai* 耶律楚材とその時代. Tokyo: Hakuteisha, 1996.

——. *Mongoru teikoku to Daigen urusu* モンゴル帝国と大元ウルス. Kyoto: Kyoto daigaku gakujutsu shuppankai, 2004.

Sugiyama Masaaki 杉山正明 and Kitagawa Seiichi 北川誠一. *Sekai no rekishi: Dai Mongoru no jidai* 世界の歴史: 大モンゴルの時代. Tokyo: Chūō kōronsha, 1997.

Sun Jiang 孙江. "Fanyi zongjiao" 翻译宗教. In *Yazhou gai'nian shi yanjiu di 1 ji* 亚洲概念史研究 第1辑. ed. Sun Jiang 孙江 and Liu Jianhui 刘建辉, 84–108. Beijing: Shenghuo, Dushu, Xinzhi Sanliang shudian, 2013.

Sun Simiao 孫思邈. *Essential Subtleties on the Silver Sea: The Yin-hai jing-wei: A Chinese Classic on Ophthalmology*. Translated and annotated by Jürgen Kovacs and Paul U. Unschuld. Berkeley: University of California Press, 1998.

Sun Yingshi 孫應時. *Chongxiu Qinchuan zhi* 重修琴川志. 15 *juan*. 1363. Sanshiqi (titled *Qinchuan zhi*). Also SYD Xubian.

Sutō Yoshiyuki 周藤吉之. *Sōdai kanryōsei to daitochishoyū* 宋代官僚制と大土地所有. Tokyo: Nihon Hyōronsha, 1950.

Taga Akigorō 多賀秋五郎. *Tōdai kyōiku shi no kenkyū: Nihon gakkō kyōiku no genryū* 唐代教育史の研究:日本学校教育の源流. Fumaido, 1953.

Takano Shigeo 高野繁男. "*Meiroku zasshi* no goi kōzō: niji kango o chūshin ni (sono 1)" 『明六雑誌』の語彙構造：2 字漢語を中心に（その1）. *Jinbungaku kenkyūjo hō* 人文学学研究所報. Kanagawa Daigaku 神奈川大学 34 (2001): 39–52.

――. "*Meiroku zasshi* no wasei kango: gendaigo ni natta go to shōmetsu shita go" 『明六雑誌』の和製漢語: 現代語になった語と消滅した語. In *Meiroku zasshi to sono shūhen* 『明六雑誌』とその周辺, ed. Kanagawa Daigaku Jinbungaku Kenkyūjo 神奈川大学人文学研究所, 175–207. Tokyo: Ochanomizu shobō, 2004.

Taki Motoyasu 多紀元簡. *I yō* 醫賸. Shanghai: Shanghai Zhongyi xueyuan chubanshe, 1993.

Tan Yao 談鑰. *Jiatai Wuxingzhi* 嘉泰吳興志. 20 *juan*. 1201. Sanshiqi.

Tanaka Kenji 田中謙二. "Mōbun chokuyakutai ni okeru hakuwa ni tsuite: Gen tenshō oboegaki" 蒙文直譯體における白話について: 元典章覚書. *Tōyōshi kenkyū* 東洋史研究 19.4 (1961): 483–501.

――. "*Gen tenshō* ni okeru Mōbun chokuyakutai no bunshō" 元典章における蒙文直譯體の文體. In *Gen Tenshō no buntai* 元典章の文體, by Yoshikawa Kōjirō and Tanaka Kenji, a supplement (*furoku* 付録) to *Kōteibon Gen Tenshō keibu dai 1 satsu* 校定本元典章刑部第一冊, by Iwamura Shinobu and Tanaka Kenji, 1964.

――. "*Gen tenshō* bunshō no kōsei" 元典章文章の構成. *Tōyōshi kenkyū* 東洋史研究 23.4 (March, 1965): 452–77.

Tanba Mototane 丹波元胤. *Chūgoku iseki kō* 中國醫籍考. Beijing: Renmin weisheng chubanshe, 1956.

Tao Yuanming 陶淵明. "Yinjiu qishiyi 飲酒其十一." In *To Enmei shū zenshaku* 陶淵明集全釈, translated and annotated by Tabei Fumio 田部井文雄 and Ueda Takeshi 上田武, 175–77. Tokyo: Meiji Shoin, 2001.

Tao Zongyi 陶宗儀. *Nancun chuogeng lu* 南村輟耕錄. Beijing: Zhonghua shuju, 1959.

Tillman, Hoyt Cleveland. *Confucian Discourse and Chu Hsi's Ascendancy*. Honolulu: University of Hawai'i Press, 1992.

――. "Confucianism under the Chin and the Impact of Sung Confucian Tao-Hsüeh." In *China under the Jurchen Rule: Essays on Chin Intellectual and Cultural History,* ed. Hoyt Cleveland Tillman and Stephen H. West, 71–114. Albany: State University of New York Press, 1995.

Tillman, Hoyt Cleveland, and Stephen H. West, eds. *China under the Jurchen Rule: Essays on Chin Intellectual and Cultural History*. Albany: State University of New York Press, 1995.

Tonami Mamoru 礪波護, Kishimoto Mio 岸本美緒, Sugiyama Masaaki 杉山正明, eds. *Chūgoku Rekishi kenkyū nyūmon* 中国歴史研究入門. Nagoya: Nagoya daigaku shuppankai, 2006.

Tongzhi tiaoge 通制條格. Nanjing: Zhejiang guji chubanshe, 1986.

Tsuchiya Yūko 土屋悠子. "Mindai no tai'i in seki ni tsuite" 明代の太醫院籍について. *Ajia shi kenkyū* アジア史研究 34 (2010): 159–92.

Tuotuo 脱脱 et al. *Jinshi* 金史. Beijing: Zhonghua shuju, 1975.

—— et al. *Songshi* 宋史. Beijing: Zhonghua shuju, 1977.

Twitchett, Denis Crispin. *Financial Administration Under the T'ang dynasty*. 2nd ed. Cambridge: Cambridge Unversity Press, 1970.

Uematsu Tadashi 植松正. "Gendai no shiden ni tsuite no ichi kōsatsu" 元代の賜田についての一考察. In *Chūgoku no dentō shakai to kazoku* 中国の伝統社会と家族, ed. Yanagida setsuko sensei kokikinen ronshū henshū iinkai 柳田節子先生古稀記念論集編集委員会, 231–52. Tokyo: Kyūko shoin, 1993.

——. "Gendai Kōnan no chihōkan nin'yō ni tsuite" 元代江南の地方官任用について. *Hōseishi kenkyū* 法制史研究 38 (1988): 1–42. Also reprinted in *Gendai kōnan seiji shakaishi kenkyū* 元代江南政治社会史研究, 222–70, Tokyo: Kyūko shoin, 1997.

——. *Gendai Kōnan seiji shakaishi kenkyū* 元代江南政治社会史研究. Tokyo: Kyūko shoin, 1997.

Umehara Kaoru 梅原郁. "Gendai saeki hō shōron" 元代差役法小論. *Tōyōshi kenkyū* 東洋史研究 23.4 (March, 1965): 39–67.

——. *Sōdai kanryō seido kenkyū* 宋代官僚制度研究. Kyoto: Dōhōsha, 1985.

Unschuld, Paul U. *Medicine in China: A History of Ideas*. Berkeley: University of California Press, 1985.

——. *Medicine in China: A History of Pharmacology*. Berkeley: University of California Press, 1986.

Unschuld, Ulrike. "Traditional Chinese Pharmacology: An Analysis of Its Development in the Thirteenth Century." *Isis* 68.2 (1977): 224–48.

Urayama Kika 浦山きか. *Chūgoku isho no bunkengaku teki kenkyū* 中國醫書の文獻學的研究. Tokyo: Kyūko shoin, 2014.

Walton, Linda. "The Institutional Context of Neo-Confucianism: Scholars, Schools, and *Shu-yüan* in Sung-Yüan China." In *Neo-Confucian Education: The Formative Stage*, ed. Wm. Theodore de Bary and John W. Chaffee, 457–92. Berkeley: University of California Press, 1989.

——. "Southern Song Academies as Sacred Places." In *Religion and Society in T'ang and Sung China*, ed. Patricia Buckley Ebrey and Peter N. Gregory, 335–63. Honolulu: University of Hawai'i Press, 1993.

Walton-Vargö, Linda Ann. "Education, Social Change, and Neo-Confucianism in Sung-Yuan China: Academies and the Local Elite in Ming Prefecture (Ningpo)." Ph.D. diss., University of Pennsylvania, 1978.

Wang Deyi 王德毅 et al., eds. *Yuanren zhuanji ziliao suoyin* 元人傳記資料索引. 5 vols. Taibei: Xinwenfeng chuban gongsi, 1979–82.

Wang Feng 王逢. *Wuxi ji* 梧溪集. Beitu.

Wang Haogu 王好古. *Wang Haogu yixue quanshu* 王好古醫學全書. Beijing: Zhongguo Zhong yiyao chubanshe, 2006.

Wang Pu 王溥. *Tang huiyao* 唐會要. CSJC chubian.

Wang Qi 王圻. *Xu wenxian tongkao* 續文獻通考. Beijing: Xiandai chubanshe, 1986.

Wang Yinglin 王應麟. *Xiaoxue ganzhu* 小學紺珠. CSJC.

——. *Yuhai* 玉海. Taibei: Taiwan huawen shuju.

Wang Yuangong 王元恭. *Zhizheng Siming xuzhi* 至正四明續志. 12 *juan*. 1342. ZGFZCS.

Wang Yun 王惲. *Qiujian ji* 秋澗集. SKQS.

——. *Qiujian xiansheng daquan wenji* 秋澗先生大全文集. SBCK chubian.

Watson, James L. "Chinese Kinship Reconsidered: Anthropological Perspectives on Historical Research." *China Quarterly* 92 (1982): 589–622.

Wei Chu 魏初. *Qingya ji* 青崖集. SKQS.

Wei Su 危素. *Wei Taipu wen xuji* 危太樸文續集. 10 *juan*. YRCK.

Wei Yilin 危亦林. *Shiyi dexiao fang* 世醫得効方. Beijing: Renmin weisheng chubanshe, 1990.

——. *Wei Yilin yixue quanshu* 危亦林醫學全書. Beijing: Zhongguo Zhong yiyao chubanshe, 2006.

Wei Zheng 魏徵 et al. *Suishu* 隋書. Beijing: Zhonghua shuju, 1973.

Wilson, Thomas A. *Genealogy of the Way: The Construction and Uses of the Confucian Tradition in Late Imperial China*. Stanford, CA: Stanford University Press, 1995.

Wu Cheng 吳澄. *Wu Wenzheng gong ji* 吳文正公集, 49 *juan* and *waiji* 外集 3 *juan*. YRCK.

——. *Wu Wenzheng ji* 吳文正集. SKQS.

Wu Hai 吳海. *Wenguozhai ji* 聞過齋集. SKQS.

Wu Sidao 烏斯道. *Chuncaozhai ji* 春草齋集. SKQS.

Wu Xianglan 武香兰. "Yuandai yizheng yanjiu" 元代医政研究. Ph.D. diss., Jinan daxue 暨南大学, 2008.

Wu, Yi-Li. *Reproducing Women: Medicine, Metaphor, and Childbirth in Late Imperial China*. Berkeley: University of California Press, 2010.

Wu Yiyi. "A Medical Line of Many Masters: A Prosopographical Study of Liu Wansu and His Disciples from the Jin to the Early Ming." *Chinese Science* 11 (1993–94): 36–65.

Wuxi zhi 無錫志. 4 *juan*. SYD Xubian.

Xiong Mengxiang 熊夢祥. *Xijin zhi jiyi* 析津志輯佚. Bejing guji chubanshe, 1983.

Xiong, Victor C. "The Land Tenure System of Tang China: A Study of Equal Field System and the Turfan Documents." *T'oung Pao* 85.4 & 5 (1999): 328–90.

Xu Guozhen 許國禎. *Yu yaoyuan fang* 御藥院方. Zhongyi guji zhengli congshu 中醫古籍整理叢書 series. Beijing: Renmin weisheng chubanshe, 1992.

Xu Heng 許衡. *Luzhai yishu* 魯齋遺書. SKQS.

Xu Shidong 徐時棟. *Song-Yuan Siming liuzhi jiaokan ji* 宋元四明六志校勘記. ZGFZCS (vol. 580).

Xu Shuwei 許叔微. *Puji benshifang* 普濟本事方. In his *Xu Shuwei yixue quanshu* 許叔微醫學全書. Beijing: Zhongguo Zhongyiyao chubanshe, 2006.

Xu Song 徐松, ed. *Song huiyao jigao* 宋會要輯稿. Beijing: Zhonghua shuju, 1957.

Xu Suo 徐碩. *Zhiyuan Jiahe zhi* 至元嘉禾志. 32 *juan*. Sanshiqi. Also SYD Xubian.

Xu wenxian tongkao 續文獻通考. Commissioned by the Qianlong emperor (Qing dynasty). Shanghai: Shangwu yinshuguan, 1936.

Xu Youren 許有壬. *Zhizheng ji* 至正集. SKQS.

——. *Zhizheng ji* 至正集. YRCK.

Yamamoto Takayoshi 山本隆義. "Gendai ni okeru kanrin gakushiin ni tsuite" 元代に於ける翰林学士院について. *Tōhōgaku* 東方學 12 (1955): 81–99.

Yan Fu 閻復. *Jingxuan ji* 靜軒集. 6 *juan*. YRCK.

Yanagida Setsuko 柳田節子. "Sōdai chūō shūkenteki bunshin kanryō shihai no seiritsu o megutte" 宋代中央集権的文臣官僚支配の成立をめぐって. *Rekishigaku kenkyū* 288 (May 1964): 2–5.

——. "Sōdai kokka kenryoku to nōson chitsujo: kotōsei shihai to kyakko" 宋代国家権力と農村秩序: 戸等制支配と客戸. In *Niida Noboru hakushi tsuitō ronbunshū* 仁井田陞博士追悼論文集, ed. Fukushima Masao 福島正夫 et al., 337–64. Tokyo: Keisō Shobō, 1967.

——. "Gendai kyōson no kotōsei" 元代郷村の戸等制. *Tōyō bunka kenkyūjo kiyō* 東洋文化研究所紀要 73 (March, 1977): 1–43.

Yang Hui 楊譓. *Zhizheng Kunshan zhi* 至正崑山志. 6 *juan*. Sanshiqi.

Yang Jian 楊僭. *Shaoxi Yunjian zhi* 紹熙雲間志. 3 *juan*. 1193. Sanshiqi.

Yang Jizhou 楊繼洲. *Zhenjiu dacheng* 鍼灸大成. Beijing: Zhongyi guji chubanshe, 1998.

Yang Kuan 楊寬. "Zhongguo shanggushi daolun" 中國上古史導論. In *Gushi bian* 古史辨 7.1, ed. Lu Simian 呂思勉 and Tong Shuye 童書業. Shanghai: Kaiming shudian, 1941.

Yang Shou-zhong and Duan Wu-jin. *Extra Treatises Based on Investigation and Inquiry: A Translation of Zhu Dan-xi's Ge Zhi Yu Lun*. Boulder, CO: Blue Poppy Press, 1994.

Yao Sui 姚燧. *Mu'an ji* 牧庵集. SBCK chubian.

Yokote Yutaka 横手裕. *Chūgoku dōkyō no tenkai* 中国道教の展開. Tokyo: Yamakawa Shuppansha, 2008.

Yoshikawa Kōjirō 吉川幸次郎. *Sō-Min shi gaisetsu* 宋明詩概説. Tokyo: Iwanami Shoten, 1963.

——. "Gen Tenshō ni mieta Kanbun ritoku no buntai 元典章に見えた漢文吏牘の文體." In Yoshikawa Kōjirō and Tanaka Kenji, *Gen Tenshō no buntai* 元典章の文體, a supplement (*furoku* 付録) to Iwamura Shinobu and Tanaka Kenji, *Kōteibon Gen Tenshō keibu dai 1 satsu* 校定本元典章刑部第一冊, 1964.

——. "Shushigaku hokuden zenshi: Kinchō to Shushigaku" 朱子学北伝前史: 金朝と朱子学. In *Uno Tetsuto sensei hakuju shukuga kinen Tōyōgaku ronsō* 宇野哲人先生白寿祝賀記念東洋学論叢, ed. Uno Tetsuto hakuju shukuga kinenkai, 1237–58. Tokyo: Uno Tetsujin hakuju shukuga kinenkai, 1974.

Yu Ji 虞集. *Daoyuan leigao* 道園類藁. 50 *juan*. YRCK.

——. *Daoyuan xuegulu* 道園學古錄. SKQS.

——. *Yu Ji Quanji* 虞集全集. Tianjin: Tianjin guji chubanshe, 2007.

Yu Qin 于欽. *Qisheng* 齊乘. 6 *juan*. Sanshiqi.

Yu Xilu 俞希魯. *Zhishun Zhenjiang zhi* 至順鎮江志. Taibei: Huawen Shuju, 1968.

——. *Zhishun Zhenjiang zhi*. Nanjing: Jiangsu guji chubanshe, 1999.

Yuan Haowen 元好問. *Yishan ji* 遺山集. SKQS.

——. *Yuan Haowen quanji* 元好問全集. Expanded edition. Taiyuan: Shanxi guji chubanshe, 2004.

Yuan Henan zhi 元河南志. 4 *juan*. Sanshiqi.

Yuan Jue 袁桷. *Qingrong jushi ji* 清容居士集. SKQS.

——. *Yanyou Siming zhi* 延祐四明志. 20 *juan*. 1320. ZGFZCS (vol. 578).

Zhang Gao 張杲. *Yishuo* 醫説. SKQS.

Zhang Hao 張淏. *Kuaiji xuzhi* 會稽續志. 8 *juan*. Sanshiqi.

Zhang Ji 張機. *Jinkui yaolüe jiaozhu* 金匱要略校注. Ed. He Ren 何任, et al. Beijing: Renmin weisheng chubanshe, 1990.

——. *Shanghan lun jiaozhu* 傷寒論校注, ed. Liu Duzhou 劉度舟 et al. Beijng: Renmin weisheng chubanshe, 1990.

Zhang Jin 張津 et al. *Qiandao Siming tujing* 乾道四明圖經. 12 *juan*. 1169. Sanshiqi.

Zhang Jinwu 張金吾. *Airi jinglu cangshu zhi* 愛日精廬藏書志. In *Qian Zunwang Dushu minqiuji jiaozheng, Airi jinglu canshu zhi* 錢遵王讀書敏求記校證, 愛日精廬藏書志. Beijing: Zhonghua shuju, 1990.

Zhang Tingyu 張廷玉 et al. *Mingshi* 明史. Beijing: Zhonghua shuju, 1975.

Zhang Xuan 張鉉. *Zhizheng Jinling xinzhi* 至正金陵新志. 15 *juan*. 1344. Sanshiqi.

——. *Zhizheng Jinling xinzhi*. 15 *juan*. 1344. Song-Yuan fangzhi congkan, Beijing: Zhonghua shuju.

Zhang Xueqian 張學謙. "Yuan-Ming ruyi sixiang yu shijian de shehuishi: yi Zhu Zhenheng ji 'Danxi xuepai' wei zhongxin" 元明儒醫思想與實踐的社會史: 以朱震亨及《丹溪學派》爲中心. Ph.D. diss., Xianggang Zhongwen Daxue 香港中文大學, 2012.

Zhang Yanghao 張養浩. *Guitian leigao* 歸田類稿. SKQS.

Zhang Yuansu 張元素. *Zhang Yuansu yixue quanshu* 張元素醫學全書. Beijing: Zhongguo Zhong yiyao chubanshe, 2006.

Zhao Erxun 趙爾巽 et al. *Qingshi gao* 清史稿. Beijing: Zhonghua shuju, 1976.

Zhao Fu 趙復. *Xianru Zhaozi yangxing lu* 先儒趙子言行録. Compiled by Chen Tingjun 陳廷鈞. 1856.

Zheng Sixiao 鄭思肖. *Xinshi* 心史. A punctuated version published with Liang Qichao's preface dated 1905. Beijing: Wendiange shuzhuan.

Zheng Yao 鄭瑶. *Jingding Yanzhou xuzhi* 景定嚴州續志. 10 *juan*. 1262. Sanshiqi.

Zheng Yu 鄭玉. *Shishan ji* 師山集. SKQS.

Zhengde Songjiang fu zhi 正徳松江府志. TYG Xubian.

Zhou Cong 周淙. *Qiandao Lin'an zhi* 乾道臨安志. 3 *juan* (incomplete). 1169. Sanshiqi.

Zhou li 周禮. SBCK chubian. Annotated by Zheng Xuan 鄭玄 and Lu Deming 陸徳明.

Zhou Xizhe 周希哲 et al. *Ningbofu zhi* 寧波府志. FZCS (vol. 495).

Zhou Yinghe 周應合. *Jingding Jiankang zhi* 景定建康志. 50 *juan*. 1261. Sanshiqi.

Zhu Changwen 朱長文. *Wujun tujing duji* 吳郡圖經讀記. 3 *juan*. Sanshiqi.

Zhu Gong 朱肱 and Pang Anshi 龐安時. *Zhu Gong Pang Anshi yixue quanshu* 朱肱龐安時醫學全書. Beijing: Zhongguo Zhongyiyao chubanshe, 2006.

Zhu Xi 朱熹. *Daxue zhangju* 大学章句. Collected in *Sishu zhangju jizhu* 四書章句集注. Beijing: Zhonghua shuju chubanshe, 1983.

Zhu Xi 朱熹 and Li Youwu 李幼武. *Song Mingchen yanxing lu wuji* 宋名臣言行録五集. Taibei: Wenhai chubanshe, 1967.

Zhu Zhenheng 朱震亨. *Danxi yiji* 丹溪醫集. Compiled by Zhejiang sheng Zhongyiyao yanjiuyuan wenxian yanjiushi 浙江省中醫藥研究院文献研究室. Beijing: Renmin weisheng chubanshe, 1993.

——. *Gezhi Yulun* 格致餘論. In his *Danxi yiji*. Compiled by Zhejiang sheng Zhongyiyao yanjiuyuan wenxian yanjiushi. Beijing: Renmin weisheng chubanshe, 1993.

——. *Jufang fahui* 局方發揮. In his *Danxi yiji*. Compiled by Zhejiang sheng Zhongyiyao yanjiuyuan wenxian yanjiushi. Beijing: Renmin weisheng chubanshe, 1993.

Zuantu huzhu Li ji 纂图互註禮記. SBCK chubian. Annotated by Zheng Xuan 鄭玄 and Lu Deming 陸徳明.

Index